Case Studies in Pediatric Anesthesia

Case Studies in Pediatric Anesthesia

Edited by

Adam C. Adler

Assistant Professor of Anesthesiology, Texas Children's Hospital

Arvind Chandrakantan

Assistant Professor of Anesthesiology, Texas Children's Hospital

Ronald S. Litman

Professor of Anesthesiology, The Children's Hospital of Philadelphia

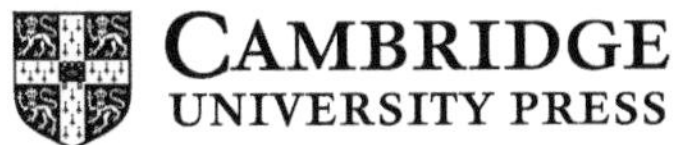

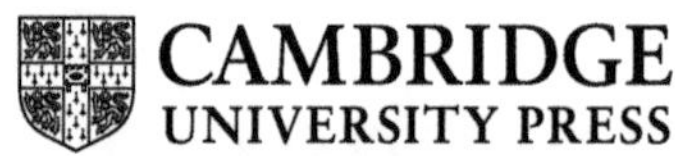

Shaftesbury Road, Cambridge CB2 8EA, United Kingdom

One Liberty Plaza, 20th Floor, New York, NY 10006, USA

477 Williamstown Road, Port Melbourne, VIC 3207, Australia

314–321, 3rd Floor, Plot 3, Splendor Forum, Jasola District Centre, New Delhi – 110025, India

103 Penang Road, #0506/07, Visioncrest Commercial, Singapore 238467

Cambridge University Press & Assessment is a department of the University of Cambridge.

We share the University's mission to contribute to society through the pursuit of education, learning and research at the highest international levels of excellence

www.cambridge.org
Information on this title: www.cambridge.org/9781108465519
DOI: 10.1017/9781108668736

First published 2019 (version 2, September 2023)

Printed in the United Kingdom by TJ Books Ltd, Padstow Cornwall

A catalog record for this publication is available from the British Library.

Library of Congress Cataloging-in-Publication Data
Names: Adler, Adam C., 1983– editor. | Chandrakantan, Arvind, 1977– editor. | Litman, Ronald S., editor.
Title: Case studies in pediatric anesthesia / edited by Adam C. Adler, Arvind Chandrakantan, Ronald S. Litman.
Description: Cambridge, United Kingdom ; New York, NY : University Printing House, 2019. | Includes bibliographical references and index.
Identifiers: LCCN 2019002065 | ISBN 9781108465519 (pbk. : alk. paper)
Subjects: | MESH: Anesthesia–methods | Pediatrics–methods | Case Reports
Classification: LCC RD139 | NLM WO 440 | DDC 617.9/6083–dc23
LC record available at https://lccn.loc.gov/2019002065

ISBN 978-1-108-46551-9 Paperback

Every effort has been made in preparing this book to provide accurate and up-to-date information that is in accord with accepted standards and practice at the time of publication. Although case histories are drawn from actual cases, every effort has been made to disguise the identities of the individuals involved. Nevertheless, the authors, editors, and publishers can make no warranties that the information contained herein is totally free from error, not least because clinical standards are constantly changing through research and regulation. The authors, editors, and publishers therefore disclaim all liability for direct or consequential damages resulting from the use of material contained in this book. Readers are strongly advised to pay careful attention to information provided by the manufacturer of any drugs or equipment that they plan to use.

To my parents for their continued support throughout my medical journey and to my wonderful wife Lindsay.
To Max: With hard work, dedication, and passion you can accomplish anything!
– Adam

To my wife, Kripa, and daughters, Anikah, Mayuri, and Vinayaa Chandrakantan.
– Arvind

To all my past, present, and future residents and fellows who keep me intellectually stimulated and motivated to continue to teach and write about pediatric anesthesia. I have confidence that you will be the unwavering and committed guardians of children under your care.
– Ron

Contents

Contributors

Adam C. Adler, MS, MD, FAAP, FASE
Assistant Professor of Anesthesiology, Baylor College of Medicine and Department of Anesthesiology, Perioperative and Pain Medicine, Texas Children's Hospital, Houston, TX, USA

Titilopemi A.O. Aina, MD
Assistant Professor of Anesthesiology, Baylor College of Medicine and Department of Anesthesiology, Perioperative and Pain Medicine, Texas Children's Hospital, Houston, TX, USA

Dean B. Andropoulos, MD, MHCM
Anesthesiologist-in-Chief, Department of Anesthesiology, Perioperative and Pain Medicine, Texas Children's Hospital and Professor, Anesthesiology and Pediatrics and Vice Chair for Clinical Affairs, Department of Anesthesiology, Baylor College of Medicine, Houston, TX, USA

Rahul G. Baijal, MD
Associate Professor of Anesthesiology, Baylor College of Medicine and Department of Anesthesiology, Perioperative and Pain Medicine, Texas Children's Hospital, Houston, TX, USA

Christian Balabanoff-Acosta, MD
Fellow in Critical Care and Cardiovascular Anesthesiology, the University of Miami Miller School of Medicine, Miami, FL, USA

Maura Berkelhamer, MD
Assistant Professor of Anesthesiology and Pediatrics, Case Western Reserve University School of Medicine and Department of Pediatric Anesthesiology and Perioperative Medicine, Rainbow Babies and Children's Hospital, Cleveland, OH, USA

Sudha Bidani, MBBS
Assistant Professor of Anesthesiology, Baylor College of Medicine and Department of Anesthesiology, Perioperative and Pain Medicine, Texas Children's Hospital, Houston, TX, USA

Jaime Bozentka, MD
Assistant Professor of Clinical Anesthesiology, University of Cincinnati College of Medicine and Cincinnati Children's Hospital Medical Center, Cincinnati, OH, USA

Arvind Chandrakantan, MD, MBA, FAAP, FASA
Assistant Professor of Anesthesiology and Pediatrics, Baylor College of Medicine and Department of Anesthesiology, Perioperative and Pain Medicine, Texas Children's Hospital, Houston, TX, USA

Julia H. Chen, MD
Assistant Professor of Anesthesiology, Baylor College of Medicine and Department of Anesthesiology, Perioperative and Pain Medicine, Texas Children's Hospital, Houston, TX, USA

Kathleen Chen, MD
Assistant Professor of Anesthesiology, Baylor College of Medicine and Department of Anesthesiology, Perioperative and Pain Medicine, Texas Children's Hospital, Houston, TX, USA

Monica Chen, MD
Assistant Professor of Anesthesiology, Baylor College of Medicine and Department of Anesthesiology, Perioperative and Pain Medicine, Texas Children's Hospital, Houston, TX, USA

Devyani Chowdhury, MBBS, FACC, FASE
Director, Cardiology Care for Children, Lancaster, PA, USA

Yeona Chun, MD
Resident in Anesthesiology, Department of Anesthesiology, Rush University Medical Center, Chicago, IL, USA

Laura Diaz-Berenstain, MD
Associate Professor of Clinical Anesthesiology, University of Cincinnati College of Medicine and Cincinnati Children's Hospital Medical Center, Cincinnati, OH, USA

Rebecca Evans, MD
Assistant Professor of Anesthesiology, Larner College of Medicine and Department of Anesthesiology, University of Vermont Medical Center, Burlington, VT, USA

Giuliana Geng-Ramos, MD
Assistant Professor, The George Washington University School of Medicine, Division of Anesthesiology, Pain and Perioperative Medicine, Children's National Health System, District of Columbia, USA

Chris D. Glover, MD, MBA
Associate Professor of Anesthesiology, Baylor College of Medicine and Department of Anesthesiology, Perioperative and Pain Medicine, Texas Children's Hospital, Houston, TX, USA

Aysha Hasan, MD
Division Chief of Acute Pain and Regional Anesthesiology, Pediatric Anesthesiologist, St. Christopher's Hospital for Children and Assistant Professor, Drexel University College of Medicine, Philadelphia, PA, USA

Lisa D. Heyden, MD
Assistant Professor of Anesthesiology, Baylor College of Medicine and Department of Anesthesiology, Perioperative and Pain Medicine, Texas Children's Hospital, Houston, TX, USA

Grace Hsu, MD
Assistant Professor of Clinical Anesthesiology and Critical Care Medicine, Department of Anesthesiology and Critical Care Medicine, the Children's Hospital of Philadelphia, University of Pennsylvania School of Medicine, Philadelphia, PA, USA

Matthew D. James, MD
Assistant Professor of Anesthesiology, Baylor College of Medicine and Department of Anesthesiology, Perioperative and Pain Medicine, Texas Children's Hospital, Houston, TX, USA

Megha K. Kanjia, MD
Assistant Professor of Anesthesiology, Baylor College of Medicine and Department of Anesthesiology, Perioperative and Pain Medicine, Texas Children's Hospital, Houston, TX, USA

Grace S. Kao, PhD
Assistant Professor, Baylor College of Medicine and Pediatric Pain Psychologist, Department of Anesthesiology, Perioperative and Pain Medicine, Texas Children's Hospital, Houston, TX, USA

Michael R. King, MD
Assistant Professor, Northwestern University Feinberg School of Medicine and Department of Pediatric Anesthesiology, Ann and Robert H. Lurie Children's Hospital of Chicago, Chicago, IL, USA

Ramesh Kodavatiganti, MD
Assistant Professor of Anesthesiology, University of Pennsylvania Perelman School of Medicine and Department of Anesthesiology and Critical Care Medicine, the Children's Hospital of Philadelphia and Program Director, Pediatric Cardiac Anesthesia Fellowship, Philadelphia, PA, USA

Ronald S. Litman, DO, ML
Professor of Anesthesiology and Pediatrics, Department of Anesthesiology and Critical Care Medicine, the Children's Hospital of Philadelphia, University of Pennsylvania School of Medicine, Philadelphia, PA, USA

Yang Liu, MD
Assistant Professor of Anesthesiology, Baylor College of Medicine and Department of Anesthesiology, Perioperative and Pain Medicine, Texas Children's Hospital, Houston, TX, USA

Vibha Mahendra, MD
Fellow in Obstetric Anesthesiology, Department of Anesthesiology, Baylor College of Medicine, Ben Taub Hospital, Houston, TX, USA

Kayla McGrath, MD
Fellow in Pediatric Anesthesiology, Baylor College of Medicine and Department of Anesthesiology, Perioperative and Pain Medicine, Texas Children's Hospital, Houston, TX, USA

Deepak K. Mehta, MD
Professor of Otolaryngology, Baylor College of Medicine and Director, Pediatric Aerodigestive Center, Texas Children's Hospital, Houston, TX, USA

Sheryl Modlin, MD
Associate Professor of Anesthesiology and Pediatrics, Case Western Reserve University School of Medicine and Department of Pediatric Anesthesiology and Perioperative Medicine, Rainbow Babies and Children's Hospital, Cleveland, OH, USA

Caro Monico, MD
Assistant Professor of Anesthesiology, Baylor College of Medicine and Department of Anesthesiology, Perioperative and Pain Medicine, Division of Pain Medicine, Texas Children's Hospital, Houston, TX, USA

Ann Ng, MD
Assistant Professor of Anesthesiology, Baylor College of Medicine and Department of Anesthesiology, Perioperative and Pain Medicine, Texas Children's Hospital, Houston, TX, USA

Kim-Phuong Nguyen, MD
Associate Professor of Anesthesiology, Baylor College of Medicine and Department of Anesthesiology, Perioperative and Pain Medicine, Texas Children's Hospital, Houston, TX, USA

Elyse C. Parchmont, CRNA, MSN
Instructor, Baylor College of Medicine and Department of Anesthesiology, Perioperative and Pain Medicine, Texas Children's Hospital, Houston, TX, USA

Nihar V. Patel, MD
Associate Professor of Anesthesiology and Pediatrics, Baylor College of Medicine and Department of Anesthesiology, Perioperative and Pain Medicine, Texas Children's Hospital, Houston, TX, USA

Mario Patino, MD
Associate Professor of Anesthesiology, Baylor College of Medicine and Department of Anesthesiology, Perioperative and Pain Medicine, Texas Children's Hospital, Houston, TX, USA

Miguel R. Prada, MD
Assistant Professor of Anesthesiology, Baylor College of Medicine and Department of Anesthesiology, Perioperative and Pain Medicine, Texas Children's Hospital, Houston, TX, USA

Kriti Puri, MBBS
Pediatric Cardiologist, Fellow in Pediatric Critical Care Medicine, Departments of Pediatrics and Cardiology, Texas Children's Hospital, Houston, TX, USA

Zoel A. Quiñónez, MD
Assistant Professor of Pediatric Anesthesiology, Baylor College of Medicine and Department of Anesthesiology, Perioperative and Pain Medicine, Texas Children's Hospital, Houston, TX, USA

Kasia Rubin, MD
Division Chief, Pediatric Anesthesiology and Perioperative Medicine, Rainbow Babies and Children's Hospital and Associate Professor of Anesthesiology and Pediatrics, Case Western Reserve University School of Medicine, Cleveland, OH, USA

William D. Ryan
Drexel University, Philadelphia, PA, USA

Donald A. Schwartz, MD
Associate Professor, Tufts University School of Medicine and Department of Anesthesiology and Pain Medicine, Baystate Medical Center, Springfield, MA, USA

Emily R. Schwartz, BS, BA
Research Assistant, Harvard Medical School, Boston, MA, USA

Maureen E. Scollon-McCarthy, MSN, CRNP, FNP-BC
Nurse Practitioner, Pain Management Program, The Children's Hospital of Philadelphia, Department of Anesthesiology and Critical Care Medicine, Philadelphia, PA, USA

Jamie W. Sinton, MD
Assistant Professor of Anesthesiology, Baylor College of Medicine and Department of Anesthesiology, Perioperative and Pain Medicine, Texas Children's Hospital, Houston, TX, USA

Paulus Steyn, MD
Resident in Anesthesiology, Temple University Hospital, Philadelphia, PA, USA

Caitlin D. Sutton, MD
Assistant Professor of Anesthesiology, Pediatrics and Obstetrics, Baylor College of Medicine and Department of Anesthesiology, Perioperative and Pain Medicine, Texas Children's Hospital, Houston, TX, USA

Stephen A. Stayer, MD
Professor of Anesthesiology and Pediatrics, Texas Children's Hospital, Houston, TX, USA

Matthew Taylor, MD
Assistant Professor of Pediatrics, Donald and Barbara Zucker School of Medicine at Hofstra/Northwell, Cohen Children's Medical Center, Hyde Park, NY, USA

Howard Teng, MD
Assistant Attending, Department of Anesthesiology and Critical Care Medicine, Memorial Sloan Kettering Cancer Center, New York, NY, USA

Giselle Torres, MD
Anesthesiologist, Hackensack University Medical Center, Hackensack, NJ, USA

Premal M. Trivedi, MD
Assistant Professor of Pediatric Cardiovascular Anesthesiology, Baylor College of Medicine and Department of Anesthesiology, Perioperative and Pain Medicine, Texas Children's Hospital, Houston, TX, USA

Eric L. Vu, MD
Assistant Professor of Pediatric Anesthesiology, Baylor College of Medicine and Department of Anesthesiology, Perioperative and Pain Medicine, Texas Children's Hospital, Houston, TX, USA

Karla E.K. Wyatt, MD, MS, FAAP
Assistant Professor of Anesthesiology, Baylor College of Medicine and Department of Anesthesiology, Perioperative and Pain Medicine, Texas Children's Hospital, Houston, TX, USA

Esther Y. Yang, DDS
Assistant Professor, Baylor College of Medicine and Department of Plastic Surgery, Texas Children's Hospital, Houston, TX, USA

Foreword

Case Studies in Pediatric Anesthesia is a new text edited by Adam C. Adler MS, MD, FAAP, FASE; Arvind Chandrakantan MD, MBA, FAAP, FASA; and Ronald S. Litman, DO, ML. These three academic pediatric anesthesiologists are passionate educators who have a talent for synthesizing information in a way that learners find easy to digest and remember. They all work full time in a busy children's hospital where they teach medical students, residents, and fellows. In addition, they all are active investigators working with both basic scientists and clinical scientists. Their experience as scientists and educators is reflected in their writing. They have chosen to use case studies to teach the practice of pediatric anesthesiology. Each chapter begins with a brief case presentation followed by key questions regarding the case, which are then answered in the text, and the evidence for decision making is presented. As the case progresses, similar to a mystery novel, readers are intrigued to determine the outcome. Learners are more likely to retain the information because of the feeling of being involved with an actual patient.

The editors have assembled a large number of experts in pediatric anesthesiology, pediatric surgery, and pediatric cardiology to author the chapters. These authors present information that is up-to-date and practical. Most importantly, as chief editors they have actively edited the individual chapters to ensure that the information flows in the same way throughout each chapter and that there is a similar voice for each chapter, making it much easier for readers to digest. I feel that readers of this textbook will find this format and writing style fun and informative to read and easy to retain. Lastly, I must admit my personal bias; I have worked with all three editors and find each of them to have a great sense of humor and broad interests outside medicine.

Stephen A. Stayer

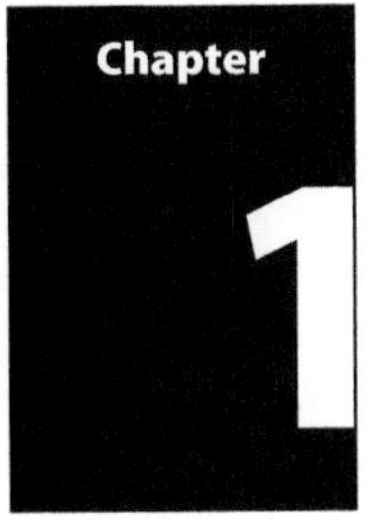

Normal Parameters for Pediatric Anesthesia

Adam C. Adler

As compared to adults, the "normal values" for a variety of physiologic measurements change throughout development. Listed in this chapter is a rough guide to be used in the anesthesia care of children. As always, the patients' baseline and co-existing illness should be carefully considered when choosing a baseline.

Table 1.1 What are the normal values for heart rate in children?

Age	Awake heart rate	Asleep heart rate
Neonates <1 month	100–125	90–160
Infants (1–12 months)	100–180	90–160
Toddlers (1–2 years)	100–140	80–120
Preschool aged (3–5 years)	80–120	65–100
School aged (6–12 years)	75–120	60–90
Adolescents (12–15 years)	60–100	50–90

Table 1.2 What are the normal values for blood pressure in children?

Age	Systolic blood pressure (mmHg)	Diastolic blood pressure (mmHg)	Mean arterial pressure (mmHg)
Birth (LBW)	40–60	15–35	30–40
Birth (3 kg, term)	60–75	31–45	45–60
Neonates	65–85	35–55	45–60
Infants (1–12 months)	70–105	35-55	50–65
Toddlers (1–2 years)	85–105	40–65	50–60
Preschool aged (3–5 years)	90–110	45–70	60–70
School aged (6–12 years)	95–115	55–75	65–70
Preadolescents (10–12 years)	100–120	60–80	70–80
Adolescents (12–15 years)	110–130	65–85	75–85

Table 1.3 What are the normal values for respiratory rate in children?

Age	Respiratory rate (breaths/min)
Infants	30–55
Toddlers	22–35
Preschool aged	20–28
School aged	18–25
Adolescents	12–20

Table 1.4 What are normal values for estimated blood volume in children?

Age	Estimated blood volume (mL/kg)
Premature infants	**100**
Term neonates (<1 month)	**90**
1–12 months	**80**
Older children	**75**
Adolescents/Adults	**70**

Table 1.5 Basic equipment sizes in children

Age	ETT size	Laryngoscope	Oral airway	Mask size	BP cuff size
<1 month 3–5 kg	3.0	Miller 0–1	40	1	Neonate/#5
1–5 months 6–7 kg	3.0/3.5	Miller 1–1.5	40/50	1,2	Pediatric
6–11 months 10–11 kg	3.5/4.0	Miller 1–1.5	50/60	2	Pediatric
1–3 years 12–14 kg	4.0/4.5	Miller 1–1.5	60	3	Pediatric
4–5 years 15–18 kg	5.0/5.5	Miller 1.5–2	60	3,4	Pediatric
6–7 years 15–18 kg	5.5/6.0	Miller 1.5–2	60	4	Pediatric
8–9 years 19–23 kg	6.0/6.5	Miller 2, MAC 2	60/70	4	Pediatric
10–12 years 24–29 kg	6.0/6.5	Miller 2, MAC 2	70/80	4,5	Pediatric
>12 years 30–35 kg	5.5/6.0/6.5	Miller 2, MAC 3	70/80	5	Pediatric/small adult

Table 1.6 Perioperative NPO guidelines

Clear liquids	**2 hours**
Breast milk (nonfortified)	**4 hours**
Nonhuman milk	**6 hours**
Light meal	**6 hours**
Full meal	**8 hours**

Table 1.7 Minimum alveolar concentration of anesthetic agents

	Infant	Child	Adult
Isoflurane	1.6	1.3–1.5	1.1
Desflurane	9.2	8.1	6.0
Sevoflurane	3.3	2.5	2.0

Table 1.8 Analgesics

Agent	Oral dose	IV dose	Continuous infusion
Morphine	0.2 mg/kg	0.1–0.2 mg/kg	0.01–0.05 mg/kg/h
Hydromorphone	-	0.01–0.03 mg/kg	0.25–6 mcg/kg/h
Fentanyl	-	1–2 mcg/kg	0.25–2 mcg/kg/h
Sufentanil	-		0.2–1 mcg/kg/h
Remifentanil	-	-	0.05–0.2 mcg/kg/min
Hydrocodone	0.1–0.15 mg/kg	-	-
Methadone	-	0.05–0.1 mg/kg	-
Acetaminophen	10–15 mg/kg		
Ibuprofen	5–10 mg/kg		
Codeine	**Not recommended for use in children**		
Ketorolac	0.5 mg/kg Max 30 mg	0.5 mg/kg Max 30 mg	-
Ketamine	-	0.5–2 mg/kg	5–20 mg/kg/h

Table 1.9 Commonly used drugs

Medication	Dose	Notes
Adenosine	0.1 mg/kg	May repeat × 2 at 0.2 mg/kg
	Maximum 6 mg	Maximum 12 mg
Amiodarone	5 mg/kg	Bolus for VF or pulseless VT
		Over 30–60 min for stable SVT/VT
Atropine	0.02 mg/kg	
Calcium chloride	10–50 mg/kg	
Cisatracurium	0.1–0.2 mg/kg	
Dexamethasone	0.5 mg/kg PO/IM/IV	Max 16 mg
Dexmedetomidine	0.2–0.5 mg/kg/h	0.25–1 mcg/kg bolus
Diazepam	0.05–0.1 mg/kg q6–8 hrs	
Epinephrine	0.01 mL/kg	Anaphylaxis
	0.1 mg/kg	Cardiac arrest
Furosemide	0.5–2 mg/kg	
Glycopyrrolate	0.01–0.02 mg/kg	
Hydrocortisone	100 mg/m^2 BSA	Adrenal insufficiency
Insulin	0.05–0.1 Units/kg bolus	0.05–0.1 Units/kg/h
Magnesium sulfate	25–50 mg/kg	
Methylprednisolone	1–2 mg/kg	
Metoclopramide	0.1 mg/kg q 6 hrs	
Midazolam IV	0.02–0.1 mg/kg/h	0.1–0.2 mg/kg bolus
Midazolam PO	0.5–1.0 mg/kg	15–20 mg/kg Max
Nicardipine	0.5–4 mcg/kg/min	
Ondansetron	0.1 mg/kg q 6 hrs prn	
Sodium bicarbonate	0.5–1 mEq/kg	
Rocuronium	0.5–1.2 mg/kg	
Vecuronium	0.05–0.2 mg/kg	

Table 1.10 Antibiotics (defer to institutional dosing for perioperative antibiotic administration)

	Dose	Max dosing	Redosing schedule
Ampicillin	50 mg/kg*	2 grams	q2 hrs × 2 then q6 hrs
Cefazolin	25–30 mg/kg	2 grams	q4 hrs × 2 then q8 hrs
Cefoxitin	30–40 mg/kg	2 grams	q2 hrs × 2 then q6 hrs
Clindamycin	10 mg/kg	900 mg	q6 hrs × 2 then q8 hrs
Gentamicin	2.5 mg/kg	120 mg	per institutional protocol
Piperacillin-Tazobactam	100 mg/kg	3 grams	q2 hrs × 2 then q6 hrs
Vancomycin	10–15 mg/kg over 60 minutes	1 gram	per institutional protocol

*** 50 mg/kg for infective endocarditis prophylaxis**

Table 1.11 Commonly used doses of blood, fluid, and factors

	Dose
Packed red blood cells	10–20 cc/kg
Platelets	10–20 cc/kg
Plasma	10–20 cc/kg
Factor 7 concentrate	90 mcg/kg/dose may repeat twice
Vitamin K	Adults 10 mg IM, infants 1 mg IM
Albumin 5%	5–10 cc/kg
Lactated Ringer's, 0.9% saline	10–30 cc/kg initial bolus

Table 1.12 Commonly used doses for neurologic surgery

	Dose
Phenytoin	15–20 mg/kg IV loading dose over 15 minutes
Levetiracetam (Keppra)	10 mg/kg IV loading dose over 15 minutes
Mannitol	0.5–1 g/kg
Furosemide	1–2 mg/kg
3% Saline – Hypertonic Saline	3 cc/kg over 30 minutes – with Na^+ monitoring following

Table 1.13 Commonly used doses of cardiovascular drugs

	Dose
Atropine	0.02 mg/kg
Alprostadil	0.01–0.1 mcg/kg/min
Calcium chloride	10–50 mg/kg
Dopamine	1–10 mcg/kg/min
Epinephrine	0.01–0.5 mcg/kg/min
Esmolol	50–1000 mcg/kg/min
Lidocaine	10–50 mcg/kg/min
Milrinone	0.25–1 mcg/kg/min
Nicardipine	0.5–4 mcg/kg/min
Nitroglycerin	0.5–20 mcg/kg/min
Nitroprusside	0.3–10 mcg/kg/min
Norepinephrine	0.01–2 mcg/kg/min
Phenylephrine	0.1–10 mcg/kg/min
Vasopressin	0.1–0.5 milli-Units/kg/min

Table 1.14 Patient controlled analgesia

	Morphine	Fentanyl	Hydromorphone
Loading dose	0.1 mg/kg	0.5–1 mcg/kg (max 25 mcg)	5–15 mcg/kg
Continuous infusion	0.01–0.03 mg/kg/h	0.1 mcg/kg/h	1.5 mcg/kg/h
Bolus dose (PCA)	0.015–0.025 mg/kg	0.14–0.28 mcg/kg	3–5 mcg/kg
Lockout interval	6–12 minutes	6–10 minutes	6–15 minutes
4-hour max dose	0.25–0.35 mg/kg	2.8 mcg/kg	50–60 mcg/kg

Suggestions for opioid naïve patients
Bolus dosing should be adjusted for degree of pain reduction with bolus
Lockout interval should be adjusted for duration of pain control following bolus
Nalbuphine: 10–20 mcg/kg IV every 6 hrs for opioid induced pruritus
Naloxone infusion: for opioid induced pruritus 0.1–0.25 mcg/kg/h; consider switching opioid
Naloxone bolus: for respiratory depression 0.01 mg/kg – stop opioid infusion – continuous SpO_2 monitoring.

Pharmacology and Physiology in the Term Neonate

Adam C. Adler and Ronald S. Litman

> A one-day-old male child presents for omphalocele repair. He was born to a 30-year-old G3P1 mother at 37 weeks of gestation via a planned Cesarean section for a prenatal ultrasonographic diagnosis of omphalocele. The mother was treated for gestational diabetes with daily insulin and has a history of hypothyroidism, for which she is prescribed L-thyroxin.
>
> Pertinent findings on physical examination include midfacial hypoplasia and macroglossia. An intestinal sac is present and appears to be herniating through a defect in the umbilicus.
>
> Vital signs: BP 60/32, P 164, T 35.8, RR 36, Sat 98% on room air. Weight: 4.4 kg, Apgar scores: 8, 8, 9.

What Are the Differences Between Gastroschisis and Omphalocele?

Gastroschisis and omphalocele are the most common congenital abdominal wall defects with a prevalence of approximately 1:2,000–1:5,000 live births in the United States. Although each represents a distinct anatomical defect, their anesthetic considerations are the same. Each is a congenital defect that allows a portion of the intestinal viscera to extrude outside the abdominal cavity and both require surgical repair in the newborn period (Figure 2.1). Large defects are managed with a staged approach if primary closure is not possible.

An omphalocele occurs when the visceral organs fail to migrate from the yolk sac back into the abdomen early in gestation and the umbilical ring remains open; the defect is a central lesion and occurs at the insertion of the umbilicus. Gastroschisis is thought to result from an occlusion of the omphalomesenteric artery during early development. As a result, the abdominal viscera herniate through a rent in the abdominal wall, usually to the right of the umbilicus. Omphalocele is more likely than gastroschisis to be associated with additional congenital defects. These occur in 25–50% of cases and include chromosome anomalies and cardiac defects. Omphalocele may be a component of the Beckwith–Wiedemann syndrome, which consists of hypertrophy of multiple organs. This syndrome is particularly relevant to the anesthesiologist as enlargement of the tongue may compromise the upper airway and be associated with difficult intubation. Pancreatic enlargement causes hyperinsulinism, which results in hypoglycemia and needs to be monitored intraoperatively. The key characteristic differences are summarized in Table 2.1.

Infants with gastroschisis are usually born at full term without additional isolated defects. The major pathophysiological difference between the two is that, in omphalocele, the intestinal contents remain covered with the peritoneal membrane, which protects the intestinal mucosa from the irritative effects of amniotic fluid and protects the infant from excessive evaporative fluid and temperature loss after delivery. Infants with gastroschisis lack this natural protective covering, and thus are more prone to dehydration, hypoglycemia, hypothermia, third-space fluid accumulation, electrolyte imbalance, acidosis, bleeding, and sepsis.

Management of omphalocele or gastroschisis begins immediately after birth. The extruded abdominal contents are covered with warm saline dressings and are encased in a sterile plastic bag or wrap to decrease fluid and temperature loss and discourage infection (Figure 2.2). A naso- or orogastric tube is placed for gastric decompression, normovolemia is maintained with intravenous hydration, and associated comorbidities are addressed prior to surgical repair. Antibiotics may be necessary if intestinal abnormalities are suspected.

Achieving a primary repair is the goal of surgery as failure to replace all of the intestinal contents back into the abdominal cavity increases postoperative

Table 2.1 Characteristic differences between omphalocele and gastroschisis

	Omphalocele	Gastroschisis
Associated anomalies	Common	Rare
Defect location	Umbilicus	Right of umbilicus
Maternal age	Average	Young
Method of delivery	Cesarean/ vaginal	Vaginal
Prognostic factors	Associated anomalies	Condition of bowel
Sac	Present	Absent
Surgical management	Not emergent	Emergent

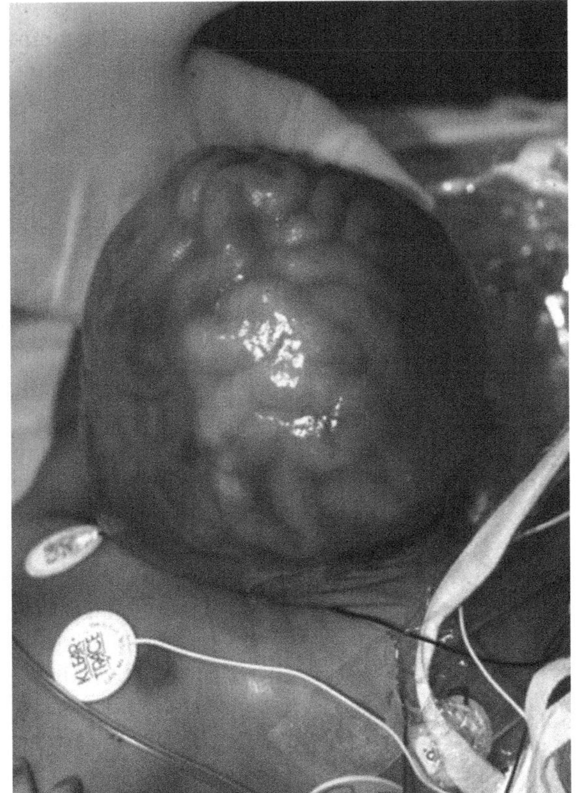

Figure 2.1 Omphalocele prior to surgery. Photograph: Ronald S. Litman, reproduced with parental permission.

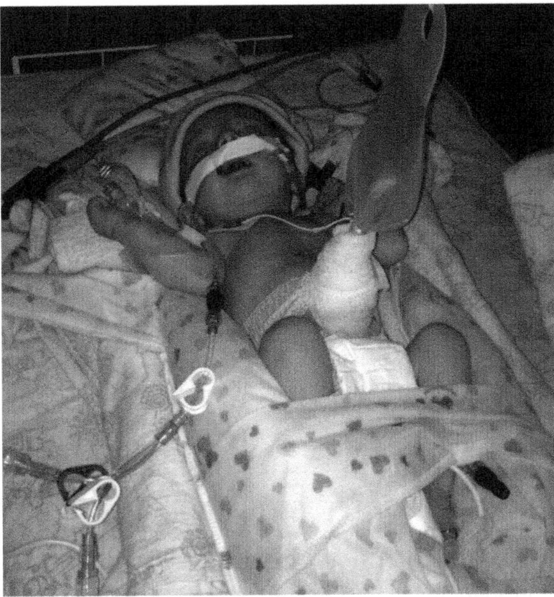

Figure 2.2 Omphalocele silo. Large omphaloceles are treated with a silo and progressive constriction until primary repair. Photograph: Ronald S. Litman, reproduced with parental permission.

morbidity. However, in many cases where the abdominal cavity is too restrictive or when there is not enough skin to close the underlying defect, a partial replacement is performed, and the remaining external viscera are encased in a synthetic silo mesh allowing for complete repair to occur as a staged procedure.

In addition to its impact on intrathoracic pressure, increased intra-abdominal pressure may result in an abdominal compartment syndrome. When this occurs, venous compression leads to a decrease in preload and hypotension as well as lower limb venous congestion. High intra-abdominal pressures may lead to renal artery compression resulting in oliguria as well as decreased perfusion to the lower extremities. Bowel ischemia may also result, secondary to decreased perfusion. Adequate volume and blood replacement and full neuromuscular blockade must be maintained throughout the procedure to optimize the chances for successful primary closure.

What Are the Risks and Benefits of Staged Versus Primary Abdominal Wall Closure?

The optimal surgical management is related to the degree of bowel extrusion and the ability of the abdominal cavity to accept bowel replacement. Infants undergoing primary closure generally require a shorter length of hospitalization and decreased utilization of parenteral nutrition.

Secondary closure techniques have evolved over the past few decades. The extruded bowel is maintained in a spring-loaded silo bag. The bag keeps the bowel intact and protected from environmental contact. This mechanism allows for daily bedside reduction of the bowel over one to two weeks providing time for the abdominal cavity to expand and accommodate without elevating abdominal pressures and interfering with ventilation.

What Are the Anesthetic Considerations for Surgical Intervention of Patients with Gastroschisis or Omphalocele?

Considerations for induction of general anesthesia are similar to those for any newborn infant with a presumed increased risk of a "full stomach" secondary to intestinal obstruction. A modified rapid sequence intubation (RSI) is performed using gentle breaths. Some pediatric anesthesiologists will prefer to temporarily remove the nasogastric tube during induction to facilitate airway management.

There are several intraoperative adverse physiologic derangements that may occur when the surgeon attempts to place a large volume of abdominal contents back into a small, restrictive abdominal cavity. Cephalad displacement of the diaphragm due to the increase in abdominal contents may significantly decrease functional residual capacity (FRC) and tidal volume, which can lead to difficult ventilation, development of atelectasis, and hypoxemia. During the repair, the anesthetist may frequently need to use manual ventilation to maintain adequate tidal volumes in response to rapid changes in lung compliance. The presence of hypoxemia despite maximal ventilation may preclude completion of a primary repair. Therefore, intraoperative management should focus on ventilatory pressures, temperature regulation, and volume status. Rapidly increasing peak pressures (when using volume-controlled ventilation) or a significant decline in tidal volume (when using pressure-controlled ventilation) should raise suspicion of abdominal pressure elevation that will compete with the ability to provide adequate minute ventilation. Fluid administration, postoperative fluid shifts, and associated bowel edema can lead to increases in abdominal compartment pressure, low cardiac output, and renal hypoperfusion.

These patients are at risk of hypothermia from exposed abdominal contents. Similarly, fluid evaporative losses are common, especially with gastroschisis where the surface of the intestine is uncovered and exposed to the atmosphere.

All infants, except those with the most trivial repairs, remain intubated and mechanically ventilated in the postoperative period. Abdominal compartment syndrome and respiratory compromise may continue postoperatively; therefore, paralysis and adequate sedation with an opioid infusion are essential for optimal management.

What Are the Pertinent Preoperative Diagnostic and Laboratory Evaluations Suggested for These Patients?

The diagnosis of omphalocele should alert the clinician to the possibility of numerous coexisting congenital defects. Intrapartum diagnosis should prompt fetal echocardiography and even postnatal echocardiographic evaluation, as the incidence of concomitant cardiac anomalies is as high as 25%. Pulmonary hypoplasia often necessitating ventilatory support, cloacal exstrophy, and anomalies associated with VACTERL syndrome may be present. Normal karyotype patients have an incidence of other abnormalities that is as high as 80%, stressing the importance of a complete perioperative evaluation. Chromosomal abnormalities (especially trisomies 13, 18, and 21) exist in nearly 50% of patients with omphalocele. Unlike gastroschisis, the herniation in omphalocele patients is enclosed and amenable to supportive therapy while workup is obtained. Intravenous access should be obtained, and fluid resuscitation initiated. Glucose should be evaluated frequently, and if low, it should raise suspicion for Beckwith–Wiedemann syndrome. Careful cardiopulmonary workup should ensue prior to closure in a stable neonate. The bowel should be wrapped to minimize heat and evaporative loss, which, while less extreme compared with gastroschisis patients, remains greater than in patients with a closed abdomen. Naso- or orogastric tubes should be placed for decompression.

The assessment for comorbidities, while less common in patients with gastroschisis, should include evaluation for meningocele, limb abnormalities, and intestinal atresia. Intravenous access and maintenance of fluid homeostasis is vital as well as frequent evaluation of electrolytes. In the interim, exposed bowel should be wrapped with sterile dressing and plastic to minimize infection, evaporative fluid loss, and temperature loss. The bowel should be evaluated frequently for early recognition of ischemic changes possibly due to mesenteric kinking.

What Is the Prognosis for Patients with Gastroschisis and Omphalocele?

The prognosis for omphalocele is related to the number and severity of associated congenital anomalies. The optimal mode and timing of delivery is debated although most neonates with omphalocele are delivered via cesarean section for fear of abdominal sac rupture with labor.

Prognosis for gastroschisis is generally determined by the degree of bowel injury and bowel atresia. Exposure of the bowel to amniotic fluid and degree of bowel constriction dictates the severity of injury. Gastroschisis patients have a greater incidence of developing necrotizing enterocolitis when compared with the general population. The optimal mode and timing of delivery is still debated.

What Is the Beckwith–Wiedemann Syndrome?

The incidence of Beckwith–Wiedemann is approximately 1 in 13,000–14,000 children without gender predominance.

What Is the General Phenotypic Appearance of Children with Beckwith–Wiedemann Syndrome?

Children with Beckwith–Wiedemann syndrome display signs of accelerated growth, including height and weight. Common facial abnormalities include prominent eyes, midfacial hypoplasia, macroglossia or hemihypertrophy, prominent mandible, and earlobe anomalies.

Macroglossia can lead to sleep disordered breathing and sleep apnea. In addition, hemihypertrophy can often pose difficulty with airway management.

What Are the Associated Malformations Found in Patients with Beckwith–Wiedemann Syndrome?

Beckwith–Wiedemann is a disorder of increased growth (somatic overgrowth) with a predisposition to development of embryonal tumors. Malformations include abdominal wall defects and visceromegaly of one or more of the following: heart, liver, spleen, pancreas, kidneys and adrenals. Neonatal hypoglycemia occurs in up to 50% of children with Beckwith–Wiedemann syndrome due to pancreatic islet cell hyperplasia and hyperinsulinemia.

Cardiac anomalies are present in approximately 20% of patients with Beckwith–Wiedemann syndrome. Renal anomalies are common, including medullary dysplasia, nephrocalcinosis, or nephrolithiasis.

Patients with Beckwith–Wiedemann syndrome are predisposed to development of embryonal tumors especially within the first decade of life. Common tumors include Wilms, hepatoblastoma, rhabdomyosarcoma, neuroblastoma, and adrenocortical carcinoma. The risk of tumor development may be greater in children with hemihypertrophy and nephromegaly.

Discuss the Anesthetic Work-Up for a Patient with Beckwith–Wiedemann Syndrome

Patients with Beckwith-Wiedemann syndrome should undergo thorough preoperative evaluation for non-emergent cases. Examination should identify comorbidities especially cardiac anomalies and renal impairment. Complete airway examination and anticipation of potentially difficult airway. Neonatal hypoglycemia is common in this population and should be addressed. Macroglossia can predispose patients to postoperative airway obstruction.

Which Patients Are at Risk for Developing Neonatal Hypoglycemia?

This patient from this case stem has significant risk factors for being unable to maintain glucose homeostasis in the perioperative period. Being the infant of a diabetic mother places a neonate at risk for perinatal hypoglycemia. This results from fetal exposure to elevated maternal serum glucose levels. Fetal insulin secretion is increased to meet the demands of this glucose load. After delivery, maternal glucose exposure declines precipitously while leaving the neonatal pancreas oversecreting insulin, resulting in perinatal hypoglycemia. These infants are monitored closely, often in a NICU setting, and may require maintenance infusions of glucose-containing solutions and frequent serum glucose checks. When the perinatal period and perioperative periods coincide, the anesthesia provider must remain vigilant to avoid periods of hypoglycemia, especially during general anesthesia when signs of low serum glucose are masked.

During the neonatal period, the ability for the immature liver to undergo gluconeogenesis and glycogenolysis is incomplete. After birth, the neonates' serum glucose concentration falls, rapidly stabilizing after 3 h. Plasma insulin levels fall and glucagon is mobilized. This leads to a marked decrease in neonatal hepatic glucagon stores and thus serum glucose must be carefully monitored.

During the Procedure, the Anesthesia Team Infuses D10 as Maintenance Fluid; Does This Reduce the Need for Repeated Glucose Checks?

Surgical stress response (causing catecholamine release), infusion of glucose-containing fluids, and administration of corticosteroids (during anesthesia) can lead to hyperglycemia. The sequelae of hyperglycemia in the perioperative period include: increased risk of surgical site infection, poor wound healing, and the potentially associated increased risk of intraventricular hemorrhage and retinopathy of prematurity (in preterm infants).

Elevated hematocrits, not uncommon in neonates, may result in abnormally low glucose levels, which is especially marked when the glucose levels are low. Additionally, arterial samples can have a 10–15% increase in glucose compared with venous samples.

On Postoperative Day 3, You Are Called to Evaluate the Patient for Visible Icterus: What Is the Mechanism for Jaundice in the Neonatal Period?

Neonatal jaundice with visible icterus occurs in up to 80% of healthy neonates born after 35 weeks of gestation. The majority of neonatal jaundice resolves spontaneously with no residual effects. A small subset of patients, if left untreated, will go on to develop significant hyperbilirubinemia and encephalopathy. If jaundice is observed within the first 24 h of life, hemolytic causes must be considered.

Total bilirubin is the difference between bilirubin production and bilirubin metabolism.

Bilirubin production is the result of heme catabolism. Heme is broken down into biliverdin, and further metabolized into bilirubin. Bilirubin is conjugated in hepatocytes by the enzyme UDP-glucuronsyltransferase 1A1 (UGT1A1) and excreted into the bile ducts and bowel for elimination. In neonates, bilirubin also enters the enterohepatic circulation where it is converted into the unconjugated form once again, is resorbed, and returns to the liver for re-processing.

Hyperbilirubinemia results from an imbalance between bilirubin production and excretion. Neonates have only 1% of the UGT1A1 enzyme activity compared with adults. This becomes the rate-limiting step and thus makes neonates prone to hyperbilirubinemia. With most neonates, elevated serum bilirubin can be attributed to immature conjugation abilities. The minority of patients have underlying conditions such as Crigler–Najjar syndrome (abnormal UGT1A1) amongst others. Additionally, patients with G6-PD and RBC membrane deficiencies may suffer from hemolysis which can contribute to hyperbilirubinemia.

For the patient in this case, on postoperative day three, hemolysis may be a contributor. Sepsis can also lead to hyperbilirubinemia and should always be excluded especially in a postoperative patient.

What Is Kernicterus, and How Is It Prevented?

Kernicterus is a potentially devastating consequence of excessive and untreated hyperbilirubinemia. The excess bilirubin damages the basal ganglia resulting in chronic athetoid movements and cerebral palsy. The risk is exponentially related to the serum bilirubin, with levels >25 mg/dL. With improved detection and treatment strategies, kernicterus is rare in the Western world. Treatment focuses on prevention with screening tests, early intervention with phototherapy to aid conjugation and exchange transfusion for recalcitrant patients.

Describe the Process of Protein Synthesis by the Neonatal Liver

The liver hepatocytes synthesize most plasma proteins including alpha-fetoprotein and albumin, which reach adult levels by term. All coagulation factors are produced in the liver with the exception of factor 8 which is produced in the liver and vascular endothelium. The serum concentration of coagulation factors remains low in the first few days following birth. In the United States, neonates receive an intramuscular injection of vitamin K, to increase the vitamin K dependent factors. Low factor levels may become a consideration in neonates undergoing immediate surgical procedures. This may be complicated by dilutional coagulopathy through crystalloid administration.

Identify the Differences in the Neonatal Hematologic System

Term neonates experience a physiologic anemia around 10–12 weeks of age with a decrease in hematocrit to approximately 30%. The neonate has a normal level of platelets at birth although with reduced clot strength. Early thrombocytopenia <72 h after birth is often due to maternal–fetal interaction while late thrombocytopenia >72 hrs should prompt evaluation of sepsis or necrotizing enterocolitis.

With respect to hemostasis, the neonate has reduced levels of factors 2, 7, 9, 11, and 12. However, there is a decrease in proteins C and S and an increase in vWF which partially offsets the decrease in factors. Neonates have a prolonged PT and PTT but a slightly shorter bleeding time.

How Does the Immaturity of the Fetal Liver Effect Drug Metabolism?

The liver metabolizes drugs through biotransformation followed by excretory transport. These pathways are immature in neonates.

Hepatic biotransformation is divided into phase 1 (oxidation, reduction, and hydrolysis) via the cytochrome P450 pathway and phase 2 (conjugation/glucuronidation). The pathways mature throughout the first year of life. The concentrations of the cytochrome P450 proteins at birth are approximately 30% of adult concentrations, reaching normal levels at 1 year of age. The neonates have limited enzymatic glucuronidation and conjugation ability, which limits their metabolic capability such as the breakdown of bilirubin and morphine.

The neonates decreased ability to metabolize drugs results in increased serum levels and increased elimination half-lives. The metabolic activity is enzyme dependent and has significant inter-patient variability.

Describe the Differences in Renal Function Between the Neonatal and Adult Patient

Kidney function undergoes constant change in the neonatal period. As such, the ability of the immature kidney to deal with hypovolemia by concentrating urine is poor as is the ability to process large solute loads (Table 2.2). The differences between neonatal and adult renal function is summarized in Table 2.2.

What Are the Determinants of Neonatal Oxygenation?

Neonatal oxygen delivery depends on the amount of inspired oxygen, V/Q matching, cardiac output, and the type, concentration, and affinity of the hemoglobin. Oxygen is transported predominantly by hemoglobin with a minimal contribution of dissolved oxygen in the plasma. Dissociation of oxygen from hemoglobin is closely related to the oxygen dissociation curve and its determinants including temperature, 2,3 DPG, $[H^+]$, and hemoglobin variants. Fetal hemoglobin (HgF) has an increased O_2 affinity allowing for greater extraction of O_2 from the placenta. HgF predominates at birth and decreases to approximately 2% of total hemoglobin by 1 year. At birth, the oxygen requirement increases by >100%. To cope with these changes, the neonate has multiple adaptive mechanisms occurring at or prior to birth. Near term the fetus begins producing hemoglobin A (HgA) which, despite its lower

Table 2.2 Characteristic differences between neonatal and adult renal function

	Neonate	Adult
Renal blood flow	10% of cardiac output	25% of cardiac output
Glomerular filtration rate (mL/min/ 1.73 m²)	<2 Weeks –40	100–125
	>2 Weeks –60	
Concentrating ability	<6–12 Months - Low 700 mOsm	1,400 mOsm
Creatinine	Active reabsorption in first days of life	Not actively reabsorbed
	Elevated serum creatinine	Serum levels related to renal function
Fractional excretion sodium (FENa)	<2 Weeks, Elevated	Relative to kidney function and hydration status
Extracellular fluid (ECF)	At Birth: 40% of TBW <6 Months: 30% of TBW	20% of TBW

affinity for oxygen promotes oxygen transport to tissues. The neonate has an increase in 2,3 DPG which, aside from decreasing pH also promotes transfer of oxygen to tissues.

The transitional mechanism from placental to pulmonary oxygenation at birth is discussed in the cardiovascular section.

How Do Lung Volumes in Children Compare to Those in Adults?

Pulmonary mechanics is related to the compliance of the chest wall and lung. In neonates, the chest wall, mostly composed of cartilage has the tendency to collapse outward while the lung is more prone to inward collapse. This imbalance is partially offset by the increase in laryngeal tone during exhalation and the increase in respiratory rate.

Resistance to flow is also significantly greater in neonates as a result of decreased airway diameter. In small children, minor inflammation or reduced airway diameter causes an exponential increase in resistance to gas flow. The characteristic differences between neonatal and adult pulmonary functions are highlighted in Table 2.3.

Table 2.3 Characteristic differences between neonatal and adult pulmonary function

	Neonate	Adult
Respiratory rate (breaths/min)	50	12
Tidal volume (cc/kg)	6–8	6–7
Minute ventilation (cc/kg/min)	200–250	90
Functional residual capacity (cc/kg)	25–30	30
VO_2 oxygen consumption (cc/kg/min)	6–8	3–4
PaO_2 (mmHg)	60–90	80–100
Dead space (cc/kg)	2	2

Neonatal Apnea

Neonatal apnea is defined as cessation in respiratory flow of greater than 15–20 seconds or <15 seconds if accompanied by oxygen desaturation <90% and bradycardia of <100 beats/min.

Central apnea is cessation of air flow in the absence of respiratory effort. In obstructive apnea, there is cessation of flow with preserved respiratory efforts. In either case, there is often a closure of the glottis with pharyngeal or laryngeal collapse.

What Are the Etiologies of Neonatal Apnea?

Neonatal apnea may have central or obstructive components or occur in combination.

The incidence of neonatal apnea is inversely related to gestational age.

Neonatal apnea is thought to result from immaturity of the central mechanism for regulation of breathing and an immature response to hypoxia and hypercarbia and exaggerated protective response to airway stimulation.

What Are the Risk Factors for Neonatal Apnea?

Risk factors for development of neonatal apnea include: airway structural anomalies, ambient temperature fluctuation, anemia, cardiac anomalies, central nervous system (CNS) disorders, chronic lung disease, infection, metabolic derangement, necrotizing enterocolitis, prematurity, and sepsis.

Neonates are exquisitely sensitive to medication effects including general anesthetics, magnesium, prostaglandin, and opioids.

What Are the Treatments for Neonatal Apnea?

Treatment should start with a focus on identifying patients at risk for apnea, avoidance of inciting factors and adjustment of anesthetic technique when appropriate. Regional anesthetics provide a lower incidence of postoperative neonatal apnea compared with general anesthesia. Continuous positive pressure, including nasal CPAP (for obstructive apnea) and caffeine supplementation are commonly used to decrease the incidence of neonatal apnea. Gentle tactile stimulation will often break the apneic cycle.

Suctioning the airway prior to extubation may help to reveal an exaggerated response to stimulation leading to breath holding. Postoperative neonatal apnea is discussed in greater detail in Chapter 18.

The preanesthesia evaluation should include:

1. Identification of neonates having received treatment for apnea.
2. Consideration of the safest anesthetic and avoidance of inciting agents.
3. Postoperative discharge planning in cases of post gestational age <60 weeks.
4. Identification and avoidance of apnea risk factors.

Review the Differences Related to Spinal Anesthetics Between Neonates and Adults

There are numerous physiologic differences that must be considered when performing a spinal anesthetic on a neonate.

At birth, the spinal cord terminates around L3 to L4 and at L1 at approximately 1 year of age. Thus, spinals in neonates should be placed at L4–5 or L5–S1 to avoid injury. The volume of local anesthetic required is greater in the neonate owing to a greater cerebrospinal fluid (CSF) volume of 4 cc/kg compared with 2 cc/kg in adults. Additionally, 50% of the neonate's CSF remains in the spinal canal compared with 25% in adults leading to dilution of local anesthetics. The neonate's spinal cord has increased blood supply compared with adults and results in increased uptake of local anesthetic and a shorter duration of action. Spinal anesthetics are discussed in greater detail in Chapter 7.

Identify the Differences in Metabolism of Fentanyl and Morphine in the Neonate Compared to the Adult

Neonates require significantly less morphine than adults or older children, as their ability to metabolize morphine is not fully complete. Following administration, a neonate will display a greater serum concentration of morphine, and its active metabolites, morphine-3 and morphine-6 glucuronide, compared with an adult. Clearance of fentanyl is also reduced in the neonatal period to 70–80% of adult clearance and normalizes at about two weeks.

How Does Minimum Alveolar Concentration Relate to Age?

The minimum alveolar concentration (MAC) for inhaled anesthetic agents is directly related to age. For isoflurane and desflurane, MAC is high in neonates, peaks during infancy, and steadily declines throughout life. The MAC for sevoflurane peaks in the neonatal period and steadily declines throughout life.

What Is the Incidence of Congenital Hypothyroidism (CH)?

The incidence of CH is approximately 1 in 2,000–4,000 live births.

What Are the Clinical Characteristics of CH?

Newborn screening programs remain one of the greatest advances in medicine aimed at reducing preventable morbidity and mortality. Children with CH are generally normal at birth, emphasizing the importance of screening. Less than half of children with CH show signs by three months and only 70% will show signs by twelve months. The incidence of CH is greatest in premature infants with nearly 50% showing signs of CH when born at <30 weeks of gestation. Low or absent thyroid hormone, if untreated leads to mental retardation, severe growth restriction and brain developmental restriction. These children often have deficits in attention, arithmetic, memory and verbal skills in addition to abnormal muscle tone, ataxia, poor coordination, and strabismus. Congenital hypothyroidism is the leading cause of preventable mental retardation.

What Risks Are Associated with Maternal Hypothyroidism?

Maternal thyroid hormone is critical to fetal neurodevelopment in early pregnancy. Infants born to mothers with untreated hypothyroidism are at risk for mental retardation, hearing loss, and a variety of motor delays. Mothers should be screened for hypothyroidism in early pregnancy. Mothers with known hypothyroidism often require increased supplementation to account for the needs of the developing fetus.

What Are the Main Disorders Screened for by the Neonatal Screening Programs?

Neonatal screening programs vary by state. These screening tests generally focus on disorders of fatty acids, amino acids, organic acids, hemoglobinopathies, hypothyroidism, adrenal hyperplasia, biotinidase deficiency, galactosemia, and cystic fibrosis.

Suggested Reading

Beardsall K. Measurement of glucose levels in the newborn. *Early Hum Dev.* 2010;86(5):263–7. PMID: 20542649.

Blazer S, Zimmer EZ, Gover A, Bronshtein M. Fetal omphalocele detected early in pregnancy: associated anomalies and outcomes. *Radiology.* 2004;232:191–5. PMID: 15220502.

Brantberg A, Blaas HG, Haugen SE, Eik-Nes SH. Characteristics and outcome of 90 cases of fetal omphalocele. *Ultrasound Obstet Gynecol.* 2005;26:527–37. PMID: 16184512.

Büyükgebiz A. Newborn screening for congenital hypothyroidism. *J Clin Res Pediatr Endocrinol.* 2013;5S1:8–12. PMID: 23154158.

Christison-Lagay ER, Kelleher CM, Langer JC. Neonatal abdominal wall defects. *Semin Fetal Neonatal Med.* 2011;16:164–72. PMID: 21474399.

Coté CJ, Zaslavsky A, Downes JJ, et al. Postoperative apnea in former preterm infants after inguinal herniorrhaphy. A combined analysis. *Anesthesiology.* 1995;82:809–22. PMID: 7717551.

Davis RP, Mychaliska GB. Neonatal pulmonary physiology. *Semin Pediatr Surg.* 2013;22:179–84. PMID: 24331091.

Diaz-Miron J, Miller J, Vogel AM. Neonatal hematology. *Semin Pediatr Surg.* 2013;22:199–204. PMID: 24331095.

Grijalva J, Vakili K. Neonatal liver physiology. *Semin Pediatr Surg.* 2013;22:185–9. PMID: 24331092.

Harris DL, Weston PJ, Harding JE. Incidence of neonatal hypoglycemia in babies identified as at risk. *J Pediatr.* 2012;161:787–91. PMID: 22727868.

Hiraki S, Green NS. Newborn screening for treatable genetic conditions: past, present and future. *Obstet Gynecol Clin North Am.* 2010;37:11–21. PMID: 22727868.

Kaplan M, Bromiker R, Hammerman C. Hyperbilirubinemia, hemolysis, and increased bilirubin neurotoxicity. *Semin Perinatol.* 2014;38:429–37. PMID: 25284470.

Lerman J, Robinson S, Willis MM, Gregory GA. Anesthetic requirements for halothane in young children 0–1 month and 1–6 months of age. *Anesthesiology.* 1983;59:421–4. PMID: 6638549.

López T, Sánchez FJ, Garzón JC, Muriel C. Spinal anesthesia in pediatric patients. *Minerva Anestesiol.* 2012;78:78–87. PMID: 22211775.

Maitra S, Baidya DK, Khanna P, et al. Acute perioperative pain in neonates: An evidence-based review of neurophysiology and management. *Acta Anaesthesiol Taiwan.* 2014;52:30–7. PMID: 24999216.

Nandi-Munshi D, Taplin CE. Thyroid-related neurological disorders and complications in children. *Pediatr Neurol.* 2015;52(4):373–82. PMID: 25661286.

Nargozian C, Ririe DG, Bennun RD, et al. Hemifacial microsomia: anatomical prediction of difficult intubation. *Paediatr Anaesth.* 1999;9:393–8. PMID: 10447900.

Sale SM. Neonatal apnoea. *Best Pract Res Clin Anaesthesiol.* 2010;24:323–36. PMID: 21033010.

Sulemanji M, Vakili K. Neonatal renal physiology. *Semin Pediatr Surg.* 2013;22:195–8. PMID: 24331094.

Weksberg R, Shuman C, Beckwith JB. Beckwith–Wiedemann syndrome. *Eur J Hum Genet.* 2010;18:8–14. PMID: 19550435.

Yaster M, Scherer TL, Stone MM, et al. Prediction of successful primary closure of congenital abdominal wall defects using intraoperative measurements. *J Pediatr Surg.* 1989;24:1217–20. PMID: 2531789.

Chapter 3

Anesthetic Neurotoxicity in Children

Adam C. Adler and Dean B. Andropoulos

A nine-month-old, 7 kg male arrived for primary repair of hypospadias. He was born at 32 weeks and required ligation of a patent ductus arteriosus at 35 weeks of age via a thoracotomy. At three months, he underwent a brain MRI after a seizure, with no critical findings. During the routine preoperative evaluation, the parents ask about the possible harmful effects of anesthesia on their child and are concerned because this is his third exposure to general anesthesia.

How Many Children Undergo Procedures with Anesthesia Annually?

In the United States, about 1.5–2 million infants under one year of age undergo anesthesia each year for a variety of surgical procedures or diagnostic tests.

What Is the 2017 Concern/Warning About General Anesthesia from the Food and Drug Administration?

In 2016, with a revision in 2017, the US Food and Drug Administration (FDA) issued a warning regarding the administration of anesthetics in children. Specifically, the warning states:

> The U.S. Food and Drug Administration (FDA) is warning that repeated or lengthy use of general anesthetic and sedation drugs during surgeries or procedures in children younger than 3 years or in pregnant women during their third trimester may affect the development of children's brains.

What Studies Led to the FDA-Issued Warning?

The initial studies concerning for neurotoxic effects of anesthetics in young children date back to 1999. Ikonomidou et al. (1999) demonstrated that administration of dizocilpine (a ketamine analog) in pregnant rats and rat pups resulted in significant neuronal cell death compared to unexposed controls.

Following this study, other groups were able to demonstrate similar neurotoxic effects using halogenated agents as well as propofol in rat and rhesus macaque brains for both neonatal and fetal animal groups.

Based on the Animal Studies, Are the Effects of Neural Toxicity Dose Dependent?

Early studies using ketamine by Ikonomidou et al. (1999) demonstrated a significant dose-dependent effect on neuroapoptosis.

Summarize the Human Studies Evaluating Neurologic Effects of Anesthetics in Children

Several studies have been presented evaluating the long-term effects of early anesthesia exposure on neurological development.

An early study by Flick et al. (2011) compared 350 children with anesthesia exposures before age two. These patients were compared with 700 propensity-matched controls evaluating for the incidence of learning disabilities and school specialized educational programs. They concluded that repeated (not a single) exposure to anesthesia prior to age two was associated with a risk for development of learning disabilities.

In 2016, Sun et al. published the Pediatric Anesthesia Neurodevelopment Assessment (PANDA) study which reported the findings of a longitudinal sibling-matched multicenter study.

They compared unexposed siblings to siblings exposed to a single anesthetic for inguinal hernia repair prior to age two. The patients underwent neuropsychological testing for IQ and neurocognitive functions at a mean age of ten years. They concluded that a single exposure to anesthesia prior to thirty-six months in age did not result in any statistically significant differences in IQ scores in childhood.

In 2016, Davidson et al. presented the findings of the General Anesthesia compared to Spinal anesthesia (GAS) trial. This multi-institutional, prospective, randomized-controlled equivalent trial compared Bayley Scales of Infant and Toddler Development III, assessed at two years in children undergoing inguinal hernia repair younger than sixty weeks post-conceptual age. Patients were randomly assigned to either awake-regional anesthesia (spinal) or sevoflurane-based general anesthesia. They found no difference in Bayley III scores in children having one hour or less of anesthesia compared with unexposed children (regional group). The primary outcome of the study released in 2019 concluded that less than 1 h of general anaesthesia in early infancy did not alter neurodevelopmental outcomes at five years of age compared with awake-regional anaesthesia

Table 3.1 What drugs are included in the 2017 concern/ warning from the US Food and Drug Administration (FDA)?

• Desflurane	• Propofol	• Ketamine
• Halothane	• Pentobarbital	• Etomidate
• Sevoflurane	• Midazolam	• Methohexital
• Isoflurane	• Lorazepam	

What Future Studies Are Occurring?

For each of the landmark studies, questions exist on the extrapolatability from animal models, use of behavioral and IQ testing as surrogates for neuroapoptosis, and the generalizability of the populations studied. Other concerns include the translatability of neurodevelopmental phases from the animals studied to humans, and the medication doses and duration of exposure.

However, conducting these studies in humans is unethical, which requires us to rely on these extrapolations.

In addition to reporting the primary outcome of the GAS trial, the Toxicity of Remifentanil – Dexmedetomidine (T-REX) study is expected to evaluate the use of dexmedetomidine and remifentanil on children undergoing anesthesia. (See https://clinicaltrials.gov/ct2/show/NCT02353182.)

What Can You Tell Parents About Neuroapoptosis?

Parents of young children should be made aware of the risks of anesthesia on the developing brain as suggested by the FDA warning. At Texas Children's

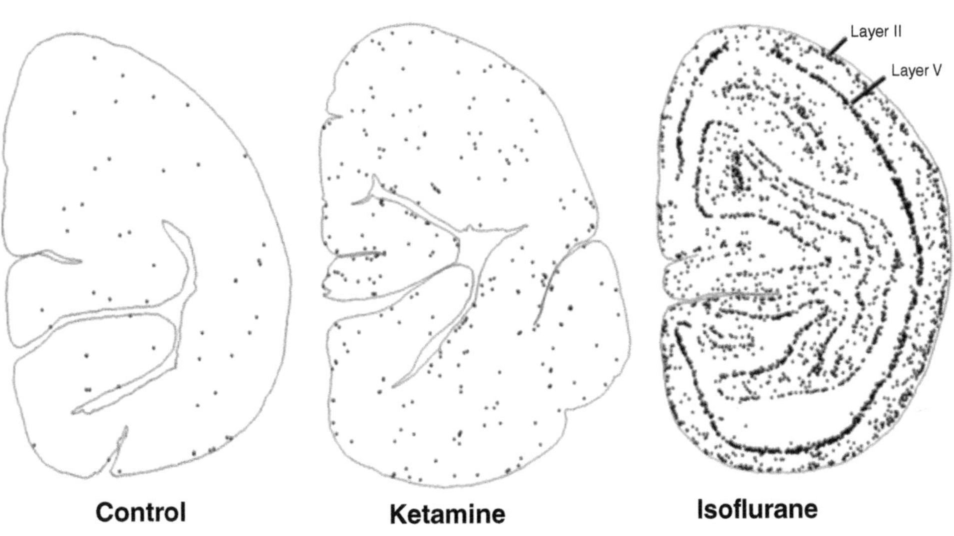

Figure 3.1 Pictorial demonstrating the degrees of neuroapoptosis seen in rhesus macaque brains in control subjects contrasted with those exposed to ketamine and isoflurane. Reproduced with permission of Wolters Kluwer Health, Inc. from Brambrink AM, et al. *Anesthesiology* 2012;116:372–384.

Hospital, in children with potentially deferrable procedures and those predicted to undergo multiple anesthetics in early childhood, the FDA warning is discussed with parents and documented. Discussion and documentation should be performed according to hospital and state guidelines.

Items to discuss with parents include:

- Human studies suggest that a short and single exposure to anesthesia appears to be safe.
- There is evidence that prolonged (>3 hours) or repeated exposures could have negative effects on behavior or learning.
- More research, especially in children, is needed to truly understand the effects of anesthesia.

We encourage parents to ask their providers:

- How long is the surgery or procedure expected to take?
- Is the procedure potentially deferrable to a later date?
- Are additional procedures likely to be needed?

What Can I Do to Limit Anesthetic Exposure in Young Children?

When evaluating children for anesthesia and surgery, it is important to identify young children scheduled for potentially deferrable procedures, and certainly procedures that are expected to exceed three hours. This is crucial in children who are likely to undergo multiple anesthetics in early childhood. Thankfully, most children do not fall into this category. However, the child presented in this chapter's case example is one in which multiple anesthetics were performed in infancy with a planned hypospadias revision that may be deferrable until later in childhood.

- When possible, perform regional anesthetic techniques.
- Minimize use of inhalation agent to reduce total exposure.
- Use opioids and dexmedetomidine to reduce the exposure to halogenated agents.

Suggested Reading

Andropoulos DB, Greene MF. Anesthesia and developing brains: implications of the FDA warning. *N Engl J Med.* 2017;376(10):905–7. PMID: 28177852.

Brambrink AM, Evers AS, Avidan MS, et al. Isoflurane-induced neuroapoptosis in the neonatal rhesus macaque brain. *Anesthesiology.* 2010;112(4):834–41. PMID: 20234312.

Brambrink AM, Evers AS, Avidan MS, et al. Ketamine-induced neuroapoptosis in the fetal and neonatal rhesus macaque brain. *Anesthesiology.* 2012;116(2):372–84. PMID: 22222480.

Creeley C, Dikranian K, Dissen G, et al. Propofol-induced apoptosis of neurones and oligodendrocytes in fetal and neonatal rhesus macaque brain. *Br J Anaesth.* 2013;110 Suppl 1:i29–38. PMID: 23722059.

Davidson AJ, Disma N, de Graaff JC, et al. Neurodevelopmental outcome at 2 years of age after general anaesthesia and awake-regional anaesthesia in infancy (GAS): an international multicentre, randomised controlled trial. *Lancet.* 2016;387:239–50. PMID: 26507180.

FDA Drug Safety Communication: FDA approves label changes for use of general anesthetic and sedation drugs in young children. www.fda.gov/Drugs/DrugSafety/ucm554634.htm.

Flick RP, Katusic SK, Colligan RC, et al. Cognitive and behavioral outcomes after early exposure to anesthesia and surgery. *Pediatrics.* 2011;128(5):e1053–61. PMID: 21969289.

Ikonomidou C, Bosch F, Miksa M, et al. Blockade of NMDA receptors and apoptotic neurodegeneration in the developing brain. *Science.* 1999;283(5398):70–4. PMID: 9872743.

McCann ME, de Graff JC, Dorris L, et al. Neurodevelopmental outcome at 5 years of age after general anaesthesia or awake-regional anaesthesia in infancy (GAS): an international, multicentre, randomised, controlled equivalence trial. *The Lancet.* 2019;393(10172): P664–677.

Sun LS, Li G, Miller TL, et al. Association between a single general anesthesia exposure before age 36 months and neurocognitive outcomes in later childhood. *JAMA.* 2016;315(21):2312–20. PMID: 27272582.

Warner DO, Zaccariello MJ, Katusic SK, et al. Neuropsychological and behavioral outcomes after exposure of young children to procedures requiring general anesthesia: the Mayo Anesthesia Safety in Kids (MASK) study. *Anesthesiology.* 2018;129(1):89–105. PMID: 29672337.

Preoperative Anxiety

Rebecca Evans and William D. Ryan

A four-year-old female presents for a tonsillectomy. She is accompanied by her mother and father. She is extremely anxious and will not separate from her parents.

At What Age Are Patients Most Likely to Develop Separation Anxiety?

Between 7–10 months of age, infants will become anxious when being separated from their parents. This separation anxiety can persist throughout all ages of childhood.

What Is the Incidence of Preoperative Anxiety in Children?

Estimates reveal that at least 60% of children develop significant fear and anxiety before surgery. Many children and families list the separation from parents and induction of anesthesia as the most stressful time during the surgical experience.

What Are the Risk Factors for Preoperative Anxiety in Children?

There are child, parent, and environmentally related risk factors for children having preoperative anxiety.

Child-Related

- Age: 1–5 years
- Poor previous experience with medical procedures
- Chronic illness
- Shy/inhibited temperament
- Lack of developmental maturity/social adaptability
- High cognitive ability
- Not enrolled in daycare

Parent-Related

- High anxiety
- Parents who use avoidance coping mechanisms
- Parents who have undergone multiple medical procedures
- Divorced parents

Environment-Related

- Sensory overload and conflicting messages
- Parental anxiety

The preoperative period is often a stressful and anxiety-provoking phase for children and their family. It is not unusual for the parents to be frightened and to project their fear and anxiety on the child, thereby unintentionally contributing to the child's fear and anxiety. Increased parental anxiety is noted in parents of children less than one year of age, and in children with repeated hospital admissions.

What Are the Overall Benefits of Reducing Preoperative Anxiety?

The most important outcomes related to preoperative distress in children are postoperative behavioral disorders. These include nightmarish sleep disturbances, feeding difficulties, apathy, withdrawal, increased level of separation anxiety, aggression toward authority, fear of subsequent medical procedures and hospital visits, and regressive behaviors such as bed wetting. Although these disturbances are primarily present within the first two postoperative weeks, in some children they may last for several months. Much has been made of this issue in the recent literature, but the concept is not new.

Children who were anxious in the preoperative period were found to have more postoperative pain, require more pain medications while hospitalized and during their first 3 days at home, and have a greater incidence of emergence delirium, postoperative anxiety, behavioral changes (apathy, withdrawal, enuresis, temper tantrums, eating disturbances), and sleep disturbances. In adults, increased preoperative anxiety is associated with poor postoperative clinical and behavior recovery.

How Should You Prepare the Parents Prior to Induction?

One of the most important preoperative responsibilities of the pediatric anesthesiologist is to allay anxiety in the parents and other family members. During the preoperative visit the anesthesiologist, while talking to the parents, should initiate contact and communication with the child. It does not matter if the child is too young to understand or is too premedicated to remember any events. The parents will key in on the anesthesiologist's manner and how he or she relates to the child. Asking children about their interests and performing a simple fist-bump will establish confidence and minimize parental anxiety.

A controversial issue in pediatric anesthesia is the extent to which the anesthesiologist should reveal the risks of anesthesia to the parents. Will this discussion increase or decrease parental (or child) anxiety? Should the anesthesiologist discuss the risk of death? What risks are appropriate to reveal? The answers to these questions are not easily found and may partly depend on the informed consent laws of the state in which one practices. Studies universally demonstrate that anxiety is decreased with more information, even though that information may allude to more harmful risks. For example, in a questionnaire study, most parents whose anesthesiologist mentioned the risk of death indicated they were satisfied to hear about this rare risk. Many parents whose anesthesiologist did not specifically mention the risk of death indicated that it should have been mentioned.

During the preoperative informed consent process, it is helpful to know the modern-day risks of general anesthesia in children. A study from the Mayo Clinic revealed an incidence of cardiac arrest in anesthetized children (for noncardiac surgery) of 2.9 per 10,000, although when attributed only to anesthetic causes, the incidence decreased to 0.65 per 10,000 anesthetics. Only a small percentage of these patients were initially healthy prior to the procedure.

What Are the Methods Used to Reduce Preoperative Anxiety?

Many different modalities have been used in an attempt to decrease fear and anxiety in patients and their families. There are two broad categories of interventions:

- ***Behavioral interventions***: preoperative preparation programs (child life therapy), distraction techniques, parental presence at induction, preoperative interview, and tour of hospital and/or operating complex.
- ***Pharmacological/premedication***: midazolam (IV, oral, nasal, or rectal routes of administration), dexmedetomidine (oral or nasal).

What Is the Efficacy of Behavioral Interventions?

In carefully performed and controlled studies, these aforementioned behavioral interventions do not fare much better than placebo in decreasing the incidence of postoperative behavioral disturbances. Although distraction techniques are often effective for allaying anxious behavior during induction of anesthesia, premedication with an anxiolytic drug is the only proven intervention to decrease these undesirable outcomes.

What Are the Benefits and Risks Associated with Parental Presence During Induction?

There is controversy surrounding the benefits to parental presence during induction of anesthesia. Potential benefits include reducing the need/amount of preoperative sedatives and avoidance of anxiety caused by parental separation. Parental presence during induction has been correlated with greater parent satisfaction with the anesthetic experience. However, parental presence can place additional stress on the anesthesiologist, crowd the OR, and may not be all that effective in decreasing the child's anxiety.

One randomized controlled trial found that only children younger than 4 years of age who have a calm baseline personality, or who have a parent with a calm baseline personality, benefit from parental presence during induction. Another study comparing parental presence versus oral midazolam found that children who were given midazolam were significantly less anxious and more compliant than children with only parental presence during induction. However, sedative and parental presence together has been shown to be more effective than sedative alone. Furthermore, many parents are terrified as they observe the placing of a mask over their child's face, watching their child become limp as consciousness is lost, and the occasional episode of upper airway obstruction that may occur. Yet when queried, parents who have been with their child in the OR during induction universally feel that they have done the right thing for their child and are happy to have experienced a sense of schadenfreude.

If a decision is made to allow a parent into the OR during induction, the anesthetist should fully explain the events that will occur during induction. Three major points should be addressed:

1. There should be an explanation of the nature of the procedure and the possible effects on the child (excitation, limpness, airway obstruction, etc.).
2. The parent must agree to leave immediately at any time when requested by an OR staff member.
3. The parent must agree to leave immediately once the child has lost consciousness. One of the surgical team members or another OR staff member should accompany the parent from the OR to the parents' smoking area.

Some institutions will ask parents to sign a written agreement to these terms, as well as a waiver of liability should parents suffer an injury secondary to fainting or other calamity.

What Premedication Can Be Used to Reduce Preoperative Anxiety?

Premedication of pediatric patients prior to induction of anesthesia can accomplish several goals, the primary one being anxiolysis, with a subsequent decrease in the incidence of postoperative negative behaviors. Other indications include preinduction of anesthesia, pain relief, drying of secretions prior to airway manipulation, vagolysis, and decreasing the risk for pulmonary aspiration of gastric contents. Preoperative sedation may be administered via any route, the most common being oral administration since the vast majority of children do not have an existing IV catheter. Rectal premedication is acceptable in toddlers, and in some centers the nasal route is preferred for midazolam. Few centers in the United States administer intramuscular premedication, or place IV catheters preoperatively.

There are various options for treatment of preoperative anxiety. None, however, are ideal; each has drawbacks. A benzodiazepine is the best treatment for preoperative anxiety. Options include midazolam, the most commonly administered premedication, and diazepam.

Midazolam

Oral midazolam is the most common preoperative anxiolytic for children. This is because it possesses most of the properties of the ideal premedication. The one exception is that it usually leaves a bitter aftertaste when administered orally, even as a specially formulated oral syrup and given with an apple juice chaser. Therefore, many children will attempt to spit it out if it is not swallowed rapidly. After oral administration, the commercially available midazolam syrup is rapidly absorbed from the stomach. The absolute bioavailability of midazolam averages 36%, within a variable and large range (9–71%). This large range in bioavailability is consistent with most oral medications administered to children. In a large study, the plasma concentration/time curves of midazolam and its α-hydroxy metabolite were highly variable, and independent of the age of the child and the dose administered. Approximately 14% of children who receive oral midazolam do not demonstrate effective anxiolysis.

Caution should be observed in children who are receiving erythromycin (or its derivatives), since it can prolong the duration of action of midazolam via cytochrome P-450 inhibition. In children who are currently receiving erythromycin, the midazolam dose should be reduced by at least 50%.

Clinical sedative effects are seen within 5–10 minutes of oral midazolam administration and appear to peak 15–30 minutes after administration. By 45 minutes, its sedative effects have dissipated in most children. Pharmacodynamic studies indicate that sedation level is directly correlated with plasma concentration of midazolam. Plasma midazolam concentrations greater than 50 ng/mL are associated with adequate preoperative sedation. However, plasma concentrations of midazolam do not correlate with anxiety scores at the time of mask induction of anesthesia.

The sedative effect of midazolam is best described as inebriation rather than sleepiness. Therefore, after administration, children should be confined to a bed or their parent's arms and be directly observed at all times by medical personnel. Clinically important cardiorespiratory side effects are not observed in healthy children but may be seen in children at risk of upper airway obstruction. Dysphoria may occur in some children. Anterograde amnesia is a favorable clinical effect following most doses of oral midazolam and may be responsible for the decrease in postoperative behavioral disturbances.

Most anesthesiologists find that an oral dose of 0.5–0.7 mg/kg results in the best clinical efficacy. However, a pharmacodynamic study showed that a dose as low as 0.25 mg/kg results in reliable preoperative anxiolysis. There are no data to indicate the most appropriate maximum dose, but most anesthesiologists use between 10 and 20 mg.

Studies are conflicting, but some evidence indicates that midazolam premedication results in longer times to discharge postoperatively following surgeries of relatively short duration. Nevertheless, its preoperative advantages outweigh this disadvantage.

Nasal administration of midazolam can be accomplished in the form of nose drops or a nasal spray. The required dose (0.2–0.3 mg/kg) is lower than with oral administration and its reliability in producing anxiolysis is excellent. However, its administration is associated with an unpleasant burning of the nasal cavity and most children are quite upset following its use. In addition, plasma concentrations of midazolam are generally higher after nasal administration when compared to the oral route. Respiratory depression has been reported on occasion following nasal administration. For these reasons, pediatric anesthesiologists tend use the nasal route of administration infrequently.

If a child has a preexisting IV catheter, it should be used to administer midazolam. Pharmacokinetic studies indicate a β-elimination half-life of less than two hours in children. The half-life of both midazolam and its major metabolite tend to increase with advancing age during childhood. The onset of IV midazolam is 2–3 minutes and the peak sedative effect is shortly thereafter. The duration of action varies between two and six hours, with most of the sedative effect dissipating within 30 minutes of a single dose. A standard dose of IV midazolam is 0.05 mg/kg, which can then be titrated to effect, depending on the clinical situation.

Diazepam

Since the advent of midazolam, diazepam has not been used routinely for premedication of children. This is primarily due to its relatively long onset of action and greater duration of action. Diazepam may be indicated for children or adolescents who require anxiolysis prior to approximately one hour before surgery. It can be administered orally at a dose of 0.3 mg/kg. It should not be given IV because of the extreme pain associated with injection.

Clonidine

Clonidine, an α_2-adrenergic agonist, has been tested as an orally administered sedative premedication in children. In doses between 2 and 4 mcg/kg, oral clonidine will produce adequate sedation and anxiolysis prior to induction of general anesthesia. A distinct advantage of clonidine is its ability to decrease intraoperative anesthetic requirements. However, its onset of action is greater than 90 minutes, so it is not suitable for use in the ambulatory setting. Furthermore, when compared with oral midazolam for children undergoing tonsillectomy, clonidine provides less anxiolysis at the time of separation of the child from the caretaker and at induction of anesthesia. An additional disadvantage of clonidine is its ability to blunt the heart rate response to administration of atropine. For these reasons, clonidine is not used routinely as a premedication in children.

Ketamine

Ketamine can be used as a premedication in children, in both oral and rectal forms. At a dose of 5 mg/kg, it reliably produces a state of sedation and disassociation within 20 minutes of its administration. Larger doses have been associated with more reliable anxiolysis at the expense of longer postoperative times to awakening and discharge. Advantages of its use include a low incidence of respiratory depression, and a possible decrease in intraoperative anesthetic requirements. It also possesses analgesic and amnestic properties. Disadvantages include increased oral and airway secretions, an increased incidence of postoperative emesis, and an occasional association with adverse psychological reactions such as delirium, dysphoria, nightmares, and hallucinations. These latter effects have not been observed when ketamine has been used as a premedication. To date, studies have not demonstrated any clear advantages of ketamine over midazolam as a premedication in children. However, it may be a useful substitute in children known to exhibit dysphoric reactions to midazolam, or as an additive to midazolam in children who may be in pain, or difficult to calm.

Intramuscular ketamine is used when children are unusually combative and refuse all attempts at medical attention, including refusal to ingest an oral premedication. It is most often used in developmentally delayed adolescents who are unable to understand their circumstances and will not cooperate with IV catheter placement or inhalational induction. To reduce the volume of the amount injected, the concentrated form (100 mg/mL) should be used, in a dose of 2–6 mg/kg. Larger doses result in greater efficacy at the expense of longer times to emergence from general anesthesia, especially for surgeries of relatively short duration. We prefer a lower dose with the modest goal of obtaining sufficient sedation to facilitate IV catheter insertion or mask induction. Some anesthesiologists will include atropine in the injectate in an attempt to reduce airway secretions.

Suggested Reading

Kain ZN, Mayes LC, Caramico LA, et al. Parental presence during induction of anesthesia: A randomized controlled trial. *Anesthesiology.* 1996;84:1060–7. PMID: 8623999.

Kain Z, Mayes L, Wang S, et al. Parental presence during induction of anesthesia vs. sedative premedication: Which intervention is more effective? *Anesthesiology.* 1998;89:1147–56. PMID: 9822003.

Kain Z, Mayes L, Wang S, et al. Parental presence and a sedative premedicant for children undergoing surgery: A hierarchical study. *Anesthesiology.* 2000;92:939–46. PMID: 10754612.

Litman RS. Allaying anxiety in children: When a funny thing happens on the way to the operating room. *Anesthesiology.* 2011;115(1):4–5. PMID: 21572313.

Litman RS, Berger AA, Chhibber A. An evaluation of preoperative anxiety in a population of parents of infants and children undergoing ambulatory surgery. *Pediatr Anaesth.* 1996;6:443–7. PMID: 8936540.

Litman RS, Perkins FM, Dawson SC. Parental knowledge and attitudes toward discussing the risk of death from anesthesia. *Anesth Analg.* 1993;77:256–60. PMID: 8346823.

Maranets I, Kain ZN. Preoperative anxiety and intraoperative anesthetic requirements. *Anesth Analg.* 1999; 89:1346–51. PMID: 10589606.

McCann ME, Kain ZN. The management of preoperative anxiety in children: An update. *Anesth Analg.* 2001;93(1): 98–105. PMID: 11429348.

Postoperative Nausea and Vomiting in Children

Arvind Chandrakantan

> A three-year-old, otherwise healthy, female presents for strabismus surgery. Her mother has a history of postoperative nausea and vomiting (PONV) and is concerned about the possibility of PONV for her child. The medical student requests to review the risk factors for PONV in children.

What Is Postoperative Nausea and Vomiting (PONV) and Postdischarge Nausea and Vomiting (PDNV)?

PONV is nausea/vomiting within 24 hours after surgery. Nausea/vomiting within the 24–72 hour time period is called PDNV.

What Is the Incidence of PONV in Children?

Multiple studies show the incidence is about 10% in outpatient ambulatory pediatric surgery. Older studies where antiemetics were not given routinely demonstrate an incidence of PONV up to 80%. There is no published incidence in pediatric inpatients.

What Are the Risk Factors for PONV in Children?

Primary risk factors for PONV in children are:

- Preoperative nausea and vomiting
- Age >3 years, and especially ages 6–13
- Surgery >30–45 minutes
- History of PONV with previous anesthesia
- Motion sickness
- ENT (tympanoplasty and adenotonsillectomy)/strabismus surgery
- Multiple doses of opioids

Why Is There a Minimal Incidence of PONV in Children under Three Years of Age?

The primary mediator of nausea/vomiting is the chemoreceptor trigger zone (CTZ) as well as the vomiting center in the medulla oblongata in the brain. The thought process is that those areas are not well developed until the age of three in humans, and therefore there is decreased susceptibility in this age group.

Is There a Multimodal PONV Model in Children? Is There a Tiered Model for PONV Based on Risk Factors?

The multimodal PONV model has not been rigorously studied in the pediatric population. Similarly, the tiered model such as the Apfel model does not have a pediatric equivalent. Given that the risk factors for adults may not translate to children, it is hard to make a recommendation at this time.

What Anesthetic Factors Can Contribute to PONV?

The incidence of PONV can be decreased by use of propofol instead of inhaled agents and minimizing use of opioids by using nonsteroidal anti-inflammatory drugs (NSAIDs) and regional analgesia. Other anesthetic considerations include limiting postoperative oral intake, increasing IV hydration, and prophylactic administration of antiemetic medications, such as ondansetron. Combination (multimodal) therapy with different classes of antiemetics (e.g., dexamethasone) more successfully prevents PONV than one type of antiemetic alone. Intraoperative evacuation of gastric contents does not reduce PONV in adults but has not been studied in pediatric patients.

Table 5.1 Incidence of postoperative and post discharge nausea and vomiting in relation to medical management by number of antiemetics administered

Antiemetics	# of patients with nausea on POD 0 (N, %)	# of patients with nausea on POD 1 (N, %)	# of patients with emesis on POD 0 (N, %)
Fluids only	9/18 (50%)	4/17 (23.5%)	4/21 (19.0%)
Ondansetron only	18/30 (60%)	6/21 (28.6%)	3/33 (9.1%)
Ondansetron & Dexamethasone	25/63 (39.7%)	11/39 (38.2%)	5/67 (7.5%)

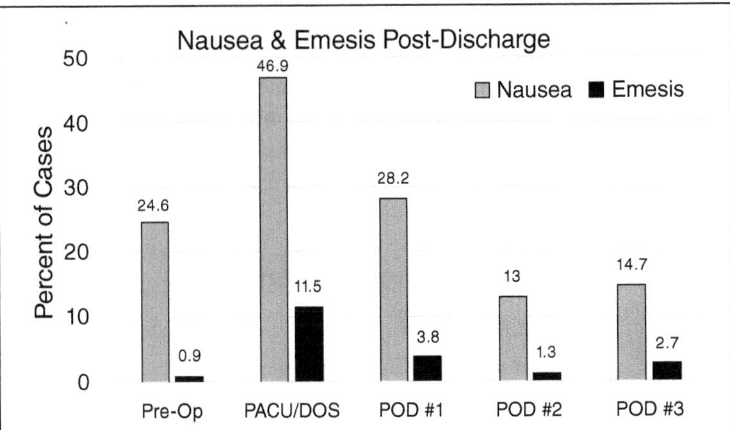

Figure 5.1 Incidence of postdischarge nausea and vomiting in children after ambulatory surgery.

Once PONV Occurs, How Is It Treated?

PONV that occurs despite intraoperative administration of prophylactic antiemetics is very difficult to treat successfully. Options include increased hydration (e.g., 30 cc/kg of intravenous crystalloids), or antihistamines such as diphenhydramine or metoclopramide. Promethazine may also be efficacious but must be given intramuscularly because of the risk of tissue damage when given into a subcutaneous IV infiltration.

What Predicts PDNV? What Is Its Incidence?

Chandrakantan and colleagues performed a study looking at pediatric PDNV. They studied ambulatory pediatric surgical patients ASA I–II for all ambulatory surgical types. Ondansetron was given to 93/113 (83.3%) of our patients, and dexamethasone was given to 65/113 (57.5%) intraoperatively. Sixty-three (55.7%) patients received both antiemetics. Children receiving only intraoperative fluids as antiemetic prophylaxis were classified as receiving zero antiemetics. There was a 10% incidence of PONV on day one, with rapid decrement thereafter (Figure 5.1 and Table 5.1).

What Are the Risk Factors for PDNV?

Presence of PONV and post anesthesia care unit pain seem to predict PDNV, although further study is needed. Number of antiemetics used intraoperatively does not seem to correlate positively or negatively with PDNV.

Suggested Reading

Apfel CC, Kranke P, Eberhart LHJ, et al. Comparison of predictive models for postoperative nausea and vomiting. *Br J Anaesth.* 2002 Feb;88(2):234–40. PMID: 11883387.

Bourdaud N, Devys JM, Bientz J, et al. Development and validation of a risk score to predict the probability of postoperative vomiting in pediatric patients: the VPOP score. *Paediatr Anaesth.* 2014 Sep;24 (9):945–52. PMID: 24823626.

Chandrakantan A, Glass PS. Multimodal therapies for postoperative nausea and vomiting, and pain. *Br J Anaesth.* 2011 Dec;107 Suppl 1:i27–40. PMID: 22156268.

Eberhart LHJ, Geldner G, Kranke P, et al. The development and validation of a risk score to predict the probability of postoperative vomiting in pediatric patients. *Anesth Analg.* 2004, 99(6);1630–7. PMID: 15562045.

Chapter 6

Emergence Delirium

Arvind Chandrakantan

> A five-year-old, otherwise healthy, boy arrives to the recovery room after his adenotonsillectomy. He is thrashing, incoherent, and inconsolable. You and the recovery room nurse are unable to obtain his vital signs.

What Is Emergence Delirium (ED)?

One clinically accepted definition of ED is the "dissociated state of consciousness in which the child is irritable, uncompromising, uncooperative, incoherent, and inconsolably crying, moaning, kicking, or thrashing" (Vlajkovic et al.) This definition lends itself to understanding that emergence disorders are a clinical spectrum, ranging from irritability (emergence agitation) to frank delirium (emergence delirium). ED may cause patient or provider injury, parental and staff distress, and parental dissatisfaction with care. The incidence varies between 10–80% in the published literature.

What Are the Risk Factors for ED, and How Is ED Measured?

Risk factors for ED include:

- Children aged 6 months to 4 years
- Preexisting anxious temperament
- Parental anxiety
- Children not in school/daycare

ED generally occurs within the first 30 minutes following anesthesia. ED seems to have a predilection for males and those children with enhanced preoperative anxiety. Proposed mechanisms include increased sympathetic nervous system activity as well as alternations in frontal lobe connectivity during the indeterminate stage of emergence. A variety of different measurement scales have been described, including the Pediatric Anesthesia Emergence Delirium (PAED) scale (Table 6.1), the Watcha scale (Table 6.2), and the Cravero scale (Table 6.3).

While each of these scales has their own strengths and limitations, a recent comparative analysis between the three concluded that the Watcha scale is simpler to use in clinical practice and may have greater sensitivity and specificity.

Can Emergence Delirium Be Prevented?

Many different pharmacological agents and approaches have been used to prevent ED. They include the avoidance of an inhalational agent and use of propofol, and a variety of other IV anesthetic adjuncts, including midazolam, clonidine, ketamine, sufentanil, and dexmedetomidine. In recent years dexmedetomidine has been gaining the most popularity because of its generally good tolerance and opioid sparing properties. Non-pharmacological approaches to ED prevention include preoperative preparation to decrease parental or child anxiety, music therapy, and distraction techniques.

What Are the Long-Term Sequelae of ED?

The long-term consequences of ED remain unknown. Currently, there exists no unequivocal data that ED leads to postoperative behavioral or other long-term disturbances. This contrasts strongly with the ICU and perioperative literature in older adults, where delirium is a known risk factor for higher morbidity and mortality on a short- and long-term basis.

What Is the Treatment of ED?

Many medications including propofol, opioids, and dexmedetomidine have been used successfully to treat ED. Their use has to be balanced against airway and hemodynamic concerns.

Table 6.1 Pediatric anesthesia emergence delirium scale (PAED)

PAED scale for evaluation of emergence delirium					
Behavior	*Not at all*	*Just a little*	*Quite a bit*	*Very much*	*Extremely*
The child makes eye contact with the caregiver	4	3	3	1	0
The child's actions are purposeful	4	3	2	1	0
The child is aware of his/her surroundings	4	3	2	1	0
The child is restless	0	1	2	3	4
The child is inconsolable	0	1	2	3	4

Scores >10 and especially >12 strongly suggest emergence delirium.

Table 6.2 Watcha scale for emergence delirium

Clinical score	Patient characteristic
1	Calm (conversation)
2	Not calm but could easily be calmed
3	Not easily calmed, moderately agitated or restless
4	Combative, excited, or disoriented

Scores >2 are suggestive of emergence agitation/delirium

Table 6.3 Cravero scale for emergence delirium

Clinical score	Patient characteristic
1	Obtunded with no response to stimulation
2	Asleep but responsive to movement or stimulation
3	Awake and responsive
4	Crying (for >3 min)
5	Thrashing behavior that requires restraint

Scores of 4 or 5 for >3 min are suggestive of emergence delirium.

Suggested Reading

Bajwa SA, et al. A comparison of emergence delirium scales following general anesthesia in children. *Paediatr Anaesth.* 2010 Aug;20(8):704–11. PMID: 20497353.

Banchs RJ, Lerman J. Preoperative anxiety management, emergence delirium, and postoperative behavior. *Anesthesiol Clin.* 2014 Mar;32(1):1–23. PMID: 24491647.

Dahmani S, Delivet H, Hilly J. Emergence delirium in children: an update. *Curr Opin Anaesthesiol.* 2014 Jun;27(3):309–15. PMID: 24784918.

Vlajkovic GP, Sindjelic RP. Emergence delirium in children: many questions, few answers. *Anesth Analg.* 2007 Jan;104(1):84–91. PMID: 17179249.

Anesthesia Care for the Premature Infant

Arvind Chandrakantan and Jamie W. Sinton

A 32-week-old baby girl presents for bilateral inguinal hernia repair. She was born at 26 weeks due to premature rupture of membranes. She had a patent ductus arteriosus (PDA) which was closed with indomethacin, as well as intubation for 1 week after birth for respiratory distress. She is currently extubated with a HR of 151, non-invasive blood pressure (NIBP) 51/33, with an O_2 sat of 95% on 2L nasal cannula (NC).

What Is a Preterm Infant? What Is a Term Baby?

A preterm infant is born between 20 weeks (viability) and 37 weeks of gestation. A term infant is born after 37 weeks of gestation. Classification is based on birth weight which can be correlated with morbidity and mortality (Table 7.1). Numerous issues are experienced by pre-term neonates affecting nearly every system (Table 7.2).

What Are the Unique Cardiovascular Issues in Preterm Infants?

Preterm infants generally have a higher total blood volume per kg than a term infant – approximately 110–120 mL/kg. However, their left ventricles are generally stiffer than term infants, and therefore very dependent on diastolic filling for generating cardiac output. As a result, very high heart rates may be deleterious as they impair diastolic filling due to shortening of the diastolic period. As such, they are less able to augment their cardiac output by increases in stroke volume when compared with older children and adults.

Patent ductus arteriosus, a highly prevalent issue in pre-term neonates, will be covered in Chapter 59.

What Is Bronchopulmonary Dysplasia?

Bronchopulmonary dysplasia (BPD) is a chronic lung disease as a result of prolonged mechanical ventilation and high O_2 concentration exposure, and is more common in preterm infants (Figure 7.1). With better lung protection strategies in premature infants, specifically surfactant and steroid utilization, the severity of BPD has declined in recent years. These children also have increased airway reactivity throughout childhood.

How Is Pulmonary Hypertension Related to Prematurity?

Elevated pulmonary artery pressure is a major source of morbidity in the preterm infant. Failure of arborization or development of the pulmonary vasculature leads to elevated pressures. Severity of illness is directly proportional to the degree of prematurity. Vasculature development may improve as the child grows but is often abnormal.

What Is Apnea of Prematurity? Can It Be Prevented?

Apnea of prematurity is a form of centrally mediated apnea which decreases in incidence with rising post-menstrual age. In the NICU, generally physical stimulation or bag mask ventilation is used to resolve the apnea. Intravenous caffeine citrate reduces the incidence of apnea, however it has other side effects which have to weighed against apnea reduction. This is discussed in greater detail in Chapter 18.

What Is Intraventricular Hemorrhage?

Intraventricular hemorrhage (IVH) has four grades of severity determined by the location of the hemorrhage. It is the most common form of neonatal hemorrhage and mainly occurs in preterm neonates, especially those <32 weeks of gestation.

Table 7.1 Gestational age and weight classifications

Gestational age	Birth weight	Classification
36–37 weeks	<2,500 grams	Low birth weight
31–36 weeks	<1,500 grams	Very low birth weight
24–30 weeks	<1,000 grams	Extremely low birth weight

Table 7.2 What are the most common problems faced by preterm infants?

Cardiovascular system	Patent ductus arteriosus, impaired ventricular diastolic filling
Respiratory system	Apnea of prematurity, bronchopulmonary dysplasia, pulmonary hypertension, laryngotracheal anomalies
Neurological system	Intraventricular hemorrhage, seizures, cerebral palsy
Integumentary system	Increased heat loss, decreased brown fat
Endocrine system	Hypoglycemia, decreased synthesis of vitamin K dependent factors
Hematopoietic system	Relative anemia, thrombocytopenia
Genitourinary system	Decreased tubular bicarbonate absorption
Gastrointestinal system	Necrotizing enterocolitis (NEC)
Ophthalmologic	Retinopathy of prematurity

What Is the Pathophysiology of Intraventricular Hemorrhage?

IVH in the preterm infant is multifactorial.

- The germinal matrix (present in children <35 weeks) is highly vascular and extremely susceptible to ischemia and hypoxic injury.
- Contributing factors may include:
  - Hypotension/reperfusion injury
  - Altered autoregulation in the neonate

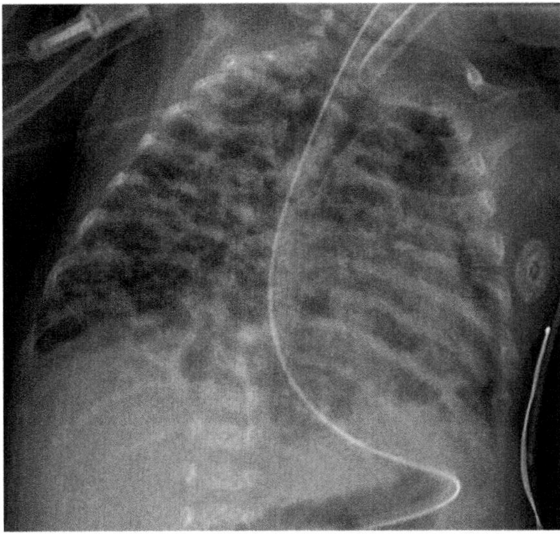

Figure 7.1 Chest X-ray demonstrating severe bronchopulmonary dysplasia. Image by Pulmonological, reproduced under the CC BY-SA 3.0 license https://creativecommons.org/licenses/by-sa/3.0/.

  - Susceptibility to hypervolemia (volume administration)
  - Underdeveloped coagulation system
  - Increased fibrinolytic activity in prematurity
  - Poorly developed arteriovenous supporting structures

What Is Retinopathy of Prematurity and How Can Anesthesia Impact This?

The cause of retinopathy of prematurity (ROP) is multifactorial and is thought to be caused by vascular injury (due to hypoxia or hyperoxia, hypotension, etc.) and resulting free radical formation. As a result, there is angiogenesis and vessel development in abnormal areas (i.e., outside the retina). To prevent further hyperoxia induced damage, most NICU babies are maintained on the minimal tolerated oxygen concentration. During transportation, oxygen/air blenders should be used to avoid prolonged periods of hyperoxia. Intra-operatively, the minimal tolerated oxygen concentration should be used. Similarly, hypoxia should also be avoided.

What Is Cerebral Palsy?

Cerebral palsy is a clinical description of non-progressive injury to the developing brain. It is characterized by upper motor neuron lesions of various

Table 7.3 Grading of interventricular hemorrhage in children by location and associated morbidity and mortality

IVH grade	Location of hemorrhage	Associated mortality (%)	Outcome	
			Progressive ventricular dilation (%)	Neurological sequelae (%)
Grade 1	Bleeding confined to periventricular area (around the germinal matrix)	5	5	5
Grade 2	Intraventricular bleeding <50% of ventricular area	10	20	15
Grade 3	Intraventricular bleeding >50% of ventricular area or resulting in ventricular enlargement	20	55	35
Grade 4	Intraparenchymal extension of bleed – Periventricular hemorrhagic/infarction	50	80	90

etiologies resulting in static encephalopathy. While the encephalopathy is static, progressive musculoskeletal pathology continues.

Cerebral palsy can be classified according to description of motor involvement and topography. Spastic and mixed motor disorders are far more common than dyskinetic cerebral palsy. Simultaneously, spastic hemiplegia, spastic diplegia, and spastic quadriplegia topographically characterize this condition. Those with spastic quadriplegia are more likely to develop scoliosis than those with either spastic hemiplegia or spastic diplegia. Scoliosis occurs secondarily due to failure of growth and ability to relax longitudinal skeletal muscle.

What Is the Incidence of Cerebral Palsy (CP)?

The incidence of CP is approximately 2–2.5/1,000 live births. The exact etiology of CP is unknown and it represents a collection of clinical symptoms rather than a single diagnosis. The causes are likely multifactorial and include antenatal factors, preterm delivery, intrauterine infections, and inherited malformations.

What Are the Consequences of CP?

Progressive musculoskeletal disease often results in hip dislocation, and fixed contractures. Failure of growth of longitudinal muscles leads to contractures, long bone torsion, and joint instability. These musculoskeletal changes eventually lead to discomfort related to degenerative joint changes. Other issues include gastroesophageal reflux and seizures.

Why Are Premature Neonates Prone to Hypothermia?

Preterm neonates have a decreased percentage of brown fat and thus, a decreased ability to generate heat by shivering thermogenesis. Since shivering is an important mechanism to maintain body temperature, this makes them more prone to hypothermia. Premature infants also have a large body surface area (BSA) which leads to evaporative heat loss. Therefore, careful attention must be paid to maintenance of body temperature in the operating room environment in these children.

Why Are Premature Neonates More Prone to Hypoglycemia? What Are the Risks of Hypoglycemia?

There are multiple etiologies for the premature infants' susceptibility to hypoglycemia. Briefly, the premature infant has increased use of glucose coupled with limited mechanisms of gluconeogenesis. This combination is potentially lethal due to the fragility of these small infants. Hypoglycemia is deleterious to the small infant because of their high dependence on glucose for basic metabolic functions. Therefore, in both NICU and operative environments, maintenance of glucose homeostasis is critical.

What Is Neonatal Acidosis?

A mild acidosis is common in neonates due to decreased renal tubular absorption of bicarbonate. This pushes the acid base curve toward increasing respiratory compensation for the acidosis. Under physiological conditions, the acidosis is limited and not harmful. However, under pathological conditions, the limited renal compensation puts even greater pressure on the respiratory component to compensate for acidosis. This explains the rapid acidosis and decompensation seen in ill premature infants.

What Is Necrotizing Enterocolitis?

Necrotizing enterocolitis (NEC) is a potentially fatal condition in which localized bacterial invasion of the intentional lumen leads to bowel perforation. Transluminal bowel perforation leads to spillage of bowel contents. There has been a shift toward medical management of NEC in preterm infants in recent years.

What Is the Preoperative Evaluation for the Premature Infant?

A systematic head to toe approach should be taken with all premature infants. Understanding the child's physiology, including temperature homeostasis, apnea and bradycardia episodes, and ventilatory impairments are important for the transport process and the operating room.

Pre- and post-ductal oxygen saturations should be employed when the ductus arteriosus is patent.

Line placement should be assessed.

Is Regional or General Anesthesia Preferred for This Procedure?

There is no uniform consensus answer to this question. The Vermont Infant Spinal Registry, which has the largest database of infant spinals in the country, has a high rate of long-standing success with the procedure in premature and term infants. Given that the spinal is done awake, however, this technique is limited to select centers that are comfortable with the procedure.

How Is a Neonatal Spinal Anesthetic Performed?

While many techniques including the use of the intercristal line (Truffier's line) have been described, other researchers typically utilize the most palpable interspace below the third lumbar vertebrae and to date have not recorded a conus puncture [personal correspondence, Robin Williams, MD, University of Vermont]. While both the sitting position and the lateral decubitus position have been described for block placement, the lateral decubitus position seems to offer the benefit of decreased risk of airway obstruction secondary to head flexion. On the other hand, it has been reported that palpation of bony landmarks seems to be easier in the sitting position. The distance from the skin to subarachnoid space has been calculated by ultrasound determination to be:

Distance from skin to subarachnoid space (cm) = 0. 03 × height (cm)

Distance from skin to subarachnoid space (cm) = (2 × weight) + 7 (mm)

A dedicated person to act as "baby holder" is requisite for preventing movement, as well as to ensure neck extension during the placement of the spinal anesthetic. A variety of needles have been utilized for this purpose from 23 gauge to 26 gauge needles. There is no current data on the efficacy of the use of different needle gauges on block success. Once the block has been placed, it is important that the patient lies supine or even in a reverse Trendelenburg position to prevent cephalad spread, especially with hyperbaric solutions. Prompt attention to the airway is critical, including adequate head support and extension after lying the neonate supine. All local anesthetics have been successfully used for infant spinals, including 0.5–0.6 mg/kg tetracaine 0.5%, 1 mg/kg 0.5% isobaric bupivacaine or ropivacaine, and 1.2 mg/kg of isobaric 0.5% levobupivacaine.

The onset of analgesia is between two to four minutes.

Is the Incidence of Postoperative Apnea Different Between Regional and General Anesthesia?

Multiple studies have looked at the incidence of regional anesthesia versus general anesthesia and are inconclusive. There are significant confounders in this vulnerable population and therefore, further studies are needed to clarify this issue. Postoperative apnea is discussed in greater detail in chapter 18.

Suggested Reading

Bax M, Goldstein M, Rosenbaum P, et al. Proposed definition and classification of cerebral palsy. *Dev Med Child Neurol.* 2005;47 (8):571–6. PMID: 16108461.

Davidson AJ, Morton NS, Arnup SJ, et al. Apnea after awake regional and general anesthesia in infants. *Anesthesiology.* 2015;123(1):55–65. PMID: 26001028.

Kidokoro H, Andersen PJ, Doyle LW, et al. Brain injury and altered brain growth in preterm infants: predictors and prognosis. *Pediatrics.* 2014;134(2):e444–53. PMID: 25070300.

Taneja B, Srivastava V, Saxena K. Physiological and anesthetic considerations for the preterm neonate undergoing surgery. *J Neonatal Surg.* 2012;1(1):14. PMID: 26023373.

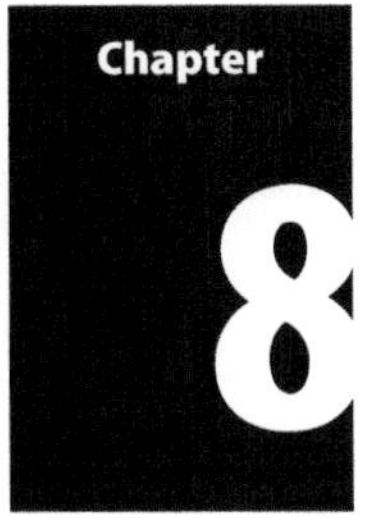

Monitoring of the Pediatric Patient

Michael R. King

A three-day-old, 3 kg female infant with transposition of the great arteries presents for an arterial switch operation. Transthoracic echo revealed an L-type transposition with an unrestrictive atrial shunt. The patient has been stable since birth in the neonatal intensive care unit receiving an alprostadil infusion.

Prior to the procedure, vitals include: temperature 37.2°C, BP 63/42, HR 130 bpm, SpO_2 88% on room air.

What Are the American Society of Anesthesiologists (ASA) Standard Monitors?

The goals of monitoring are to have consistent feedback on the patient's oxygenation, ventilation, circulation, and body temperature. This is most commonly achieved with the ASA basic monitors: 3-lead electrocardiogram, pulse oximetry, non-invasive blood pressure, capnography, temperature probe for cases lasting longer than 30 minutes or shorter cases with expected temperature changes, and oxygen/inspired gas monitoring.

What Other Monitors May Be Useful for This Case?

Neonates undergoing congenital cardiac surgery require additional monitoring beyond the ASA basic monitors. At minimum, an arterial line will be needed for continuous blood pressure monitoring on bypass as well as to facilitate blood sampling. Many centers will also assess brain oxygenation with near-infrared spectroscopy (NIRS), central/right atrial pressures with a central venous catheter, and post-surgical anatomy and function with transesophageal echocardiography (TEE).

What Is Near-Infrared Spectroscopy and What Does It Monitor?

NIRS is a monitor of oxygenation in the cerebral vessels. Using technology similar to pulse oximetry, a probe is placed on the forehead which emits light in the near-infrared spectrum. The probe then subsequently analyzes scattering and absorption to assess oxyhemoglobin and deoxyhemoglobin saturations in the cerebral vasculature. During cardiac and other procedures, sudden changes in NIRS serve to alert the anesthesiologist to decreases in cerebral oxygenation or perfusion.

How Is NIRS Different from Pulse Oximetry?

Whereas pulse oximetry takes advantage of pulsatility to distinguish between arterial and venous blood, giving a reading that reflects arterial saturation, NIRS does not incorporate pulsatility and measures both venous and arterial hemoglobin saturations. Therefore, a normal NIRS saturation will be much lower than a pulse oximeter reading, often in the 70s or 80s when the arterial saturation is 100%. Thresholds for abnormal NIRS values are thus defined by a change greater than 20% or an absolute reading of <50%.

How Should a Noninvasive Blood Pressure Cuff Be Sized?

Choosing an appropriately sized cuff is important; a small cuff tends to overestimate blood pressure while an oversized cuff tends to underestimate it. Ideally a cuff should be 2/3rds to 3/4ths the width of the upper arm.

What Is the Normal Blood Pressure in Children?

A crude estimate according to PALS may be obtained by the following formula:

$90 + (2 \times \text{age}) = 50\text{th percentile for age.}$

What Arteries Can Be Used for Invasive Blood Pressure Monitoring?

The most common arteries for arterial line placement include the radial, ulnar, femoral, dorsalis pedis, and posterior tibial arteries. In addition, in the newborn the umbilical arteries can be used for cannulation; these are most easily placed at birth, but can occasionally still be placed in the first several days of life.

What Techniques Can Be Used to Identify an Artery for Line Placement, and What Are the Limitations of Each?

Palpation is the simplest method of locating an artery for cannulation; however, numerous studies have demonstrated improved success with ultrasound utilization. Surgical cut-down allows for the direct visualization of the artery, but requires tissue dissection and may result in vessel laceration or hemorrhage.

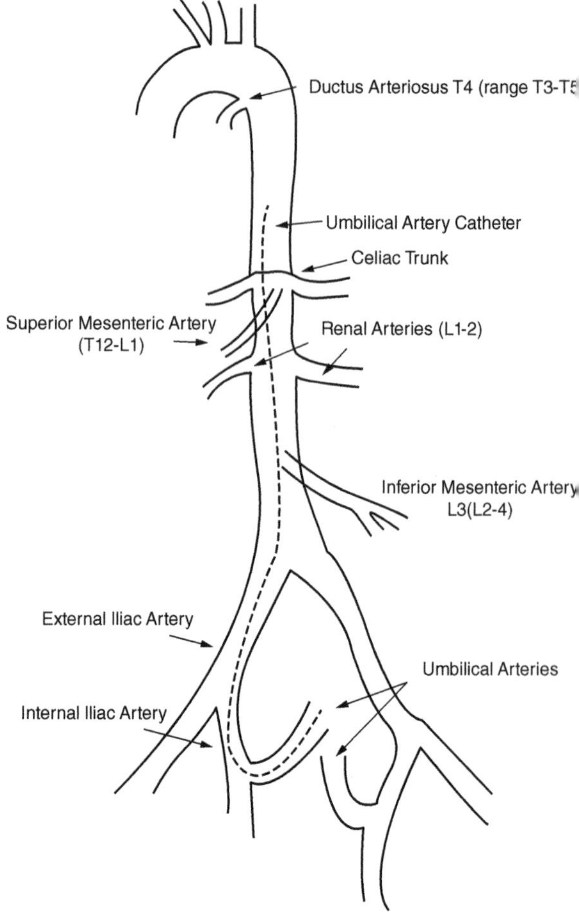

Figure 8.1 High placement of an umbilical artery catheter in relation to intraabdominal aortic branches. Illustration by Adam C. Adler, MD

Where Should the Tip of an Umbilical Artery Catheter Be Located? What Are Potential Complications of Its Migration?

Umbilical artery catheters should terminate high (T7–10) or low (below L2–3) to avoid thrombosis in one of the intra-abdominal branches off the aorta (Figure 8.1). Migration of the catheter into the femoral arteries can cause limb ischemia and migration proximally can occlude arteries leading to the kidneys, liver, or gastrointestinal tract. For umbilical vein catheters, the tip should lie at the junction of the inferior vena cava and right atrium (Figure 8.2).

How Is the Depth of Insertion Calculated for Umbilical Catheters?

In small neonates, <1,500 grams, a 3.5F catheter should be used. In larger neonates >1,500 grams a 3.5 or 5F catheter may be used.

Arterial: The depth of insertion for a "high" placement can be assessed by:

$$\text{Depth of Insertion} = (\text{weight (kg)} \times 3) + 9\ \text{cm}.$$

Venous:

$$\text{Depth of Insertion} = \frac{(\text{weight (kg)} \times 3) + 9\ \text{cm}}{2}$$

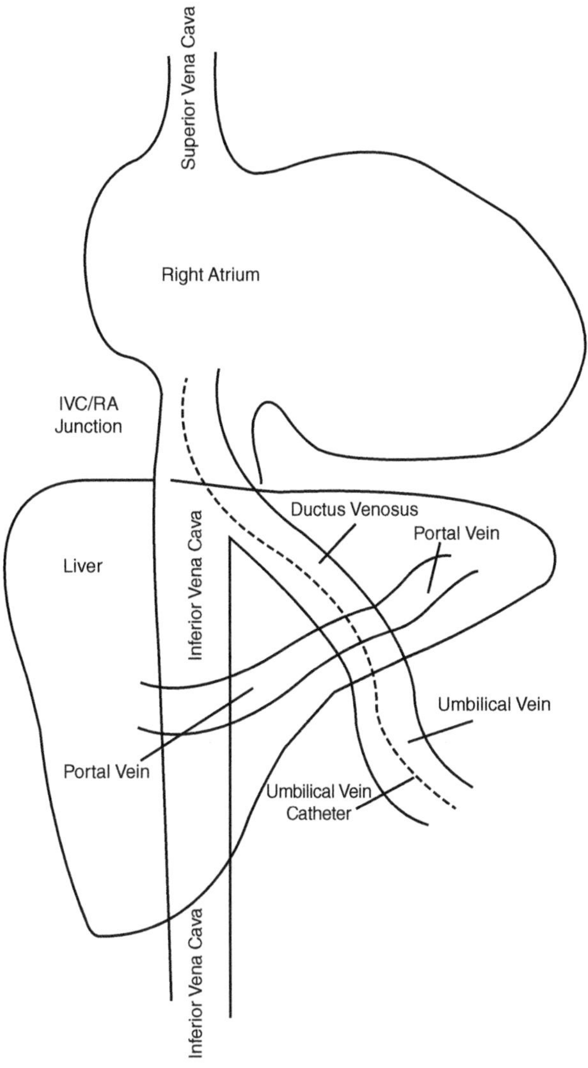

Figure 8.2 Correct placement of an umbilical venous catheter in relation to the hepatic vessels. Illustration by Adam C. Adler, MD

What Vessels Can Be Utilized for Central Line Placement?

Central venous catheters are most often placed in the internal jugular, femoral, or subclavian arteries. Peripherally inserted central lines (a.k.a., "PICC lines") can be placed through peripheral veins in the arms or legs for central medication administration and phlebotomy; however, their length and small cross-sectional area often dampen signals for central venous pressure. Similar to arterial line placement, the umbilical vein can be used for cannulation in newborns. For the catheter to reach a central location it must pass through the ductus venosus, which closes a few days after birth.

Where Should the Tip of a Central Venous Catheter Lie for Accurate Central Venous Pressure Measurement?

Central venous pressure (CVP) is measured at the junction of the superior vena cava and right atrium. Central lines placed in the inferior vena cava, such as femoral lines, may have the accuracy of their CVP readings affected by changes in intra-abdominal pressure.

What Is the Role of Pulmonary Artery Catheterization in Pediatrics?

Pulmonary artery catheters are rarely used in children, but can provide information on right heart pressures which may be particularly useful in patients with pulmonary hypertension. The ability to sample mixed venous oxygen saturation can also be useful in the management of shock. Due to small patient size, relative to available catheters, their use is virtually nonexistent in infants and neonates.

Would You Use Transesophageal Echocardiography (TEE) for This Patient? What Are Potential Complications of Its Use?

TEE provides a wealth of information at the termination of cardiopulmonary bypass in congenital heart surgery. It can be used to diagnose residual shunts, patency of valves, repaired vessels or grafts, and, of particular concern in the arterial switch operation due to the relocation of the coronary arteries, wall motion abnormalities suggestive of ischemia. Care must be taken with insertion and removal of a TEE probe in neonates as the small size of the oropharynx often puts the probe in contact with the endotracheal tube, which can lead to accidental extubation or mainstem intubation. Although rare, esophageal perforation is also a known complication. More commonly, tracheal compression may occur, leading to difficulty with ventilation (high peak inspiratory pressures), especially in neonates.

What Are Potential Sources of Error in Pulse Oximeter Readings in Neonates?

In the neonate with a patent ductus arteriosus, any site monitored distal to the ductus will report a decreased saturation if a right-to-left shunt is present. In these patients it is helpful to monitor a preductal saturation in the right arm as well as a post-ductal saturation in the left arm or legs. It is notable that pulse oximeters, depending on the brand, are calibrated for best accuracy at higher saturations, typically above 70%. A pulse oximeter may therefore be less accurate in a child with cyanotic heart disease. Fetal hemoglobin and hyperbilirubinemia do not affect pulse oximeter accuracy. Common sources of error in adults, such as methylene blue, indigo carmine, and methemoglobinemia will also affect neonates.

What Are Potential Sources of an Increased Arterial to End-Tidal Carbon Dioxide Gradient in This Patient?

In all neonates and infants with small tidal volumes, increases in dead space cause dilution of the exhaled breath as measured by capnography. This can be mitigated by placing the capnography sampling site, whether sidestream sampling or mainstream sampling, as close to the endotracheal tube as possible to minimize dead space.

Where Would You Monitor Temperature on This Patient?

Temperature is typically monitored at two sites for cases involving cardiopulmonary bypass. It is essential to monitor the temperature of the brain, as cooling is used for protection from cerebral ischemia. The nasopharynx is most commonly selected. The tympanic membrane has also been used, but is less practical. A "shell" temperature site – one that reflects the body tissues that are not in the vessel-rich group – is also typically monitored. Options for this include the bladder, skin, or rectum. While esophageal probes are useful for core temperature monitoring in most general cases, in cardiac surgery, especially where deliberate hypothermia or hypothermic circulatory arrest will occur, nasopharyngeal temperature monitoring is preferred (as a surrogate for intracranial temperature).

What Properties of Neonates Limit the Utility of Neuromuscular Blockade Monitoring?

Neonates, especially those that are premature, have immature neuromuscular junctions. As a result, neuromuscular junction monitors may reveal decreased signals even at baseline. Some neonates will have fade on a train-of-four test at baseline, and may lack sustained tetany in response to a continuous stimulus. For these reasons, the neonate should also be observed clinically for signs of full neuromuscular function recovery if muscle relaxants have been used.

Suggested Reading

Aouad-Maroun M, Raphael CK, Sayyid SK, et al. Ultrasound-guided arterial cannulation for paediatrics. *Cochrane Database of Systematic Reviews.* 2016;9:CD011364. PMID: 27627458.

Badgwell JM, McLeod ME, Lerman J, Creighton RE. End-tidal PCO_2 measurements sampled at the distal and proximal ends of the endotracheal tube in infants and children. *Anesth Analg.* 1987;66 (10):959–64. PMID: 3631591.

Goudzousian NG. Maturation of neuromuscular transmission in the infant. *Br J Anaesth.* 1980;52: 205–14. PMID: 6244843.

Tortoriello TA, Stayer SA, Mott AR, et al. A noninvasive estimation of mixed venous oxygen saturation using near-infrared spectroscopy by cerebral oximetry in pediatric cardiac surgery patients. *Paediatr Anaesth.* 2005;15:495–503. PMID: 15910351.

Chapter 9

Blood and Transfusion

Megha K. Kanjia

> A five-year-old patient with history of severe sickle cell disease presents to the operating room for a craniotomy after having suffered a fall from the roof of a home. His CT scan upon admission shows a midline shift and his last hemoglobin is 7 g/dL.

What Are the Considerations for the Perioperative Management in Patients with Hemoglobinopathies?

Common Hemoglobinopathies and Bleeding Disorders: The major hemoglobinopathies seen in the pediatric population are glucose-6-phosphate dehydrogenase deficiency, hemophilia, and sickle cell disease.

Sickle Cell Disease (SCD) is caused by a variant beta-globin gene on chromosome 11 where valine is substituted for glutamine, resulting in instability of the hemoglobin molecule when deoxygenated, causing sickling, hemolysis, and vaso-occlusive crises. Sickling can be caused by hypothermia, hyperthermia, acidemia, dehydration, and poor oxygenation. Vaso-occlusive crises are caused by a combination of inflammation, vascular endothelial adhesion, and platelet dysfunction. Sickled cells occlude microvasculature causing tissue ischemia. Chronic hemolysis is seen in SCD and results in a baseline hemoglobin of 5–9 g/dL.

Chronic SCD may affect a host of systems including pulmonary restrictive lung disease and pulmonary hypertension, stroke, chronic pain, renal abnormalities and avascular necrosis of the bone.

Treatment for severe chronic disease includes hydroxyurea, which increases the concentration of fetal hemoglobin, causing a leftward shift in the oxyhemoglobin dissociation curve (Figure 9.1). Preoperatively (except with minor, non-invasive procedures), most children with homozygous sickle type hemoglobin (HbSS) should receive a transfusion to correct their hemoglobin level to 10 g/dL and may likely require preoperative hydration, however follow up with the hematologist would be beneficial for specific recommendations.

Perioperative considerations in children with SCD include: Preoperative evaluation and management has been shown to reduce peri-anesthetic morbidity and mortality. Avoidance of hypoxia, acidosis, hyperthermia, hypothermia, and dehydration is paramount to minimizing vaso-occlusive crises. Recommendations for transfusions with most patients with SCD are to correct the anemia to around 10 g/dL. Regional anesthetics are beneficial in reducing pain which can promote sickling.

Thalassemia is a common genetic disorder resulting from a disturbance of the 1:1 alpha:beta polypeptide chains. Severity may range from an asymptomatic carrier to hydrops fetalis, resulting in death. Release of toxic agents causes an alteration of red cell membranes resulting in cells that are rigid and can disintegrate. Clinically, patients may need increased erythropoiesis and, transfusions, and may have iron overload as a result. Concomitantly, infections, splenomegaly, and bone abnormalities may be seen as a result of extramedullary hematopoiesis. Patients with chronic severe disease may require splenectomies, cholecystectomies, or vascular access placement for frequent transfusions.

von Willebrand Disease (vWD) is the most common bleeding disorder, seen in 1/10,000 people. The missing or poorly functioning glycoprotein vWF in this disease causes adherence of platelets to the subendothelium and inability to carry factor VIII properly. Typical symptoms include easy bruising, epistaxis, and menorrhagia. Type 1 (85% of cases) and type 3 (5% of cases) vWD are quantitative deficiencies, while type 2 (10% of cases) is both a qualitative and quantitative deficiency of vWF multimers.

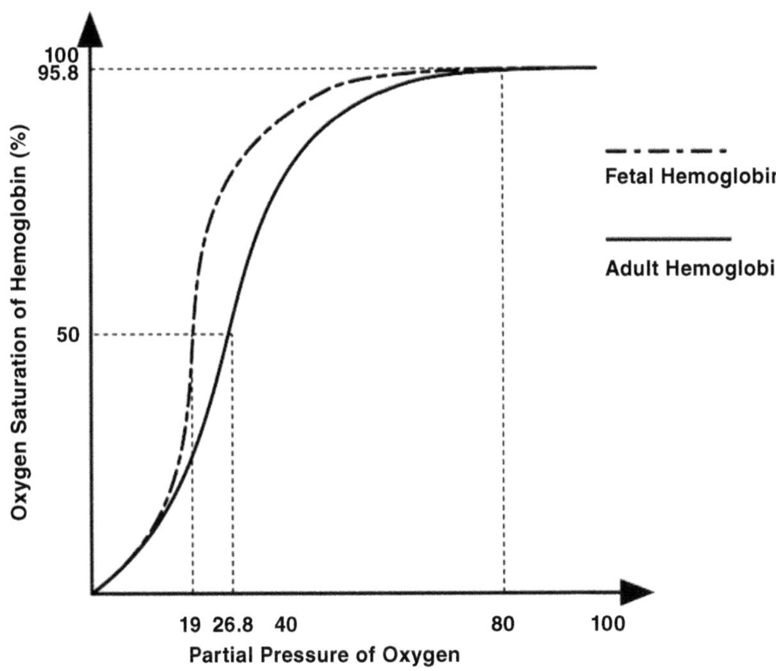

Figure 9.1 Oxyhemoglobin dissociation curve for fetal and adult hemoglobin.
Illustration by Adam C. Adler, MD

Typical coagulation studies (PT/aPTT) may be normal in patients with vWF, especially if factor VIII is normal. DDAVP is effective in type I to stimulate the release of vWF; however, it can be deleterious in type II as it may increase the level of poorly functioning vWF. Intravenous fluid hydration should be minimized after administration of exogenous factors to avoid diluting the functional factor. Additionally, acquired vWF may be seen with lymphoproliferative disorders, chronic renal failure, Wilms tumor, hypothyroidism, and certain congenital heart diseases. Caution should be used when considering regional anesthesia, intramuscular injections, nasogastric tubes, and nasal intubations. Consideration may be given to use of antifibrinolytic agents such as aminocaproic acid and tranexamic acid.

Treatment can involve use of DDAVP to encourage release of endogenous stores (types 1 and 3 only) or through use of plasma-derived factor VIII-vWF concentrates (Humate-P).

Hemophilia: Hemophilia A is a congenital bleeding disorder caused by a deficiency in factor VIII, while Hemophilia B is caused by a deficiency in factor IX; each of these bleeding disorders has wide ranges of penetrance, so mild disease may not be noted unless severe trauma occurs, while severe disease may be seen spontaneously even with minor trauma. The degree of the disease depends on the percentage of functional factor. Because hemophilia is typically X-linked, female carriers have 50% of normal factor concentrations, so they are typically asymptomatic. DDAVP may be helpful in mild cases to increase the factor VIII availability, while recombinant factor VIII may be required in other situations. Recommendations from hematology should be obtained to identify the optimal perioperative management strategy. The goal of treatment in a patient with hemophilia undergoing a surgical procedure is to obtain a factor level of 0.8–1.0 units/mL (80–100%) prior to the surgical procedure.

Patients with mild to moderate hemophilia are generally only treated prior to surgical procedures. In general, for non-life-threatening bleeding, coagulation factor activity should be raised to 40–50% of normal. For life-threatening bleeding, coagulation factor activity is raised to 80–100% of normal.

Factor replacement is continued into the postoperative period; 2–3 days after a minor procedure and 7–10 days for major procedures, especially in situations where bleeding is highly detrimental (neurological surgery). Intermittent dosing or continuous infusion factor replacement can be used to accomplish this goal.

Table 9.1 Estimated blood volume in pediatric patients

Age	Estimated blood volume (mL/kg)
Premature infants	100
Term neonates (<1 month)	90
1–12 months	80
Older children	75
Adolescents/Adults	70

$$Dose\ of\ Factor\ VIII\,(Units) = Desired\ Rise\ in\ \%\,Factor\ Activity \times Weight\ (kg) \times 0.5$$

$$Dose\ of\ Plasma-derived\ Factor\,IX\ (Units) = Desired\ Rise\ in\ \%\,Factor\ Activity \times Weight\ (kg) \times 1$$

$$Pediatric\ dose\ of\ recombinant\ Factor\,IX\,(Units) = Desired\,Rise\ in\ \%\,Factor\ Activity \times Weight\ (kg) \times 1.4$$

$$Adult\ dose\ of\ recombinant\ Factor\,IX\ (Units) = Desired\ Rise\ in\ \%\,Factor\ Activity \times Weight\ (kg) \times 1.2$$

*Dosing for modified prolonged half-life products will depend on the specific product and the patient's pharmacokinetics.

What Are the Indications for Transfusion in the Perioperative Setting?

According to the American Society of Anesthesiology Task Force on Blood Component Therapy, there is evidence to suggest that transfusion at a hemoglobin above 10 g/dL is not indicated, and that transfusion is indicated for lab values below 6 g/dL. For hemoglobin between 6 and 10 g/dL, decision to transfuse should be made based on the child's clinical picture, including vital signs, efficiency of oxygenation and perfusion, as well as degree of blood loss. Transfusion may still be indicated in a child with a Hb >10 g/dL if the clinical picture drives an indication such as baseline increased Hb, increased oxygen demand, higher concentrations of Fetal Hb, or other surgical components.

TRANSFUSION FOR THE PRETERM INFANT

What Are the Risks of Transfusion for Preterm Infants?

Significant risks include hyperkalemia and hypocalcemia. Consideration should be made to receive the freshest blood from the blood bank to minimize hyperkalemia. Often a single unit is split into multiple units over a period of time for a preterm infant, so care should be taken to ensure that the split units are administered from the same "original unit" to minimize exposure of the baby to multiple donors.

For a preterm infant, acute blood loss risks include hypovolemia, hypotension, acidosis, apnea, and hyperkalemia.

TRAUMA AND INDICATIONS FOR TRANSFUSION

What Are the Implications of Major Trauma in a Pediatric Patient?

With their relatively small blood volume (on per kg basis), pediatric patients can become unstable, hypovolemic, and anemic with what is usually considered to be small blood volumes. Twenty percent of trauma deaths are a result of coagulopathy and this is likely related to tissue hypoperfusion. The triad of hypoperfusion, hemodilution, and hypothermia increases the existing coagulopathy for poor outcomes. Hyperfibrinolysis is seen frequently in trauma, but has been found to occur more frequently in the pediatric population than seen in adults. Reliable measurement is difficult in these patients and use of rapid tests, such as rTEG (rapid thromboelastography) is helpful to guide transfusion in a timely manner. Major bleeding should trigger the anesthesiologist to consider activation of a massive transfusion protocol. Additionally, administration of recombinant Factor VIIa has been shown to increase 30-day survival rates when used within two hours of initial bleeding in addition to administration of whole blood.

What Are the Indications for Plasma/Fresh Frozen Plasma Transfusion?

Indications include replacement of a specific factor that is deficient (especially if the factor is unavailable in a recombinant or separate form), iatrogenic coagulopathy after massive transfusion, immediate need for warfarin reversal, supportive therapy in disseminated intravascular coagulation (DIC), and for children requiring heparin therapy who have an antithrombin III deficiency. Transfusion of FFP has the highest risk as it is often used unnecessarily outside of the setting of Massive Blood Transfusion (MBT) and may result in TRALI (transfusion related acute lung injury), TACO (transfusion associated circulatory overload), or TRIM (transfusion related immunomodulation). TRALI is the most common cause of transfusion related mortality.

What Are the Indications for Cryoprecipitate?

Cryoprecipitate is indicated for active/anticipated bleeding in children with fibrinogen deficiencies (congenital or as a result of massive transfusion), or von Willebrand disease in the setting of poor response to DDAVP.

One unit of cryoprecipitate contains:

- 100 IU of factor VIII
- 250 mg of fibrinogen
- von Willebrand factor (vWF)
- factor XIII

What Is the Debate of 1:1:1 Component Therapy Versus Whole Blood?

Banked whole blood should contain normal levels of all clotting factors and proteins but has 20–50% of factors V and VIII. However, a coagulopathy secondary to a deficiency of a clotting factor typically occurs if there is <30% of a normal concentration. While many experts believe that transfusion should occur in a 1:1:1 ratio (plasma:platelet:RBCs), some feel that whole blood more appropriately replaces acute blood loss during surgery. This debate has been longstanding, but it is clear that in cases where transfusion of large volumes replace significant blood loss, such as MBT, clotting factors should also be replaced. Another criticism of whole blood is the difficulty with leukocyte reduction; however newer filters have the capability to save the platelets.

How Does Heparin Resistance Play a Role in the Perioperative Setting?

Heparin is a glycosaminoglycan that binds to antithrombin III to cause a conformational change, inactivating thrombin as well as factor Xa. This is significant in the setting of heparin resistance, which is often noted over time in patients with antithrombin III deficiency, which may be treated with FFP to restore the factor, or with a recombinant antithrombin III factor. As in adults, it should be suspected if appropriate activated clotting time (ACT) levels are not achieved prior to cardiopulmonary bypass.

How Does Hydroxyethyl Starch Play a Role in Platelet Function?

Hydroxyethyl starch primarily affects coagulation by dilution, specifically factor VIII and von Willebrand factor. Additionally, the reduction of glycoprotein IIb/IIIa availability will alter platelet adhesion. Direct movement into fibrin clots will also decrease coagulability; most of these scenarios are noted when >20 mL/kg are administered.

How Does ABO Compatibility Play a Role in Transfusion?

While RBCs must only be ABO isoagglutinin compatible, any component with large volumes of plasma (FFP, whole blood, and platelets) must be compatible with the A or B surface antigens. Whole blood must be ABO identical.

What Constitutes a "Massive Blood Transfusion"?

Massive blood transfusion (MBT) is defined as administration of greater than or equal to 1 blood volume in a 24-hour period, greater than or equal to 0.5 blood volume in 12 hours, or acute administration of greater than or equal to 1.5 estimated blood volume (EBV). The goal of MBT is to minimize hemodilution of coagulation factors by replacing factors and blood products lost rather than by replacing with crystalloid and packed red blood cells.

Activation of the massive transfusion protocol through the blood bank will rely on the expertise of the blood bank/transfusion experts to assist in transfusion guidance. This may also allow transfusion to be expedited by use of type O Rh negative blood without prior sample of a cross-match. Type O Rh positive blood can be utilized for male patients. Appropriate monitoring should be established prior to surgery to ensure that adequate baseline data is available.

Additionally, a urinary catheter should allow for appropriate urine output monitoring. Arterial lines as well as central venous pressure lines will provide additional monitoring to guide transfusion as well.

How Does Hematopoietic Stem Cell Transplantation Affect Future Transfusion?

Following Hematopoietic Stem Cell Transplantation, irradiated, leukocyte reduced, cytomegalovirus (CMV)-negative blood should be used; coordination with the transplant team is prudent as the blood type of the patient may change from that of the recipient to that of the donor.

TESTS TO HELP GUIDE TRANSFUSION

How Is TEG (Thromboelastography) Useful for Guiding Transfusion?

TEG is a standardized method of quantifying the quality of a clot as well as providing information regarding fibrinolysis (Figures 9.2, 9.3, and Table 9.2). This tool is primarily used for liver transplantation and cardiac surgery as the information is more accurate and is obtained more quickly than sending prothrombin time/partial thromboplastin time/international normalized ratio (PT/PTT/INR) to the main laboratory. Some studies have found that TEG is an accurate tool for guiding transfusion of various blood products and assistance in choosing which product to transfuse.

How Is ROTEM Useful?

Both ROTEM (Rotational Thromboelastrogram) and TEG are useful in detecting hyperfibrinolysis. Some studies have found that goal directed transfusion via ROTEM has decreased cost to the patients as well, primarily by decreasing administration of FFP to patients. Additionally, clot firmness gives much more information to a clinical picture rather than the number of platelets. Very specific algorithms regarding the various factors within ROTEM have helped guide transfusion and as a result have been shown to decrease morbidity and mortality. In the setting of ongoing bleeding, ROTEM should be repeated 10–15 minutes after a specific intervention to reassess the hemostatic change.

Are PT and aPTT Interchangeable with ROTEM?

PT and PTT are not interchangeable with ROTEM according to newer studies as it appears that PT and aPTT may overestimate the need for transfusion. ROTEM also produces a faster result for treatment as opposed to the more traditional coagulation tests.

What Is a FibTEM?

FibTEM is a functional fibrinogen test that allows the examination of clot firmness based on the fibrinogen function and activity. Because fibrinogen and fibrin

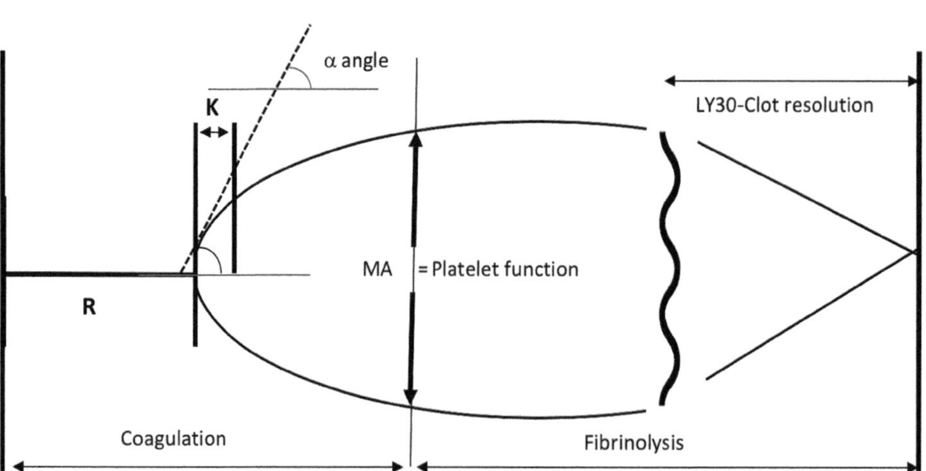

Figure 9.2 Schematic demonstrating the variables measured by thromboelastography and the corresponding portion of the cascade assessed. R=reaction time; MA=measures platelet function in mm; K=fibrin cross-linkage time; α angle=fibrinogen function. Illustration by Adam C. Adler, MD

Table 9.2 Thromboelastography variables by function

Variable	Process evaluated	Definition	Low	High
			Treatment	**Treatment**
R time	Reaction time of clotting factors	Time to formation of Fibrin	Hyperstimulation of pathway	Factor deficiency or residual heparinization
			Anticoagulation	FFP or protamine
K time	Fibrinogen function, clotting factors	Fibrin cross-linkage time (Rate of thrombin formation)	Fibrinogen/factor 8 deficiency	Platelet hypercoagulation
			Cryoprecipitate or FFP	–
α angle	Clot kinetics Fibrinogen function	Rate of clot formation	Fibrinogen/factor 8 deficiency	Platelet hypercoagulation
			Cryoprecipitate or FFP	–
MA	Platelet function, strength, and stability	Fibrin and platelet interaction	Quantitative or qualitative platelets or fibrinogen issue	Platelet hypercoagulation
			Platelet transfusion	Anti-platelet agent
LY30 Lysis 30min	Clot stability	Amount (%) of clot lysis 30 minutes after MA achieved	–	Fibrinolysis or TPA use
			–	Antifibrinolytics

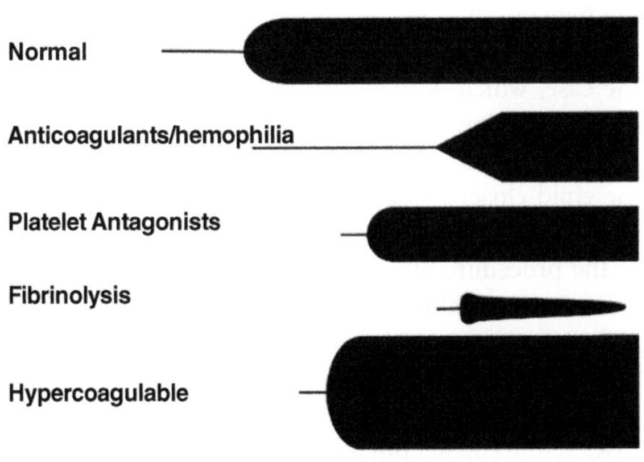

Figure 9.3 Appearance of thromboelastography maps by specific deficiencies. Illustration by Adam C. Adler, MD

are the first factors to be reduced during a significant perioperative hemorrhage, the FibTEM test allows faster examination of the fibrinogen function.

What Role Does Activated Protein C Play in Diagnosis of Coagulopathy?

A few recent studies have shown a correlation between activated protein C levels and aPTT, PT, tPA, as well as D-dimers. Activation of activated protein C signifies risk of MODS (multi-organ dysfunction syndrome), ALI (acute lung injury), as well as mortality.

How Is TRALI Diagnosed and How Significant Is It?

TRALI is diagnosed by noncardiac pulmonary edema and patchy infiltrates, and is typically indistinguishable from ARDS. It is seen in 1/5,000 transfusion and must be noted <6 hours after transfusion to be attributed to the transfusion. The highest risk of TRALI is seen in plasma rich products: FFP, platelets, whole blood. One theory is that neutrophil sequestration results in increased adhesion of molecules to pulmonary vasculature; these neutrophils are activated by donor anti-leukocyte antibodies. Acute transient leukopenia is often noted as well. For these reasons, TRALI is less likely in the neutropenic population.

Drugs

- **Meizothrombin** is inhibited by hirudin and other direct thrombin inhibitors, but is not inhibited by heparin. Specific assays may be utilized for patients with specific issues, for example, for those patients who are on extracorporeal membrane oxygenation (ECMO).

- **Tirofiban** is a nonpeptide reversible antagonist of fibrinogen binding to the GP IIb/IIIa receptor, the major platelet surface receptor involved in platelet aggregation.

When Is Factor VIIa Appropriate to Administer?

Factor VIIa is approved for hemophiliacs with high titer inhibitors or for patients with a factor VII deficiency. There has been some debate over when it is appropriate to transfuse. It should be considered that there is a 1.4–10% risk of a major embolic event in adults after transfusion of Factor VII.

What Measures Can Minimize Perioperative Blood Loss?

Erythropoietin is a pharmacologic agent that stimulates the production of endogenous RBC production. It is particularly useful in preterm infants, and for patients undergoing chemotherapy, or for children of Jehovah's witnesses. In the perioperative setting, it is typically used for major surgeries where significant blood loss is anticipated.

Preoperative Autologous Blood Donation is an alternative to allogeneic RBC transfusion, which entails the patient to place banked blood up to 35–42 days prior to the anticipated use. It is not recommended for patients with significant cardiac disease or with ongoing infections, as this will be deleterious for the patient's overall condition. Caution should be exercised when family-donated blood is given to a patient as these patients have a higher risk of graft versus host disease, so the blood should be irradiated to minimize this.

Cell Saver/Blood Recovery and Reinfusion can be used to minimize exposure to allogeneic blood thereby reducing the potential for infections and reactions. The blood is collected directly from the operative site and is washed in a centrifuge so the hematocrit of blood being infused is between 50–60%. Enough blood has to be received from the operative site to be able to convert this into a usable cell saver unit, so it is unlikely to be of help in infants and younger children. Lastly, cell saver devices and operators can have a significant cost, so are typically only financially helpful if three or fewer units of allogeneic RBCs are transfused. Contraindications to use of this equipment would include contamination of blood from bacteria (bowel, abscesses), sickle cell disease (SCD), foreign materials such as methylmethacrylate, neomycin, as well as malignancy, which is a relative contraindication.

Controlled Hypotension: This is a method whereby the systemic perfusion pressure is reduced to attempt to minimize blood loss. Techniques include vasodilators, high concentrations of volatile anesthetic, and large-dose opioid infusions. Consideration should be given to the potential of rapid blood loss, in which case a rapid reversal agent would be more beneficial to mitigate the hemodynamic response and potential collapse. Caution should be exercised because although there are no pediatric studies to support this, adult studies have shown that brain ischemia has been evident at MAP of 55 mmHg in the presence of hypocarbia.

Normovolemic Hemodilution: This is a purposeful hemodilution to minimize the need for allogenic blood transfusions. Two alternate methods are utilized to achieve normovolemic hemodilution; the first is allowing the surgical blood loss to continue until the hematocrit is in the upper teens, and then transfusing packed red blood cells (PRBCs) at the end of the case, which is theorized to allow the bleeding to occur at a lower hematocrit, lessening the loss of RBCs. The second method is to remove blood from the child closer to the initial incision while administering crystalloid and reinfusing the blood at the end of the procedure after bleeding has stopped. Normovolemic hemodilution is contraindicated in patients with cyanotic heart disease, septicemia, and SCD, and any other disease that is strongly dependent upon perfusion. Overall this can minimize the allogenic RBC requirement, but if the hematocrit is less that 15%, subendocardial myocardial ischemia is possible.

Antifibrinolytics: Aminocaproic acid and tranexamic acid (TXA) inhibit fibrinolysis primarily used to minimize bleeding. Adverse effects include anaphylaxis and risk of deep vein thrombosis, and pulmonary embolism. Some studies have found that TXA as an antifibrinolytic agent has been useful in reducing perioperative blood loss. There is evidence-based medicine suggesting that initial bolus doses with an infusion are helpful in craniofacial surgeries as well as spine surgeries to minimize blood loss.

Suggested Reading

Haas T, Goobie S, Spielmann N, et al. Improvements in patient blood management for pediatric craniosynostosis surgery using a ROTEM(®)-assisted strategy – feasibility and costs. *Paediatr Anaesth.* 2014;24(7):774–80, PMID: 24417649.

Haas T, Spielmann N, Mauch J, et al. Comparison of thromboelastometry (ROTEM®) with standard plasmatic coagulation testing in paediatric surgery. *Br J Anaesth.* 2012;108(1):36–41. PMID: 22086509.

Marques MB, Tuncer HH, Divers SG, et al. Acute transient leukopenia as a sign of TRALI. *Am J Hematol.* 2005;80(1):90–1. PMID: 16138350.

Mazzeffi MA, Stone ME. Perioperative management of von Willebrand disease: a review for the anesthesiologist. *J Clin Anesth.* 2011;23(5):418–26. PMID: 21741810.

Mehra T, Seifert B, Bravo-Reiter S, et al. Implementation of a patient blood management monitoring and feedback program significantly reduces transfusions and costs. *Transfusion.* 2015;55(12):2807–15. PMID: 26264557.

Piel FB, Steinberg MH, Rees DC. Sickle Cell Disease. *N Engl J Med.* 2017;376 (16):1561–73.

Toy P, Popovsky MA, Abraham E, et al. Transfusion-related acute lung injury: definition and review. *Crit Care Med.* 2005;33(4):721–6. PMID: 15818095.

Vogel AM, Radwan ZA, Cox CS Jr., et al. Admission rapid thrombelastography delivers real-time "actionable" data in pediatric trauma. *J Pediatr Surg.* 2013;48 (6):1371–6. PMID: 23845632.

Chapter 10

Asthma

Giuliana Geng-Ramos

A five-year-old male with a history of asthma and eczema presents for laparoscopic orchiopexy. His home regimen includes fluticasone, two puffs twice daily, and albuterol as needed. His mother reports he had an upper respiratory tract infection (URI) a few weeks ago, and since then has been using his albuterol inhaler more frequently. Ten days ago, the wheezing worsened and she took him to the emergency department where he was treated with nebulized albuterol and discharged home with a three-day course of oral corticosteroids. Since then he has returned to his usual state of activity, URI symptoms have resolved, and he has not used albuterol in the past three days. According to mom, she was told to hold all medications in preparation for surgery; therefore, he did not take fluticasone this morning.

His current vital signs are: heart rate 127, respiratory rate 28, blood pressure 101/70, SpO_2 95% on room air, with an axillary temperature of 37.0°C.

On physical exam, the child is alert and interactive. Respirations are unlabored, without nasal flaring or intercostal retractions. Chest auscultation reveals mild expiratory wheezes bilaterally.

What Is the Definition of Asthma?

Asthma is a common chronic disorder of the airways that is characterized by variable and recurring bronchial hyperresponsiveness, airflow obstruction, mucus secretion, and inflammation.

What Are the Important Differential Diagnoses to Consider?

Not all wheezing is asthma. Other diagnoses to consider include: tracheomalacia, bronchomalacia, bronchiolitis, bronchial foreign body, bronchopulmonary dysplasia, cystic fibrosis, tracheal web/stenosis, and bronchial stenosis.

What Is the Prevalence of Asthma?

Asthma is the most common chronic disease of childhood in industrialized countries, affecting more than 6 million children in the United States. The prevalence of asthma in US children is approximately 10%, and its incidence has increased by an average of 4.3% each year.

The Pathophysiology of Asthma

Although much remains unknown about the exact pathophysiologic mechanisms, the development of asthma appears to be a complex process involving the interaction of host factors and environmental exposures, leading to chronic airway inflammation and excessive airway reactivity.

One of the key drivers in the pathophysiology of asthma is inflammation, by the interaction of mast cells and eosinophils, which, when activated by interaction with antigen, release cytokines and lipid mediators that result in bronchial inflammation and airflow limitation. Airflow obstruction is caused by a combination of several factors including bronchoconstriction, airway edema, hypersecretion, and mucus plugging. This leads to increased work of breathing, ventilation-perfusion mismatch, air trapping, hyperinflation, hypoxemia, diaphragmatic fatigue, hypercapnia and, if left untreated, respiratory failure.

What Are Some Precipitating Factors of Acute Asthma?

Environmental factors, including airborne allergens and viral respiratory infections, play a crucial role in asthma exacerbation (Table 10.1). Emotional stimuli – including stress, fear, anxiety, and excitement – are also known triggers of asthma. Airway manipulation, such as occurs during induction of general anesthesia, may trigger or exacerbate asthma symptoms.

Table 10.1 Common precipitating factors for asthma

Precipitating factors of asthma
Respiratory infection (RSV)
Airway irritants (tobacco smoke, inhaled anesthetics)
Allergens
Exercise
Emotional stress
Dry/cold air
Chronic gastroesophageal reflux disease
Drugs (aspirin, beta-blockers)
Airway manipulation/stimulation

What Are the Clinical Symptoms of Asthma?

Acute exacerbations of asthma may include wheezing, dyspnea on exertion, chest tightness, or dry cough. When severe, it may be manifest as chest wall retractions, use of accessory muscles of respiration, and prolonged expiratory phase due to bronchospasm.

Are There Any Chronic Consequences of Asthma?

Airway remodeling describes permanent airway changes that develop from chronic inflammation. Structural changes include smooth muscle hypertrophy, hyperplasia, blood vessel proliferation, epithelial thickening, and fibrosis. This results in progressive loss of lung function that is not prevented or fully reversible by current available treatments.

What Are the Different Pharmacologic Agents Available for Asthma?

Medications available to treat acute exacerbations and long-term control consist of bronchodilators and anti-inflammatory drugs in six different classes:

- ***Beta$_2$-adrenergic agonists***: induce bronchial smooth muscle relaxation and bronchodilation. Short-acting beta$_2$-adrenergic agonists are the first line treatment in acute asthma exacerbation. Long-acting beta$_2$-agonists are used in combination with inhaled corticosteroids in moderate or severe persistent asthma.
- ***Corticosteroids***: the most potent and effective anti-inflammatory agents used in the long-term control of asthma. They block late-phase reactions, reduce airway hyperreactivity, and inhibit inflammatory cell activation. Most often used inhaled, with oral use reserved for severe or persistent asthma.
- ***Leukotriene inhibitors***: antagonize the leukotriene receptor leading to inhibition of leukotriene-induced bronchial smooth muscle constriction. They are mainly used as an alternative, not preferred, treatment of asthma, and often used as an adjunctive therapy to corticosteroids.
- ***Methylxanthines***: mild to moderate bronchodilator used as an alternative, not preferred, and as adjunctive therapy with corticosteroids. Monitoring of serum level is essential due to narrow therapeutic index.
- ***Cromolyn sodium***: pulmonary mast cell stabilizer that diminishes the IgE antibody-induced release of inflammatory mediators. Used as an alternative, but not preferred, medication in mild persistent asthma, or as a preventive treatment in exercise-induced asthma.
- ***Anticholinergics***: inhibit muscarinic cholinergic receptors, reducing the intrinsic vagal tone of bronchial smooth muscle. Can be used in combination with, or as an alternative to beta$_2$-adrenergic agonists.

The Preanesthetic Assessment of the Asthmatic Patient

The anesthesiologist should assess the severity and current status of disease by taking a detailed history and physical exam. Important details of the medical history include:

- Triggering factors
- Frequency and type of asthma medication used for maintenance and rescue
- Most recent use of oral corticosteroids
- History of hospitalizations, intubations, and/or emergency room visits due to asthma
- Recent upper respiratory infection, sinus infection, fever
- History of pneumothorax or respiratory arrest

The physical examination should focus on respiratory rate, signs of lung infection, air movement, detecting expiratory wheeze, and a prolonged expiratory time.

The baseline room air oxygen saturation should be determined.

What Preoperative Testing Is Indicated?

Children with well-controlled asthma who are not steroid-dependent generally do not require additional testing.

- ***Pulmonary function testing:*** Spirometry and measurement of peak flow rate can be used in older children to detect severity of airway obstruction and hyper-reactivity in an office setting. It is of limited use in assessing asthma preoperatively.
- ***Chest radiograph***: a chest radiograph may show signs of hyperinflation but is rarely useful unless looking for a condition other than asthma, such as pulmonary infection or barotrauma.
- ***Laboratory testing:*** Preoperative blood tests are not routinely indicated and should only be performed as they would be for patients without asthma.

The above emphasizes the importance of a detailed history and physical examination in the preoperative evaluation of a patient with asthma.

What Premedication Should Be Considered in Asthmatics?

Midazolam is safe to use as premedication in asthmatics to reduce anxiety; however, it does not reduce the incidence of bronchospasm. Inhaled beta$_2$-adrenergic agonists treatment should be given 20–30 minutes prior to induction of anesthesia. If the patient is on systemic corticosteroids and/or high-dose inhaled corticosteroids, the benefit of a stress dose with intravenous hydrocortisone is recommended to avoid adrenal crisis.

When Should Elective Surgery Be Delayed?

Elective surgery should be delayed if the patient's asthma symptoms do not appear to resolve with therapy, or the oxyhemoglobin saturation is below 95% on room air. Signs of a lower respiratory tract infection, such as focal wheeze or diminished air entry are also cause for concern and may warrant a chest radiograph.

URI in asthmatic children is often associated with the exacerbation of bronchospasm and increases the risk of perioperative complications. Ideally, a child with asthma should be free of URI symptoms for 4–6 weeks before an elective procedure.

Is There a Difference Between Intravenous and Inhalational Induction in Asthmatics?

The goal of induction in the asthmatic patient is to attain an adequate depth of anesthesia to prevent a response (e.g., coughing, laryngospasm or bronchospasm) to airway manipulation. Therefore, an IV induction is preferred if tolerated by the child, using either propofol or ketamine. Ketamine may also be useful in asthmatics because of its sympathomimetic bronchodilator properties and inhibition of vagal pathways. But ketamine is also associated with increased secretions, postoperative nausea and vomiting, and psychomimetic activity, and thus, is not the first line choice.

Inhaled anesthetic agents are known bronchodilators, decrease airway responsiveness, and attenuate bronchospasm. However, these agents are unable to completely abolish the bronchoconstrictive response to intubation during induction of anesthesia. Therefore, if an inhalational induction is chosen, it should be smooth and rapid, and supplemented with an IV anesthetic agent when IV access is obtained. Sevoflurane is the most effective bronchodilator and is the agent of choice in asthmatics and for pediatric inductions. Desflurane should not be used in asthmatics because of its potent airway irritating properties.

Since tracheal stimulation may trigger bronchospasm, tracheal intubation is avoided when possible, in lieu of a laryngeal mask airway (LMA) or mask ventilation.

Will the Presence of Asthma Change Your Ventilator Settings?

For children with well-controlled asthma and no signs of bronchospasm, ventilator settings should be the same as for non-asthmatics. If there are signs of bronchospasm, ventilator settings should be designed to avoid hyperinflation, air trapping, and barotrauma by:

- Reducing respiratory rate
- Reducing tidal volume
- Reducing inspiratory time and prolonging expiratory time by reducing I:E ratio (1:4)

- Using positive end-expiratory pressure 3–5 cm H_2O
- Allowing permissive hypercapnia
- Utilizing pressure regulated settings rather than volume or assist control

How Will You Manage Intraoperative Bronchospasm?

First, determine the cause of wheezing. The differential diagnosis includes a kinked endotracheal tube, mainstem bronchial intubation, airway secretions, pulmonary edema, pulmonary embolus, pulmonary aspiration, and anaphylaxis. If wheezing is thought to be due to bronchospasm, the most common causes are light anesthesia and stimulation from the endotracheal tube at the carina within the right main bronchus. Deepen the anesthetic by increasing the concentration of inhaled agent or administering IV propofol or ketamine. Lidocaine (1 mg/kg) given IV may reduce airway reactivity. If bronchospasm continues, administer a short-acting $beta_2$-adrenergic agonist, such as albuterol, via an endotracheal tube using a metered-dose inhaler. A small percentage of the administered dose will reach the end of the endotracheal tube and the lungs; therefore, multiple puffs of the $beta_2$-adrenergic agonist should be delivered and may need to be repeated.

Severe bronchospasm that impairs oxygenation requires further intervention, including:

- Maximal use of the bronchodilating properties of volatile anesthetic agents (sevoflurane or isoflurane)
- IV magnesium sulfate
- Anticholinergics, including IV atropine or glycopyrrolate, or nebulized ipratropium
- Epinephrine should be administered for refractory bronchospasm, especially if anaphylaxis is suspected
- IV terbutaline
- IV glucocorticoids (but will not be effective for 4–6 hours)
- Neuromuscular blocking agents may improve mechanics of ventilation but will not alleviate smooth muscle bronchoconstriction

How Should Emergence and Extubation Be Managed in the Asthmatic Child?

The goal is to achieve a nonairway stimulating emergence that might trigger or exacerbate bronchoconstriction. A "deep" extubation can be accomplished safely with the patient spontaneously ventilating, and the use of oropharyngeal or nasopharyngeal airway devices to manage partial airway obstruction after removal of the endotracheal tube. A successful awake extubation can be achieved by suctioning tracheal secretions, repeating a dose of inhaled $beta_2$-agonist, and IV lidocaine (1 mg/kg) to minimize tracheal stimulation.

The Surgeon Asks You to Administer IV Ketorolac to Aid with Postoperative Pain Control. Are There Any Risks Using Nonsteroidal Anti-inflammatory Drugs (NSAIDs) in Children with Asthma?

NSAIDs inhibit cyclooxygenase and result in increased leukotriene production, which can lead to bronchospasm, laryngospasm, and periorbital edema. NSAID hypersensitivity appears to be more common in asthmatic adults than children. NSAIDs are relatively contraindicated in older children with atopy and severe asthma.

Suggested Reading

Akinbami LJ, Moorman JE, Garbe PL, et al. Status of childhood asthma in the United States, 1980–2007. *Pediatrics.* 2009;123 (Suppl 3): S131–45. PMID: 19221156.

Doherty GM, Chisakuta A, Crean P, et al. Anesthesia and the child with asthma. *Paediatr Anaesth.* 2005;15:446–54. PMID: 15910343.

Hollevoet I, Herregods S, Vereecke H, et al. Medication in the perioperative period: stop or continue? A review. *Scta Anaesthesiol Belg.* 2011;62:193. PMID: 22379758.

National Heart, Lung, and Blood Institute, National Asthma Education and Prevention Program: Expert panel report 3: guidelines for the diagnosis and management of asthma. www.nhlbi.nih.gov/guidelines/asthma/asthgdln.pdf 2007 (accessed April 2016).

Stather DR, Stewart TE. Clinical review: Mechanical ventilation in severe asthma. *Crit Care.* 2005;9 (6):581–7. PMID: 16356242.

Chapter 11

Sepsis

Matthew Taylor

A six-year-old female with newly diagnosed acute lymphoblastic leukemia is in day two of induction chemotherapy. She has developed fever with diarrhea and abdominal pain. An abdominal CT demonstrates typhlitis, and a short segment of necrotic large bowel and free air under the diaphragm. She requires emergent surgery for partial bowel resection.

Her current vital signs are: blood pressure 79/31, heart rate 163/min, respiratory rate 32/min, SpO_2 89% on room air, currently on nasal cannula 2L with SpO_2 increased to 93%. Weight is 26 kg.

Chest X-ray shows bilaterally increased interstitial markings. A gallop is heard on cardiac exam. Capillary refill time is three to four seconds peripherally and she is cool in the extremities. The patient has already received 80 cc/kg in crystalloid and has not produced urine since spiking the fever. A recent arterial blood gas showed a pH 7.23, pCO_2 32, pO_2 65, bicarbonate 19, base deficit −7, and a lactate of 5.1.

What Is Sepsis?

Sepsis is a syndrome caused by over-activation of the immune response secondary to an overwhelming infection. This inflammatory reaction leads to physiologic and biochemical abnormalities in the body, which define the clinical diagnosis of sepsis and septic shock. Sepsis and septic shock are leading causes of mortality in critical care medicine and can significantly raise the risk of anesthetic and surgical mortality.

What Is Systemic Inflammatory Response Syndrome (SIRS)?

Recent revisions of the definition of the systemic inflammatory response syndrome (SIRS) have simplified the definition of the inflammation associated with infection, which, when combined, define sepsis. The new definition of SIRS includes two or more of the following: temperature >38°C or <36°C, heart rate >90/min, respiratory rate >20/min or $PaCO_2$ <32 mmHg, or white blood cell count >12,000/mm^3 or <4,000/mm^3 or >10% immature bands. This definition currently applies to adults only, but similar criteria are used for children. These were set forth along with age specific vital signs and were defined in 2005 by an international consensus conference. These vital signs, listed in Table 11.1, are used to define the SIRS response for pediatrics.

SIRS

- Temperature greater than 38.5°C or less than 36°C
- Tachycardia or, for children less than 1 year of age, bradycardia, without other explanation
- Tachypnea or requirement for mechanical ventilation without underlying respiratory disease
- Leukocytosis

Sepsis

- SIRS with suspected or proven infection

Severe Sepsis

- Sepsis plus cardiovascular dysfunction, respiratory failure, or two or more other organ failures

Septic Shock

- Sepsis with multiorgan dysfunction

What Is the Definition of Septic Shock?

When patients meet the criteria for SIRS and there are signs of end-organ dysfunction, patients meet criteria for septic shock. When patients have multiple organ systems affected, they meet the criteria for multiorgan dysfunction syndrome (MODS), a syndrome which significantly increases overall mortality.

Table 11.1 Vital sign reference by age used to define the systemic inflammatory response syndrome in children

Age	Tachycardia (beats/min)	Bradycardia (beats/min)	Respiratory rate (breaths/min)	Normal leukocyte count ($x10^3$/mm)	Systolic blood pressure (mmHg)
0 days – 1 week	>180	<100	>50	<34	<59
1 week – 1 month	>180	<100	>40	5–19.5	<79
1 month – 1 year	>180	<90	>34	5–17.5	<75
2 years – 5 years	>140	N/A	>22	6–15.5	<74
6 years – 12 years	>130	N/A	>18	4.5–13.5	<83
13 years – 18 years	>110	N/A	>14	4.5–11	<90

What Are Important Diagnoses to Consider in a Child with Sepsis?

The clinical presentation of sepsis emerges from a combination of host factors, such as genetics and predisposing conditions, and pathogenic factors, including virulence and pathogen load. The pathogen can be a wide range of infections, including all variety of viral, bacterial, and fungal disease. The likelihood of each different pathogen to cause infection varies by patient comorbidity. For example, the youngest children and babies are more vulnerable to viral illness and spontaneous bacterial infection, while older patients can have medical comorbidities such as rheumatologic or oncologic disease that can predispose to sepsis because of a weakened immune response.

Viral illnesses such as influenza, rhinovirus, and Epstein-Barr virus can all present with symptoms that can meet clinical criteria for sepsis. The most common and obvious cause of sepsis include bacterial infections. These can occur in many different sites as manifestation of pneumonia, urogenital tract infection, and blood stream infections.

Fungal infection can also cause sepsis, though the presentation of this type of disease tends to be more indolent and is significantly more dependent on a previously weakened immune response.

The patient in the vignette at the beginning of the chapter meets clinical criteria for septic shock with end-organ dysfunction including respiratory compromise, renal dysfunction, and hemodynamic failure. She also has leukemia and has recently undergone chemotherapy, leading to significant immunosuppression. Both of these represent significant predisposing comorbidities. Typhlitis is a neutropenic colitis seen in oncologic patients leading to a dilated large bowel, with high chance of perforation, which is the likely cause of septic shock in this patient.

What Are the Most Common Sites for Infection Leading to Sepsis?

The cause of severe sepsis can vary significantly by location, age, and institution. The most common site of primary infection in severe sepsis is the respiratory system followed by bloodstream infection, genitourinary tract infections, abdominal, and central nervous system infections.

What Are the Most Common Pathogens Leading to Severe Sepsis?

Common bacterial causes include both gram-negative bacteria including *Escherichia coli, Klebsiella* species and *Pseudomonas aeruginosa* and gram-positive bacteria such as *Staphylococcus* and *Streptococcus.* It is important to consider early involvement of infectious disease specialists and to follow local antibiotic guidelines for appropriate treatment of at-risk populations to ensure broad coverage to cover all likely causative agents. Without appropriate source control, septic shock will continue to worsen and will lead to severe morbidity.

What Is the Incidence and Most Common Age of Presentation of Sepsis?

Sepsis and septic shock are leading causes of worldwide morbidity and mortality and a leading cause of critical illness. Approximately 1/3 of mortality in tertiary pediatric intensive care units (PICUs) is attributable to sepsis. A recent international survey of

PICUs demonstrated a prevalence of 8.2% among patients admitted to a PICU with a median age of 3 years and a range from 0.7 years to 11 years.

What Is the Pathophysiology of Septic Shock?

The understanding of the cause of sepsis is incomplete, but the fundamental etiology is a significant release of vasoactive cytokines and bacterial derived products. Certain pathogens contain products such as lipopolysaccharides that have a higher potential to cause this cytokine storm. Similarly, certain individuals will have a more exaggerated response to pathogenic products, which will also lead to a higher cytokine response.

The specific response of each individual patient varies widely and depends on the pathogen load and virulence, and on the host with significant genetic variation and coexisting disease. The initial immune response also triggers several other cascades including complement and coagulation activation and catecholamine release.

What Are the Major Hemodynamic Consequences of Septic Shock?

Septic shock is most commonly seen in adults as warm shock with significant peripheral vasodilation leading to a high-output shock state. Tachycardia will increase total cardiac output to compensate for a greater volume of distribution secondary to vasoplegia caused by cytokine release. While warm shock is still the most common presentation in pediatrics, a considerable proportion of patients may also present in a cold shock state with decreased perfusion and delayed capillary refill. This version of septic shock is associated with depressed cardiac function and decreased cardiac output. The cause of this variation is incompletely understood but the consequences are the same as the majority of cases present with metabolic acidosis and end-organ dysfunction.

During early resuscitation, it is important to distinguish between warm and cold shock. Both instantaneous capillary refill and delayed capillary refill are seen in sepsis and management of septic shock should be adapted accordingly. Current guidelines for septic shock recommend initial volume resuscitation with crystalloid, up to 200 mL/kg, though most children will be given 40–60 mL/kg. Central venous pressure monitoring is useful to guide volume resuscitation with a common goal of approximately 8–12 cm H_2O, while monitoring for signs of fluid overload. There do not seem to be any advantages to colloid therapy.

Early initiation of inotropic support is recommended, preferably via central access if available. Epinephrine is the first-line choice for cold vasoconstricted shock, but dopamine has also been used successfully. Norepinephrine is the first-line therapy for warm vasodilatory shock. The role for other vasoactive medications in pediatrics has not been defined, though phenylephrine may provide peripheral vasoconstriction to treat hypotension secondary to warm shock, while dobutamine often provides significant inotropy.

What Treatment Options Are Available for Pressor Refractory Septic Shock?

In pressor refractory shock, consideration of adrenal insufficiency should prompt initiation of hydrocortisone stress dosing, though the evidence for or against this therapy is limited. Milrinone may effectively offload a volume overloaded heart, though this medication is long-acting and slow to titrate, making it difficult to use in rapidly changing clinical situations. Vasopressin should also be considered in pressor refractory warm shock. A final rescue therapy for pediatric septic shock is veno-arterial extracorporeal membrane oxygenation (ECMO).

Is an Arterial Line Necessary in Septic Patients?

All hemodynamic interventions should be managed with the goal of optimizing end-organ perfusion. Invasive blood pressure monitoring with arterial access should be used to obtain instantaneous determination of blood pressure, pulsatility, and pulse pressure. This also allows for repeated sampling of blood gas and lactate samples.

Lactic acidosis is a significant sign of hypoperfusion and can be used to guide blood pressure goals. Cardiac dysfunction is worsened by significant acidosis and frequent laboratory monitoring is required to detect additional end-organ dysfunction.

Is a Central Venous Line Necessary in Sepsis Patients?

Central venous access with the ability for rapid infusion of volume and blood products would be helpful for the septic patient requiring general anesthesia.

Table 11.2 Sequential Organ Failure Assessment (SOFA). Reproduced with permission of Wolters Kluwer Health, Inc. from Jones AE, et al. Crit Care Med. 2009 May;37(5):1649–54

SOFA score	1	2	3	4
Respiration[a]				
Pao_2/Fio_2 (mm Hg)	<400	<300	<200	<100
Sao_2/Fio_2	221–301	142–220	67–141	<67
Coagulation				
Platelets × $10^3/mm^3$	<150	<100	<50	<20
Liver				
Bilirubin (mg/dL)	1.2–1.9	2.0–5.9	6.0–11.9	>12.0
Cardiovascular[b]				
Hypotension	MAP <70	Dopamine ≤5 or dobutamine (any)	Dopamine >5 or norepinephrine ≤0.1	Dopamine >15 or norepinephrine >0.1
CNS				
Glasgow Coma Score	13–14	10–12	6–9	<6
Renal				
Creatinine (mg/dL) or urine output (mL/d)	1.2–1.9	2.0–3.4	3.5–4.9 or <500	>5.0 or <200

MAP, mean arterial pressure; CNS, central nervous system; Sao_2, peripheral arterial oxygen saturation.
[a]Pao_2/Fio_2 ratio was used preferentially. If not available, the Sao_2/Fio_2 ratio was used; [b]vasoactive medications administered for at least 1 h (dopamine and norepinephrine mcg/kg/min).

Many of the vasoactive medications necessary for hemodynamic modulation require central access due to the risk of soft tissue damage with infiltration.

Central venous oxygen saturation can be utilized with a goal of normalization to approximately 70%. This number reflects oxygen delivery, which is a combination of cardiac output and arterial oxygen content, and oxygen consumption. Sepsis can have decreased central venous oxygen saturation because of a combination of both increased oxygen consumption, secondary to fever and metabolic stress, and decreased oxygen delivery, secondary to decreased cardiac output, anemia, and decreased oxygenation ability from lung injury. Any decrease in central venous saturation can indicate a lack of adequate oxygenation in the end-organ capillary beds, which can lead to tissue injury and must be corrected.

What Other Monitoring Devices Are Used in Sepsis Patients?

Urine output remains an important monitor of end-organ perfusion to the kidney, with a goal of at least 0.5 mL/kg/h. NIRS may have a role in monitoring cerebral oxygen delivery but evidence-based outcome studies have not been performed. Transthoracic and transesophageal echocardiography may also be useful in monitoring cardiac function.

How Is Multiorgan Dysfunction Measured in Septic Shock?

The risk of mortality with septic shock increases with multiorgan dysfunction. A common scoring algorithm used to define organ dysfunction in septic shock is the Sequential Organ Failure Assessment (SOFA), shown in Table 11.2. This assessment tool takes into account end-organ dysfunction and demonstrates increased mortality with higher scores. The trend of this score also correlates with higher or lower mortality. This assessment tool has been shown to be effective in small cohorts of pediatric patients and is useful to monitor severity of illness. Practitioners must be prepared for severe end-organ dysfunction during progression of severe sepsis and patients undergoing surgical procedures will be at higher risk of more end-organ involvement. The cause of progression to multiorgan dysfunction syndrome is unknown, but it is likely a combination of severe inflammatory products, hypoperfusion, acidosis, hypoxemia and alterations in coagulation.

What Are the Respiratory Symptoms of Advanced Sepsis?

Acute respiratory distress syndrome (ARDS) is defined as acute hypoxemia with a P:F<300 with bilateral pulmonary infiltrates on chest radiograph not due to congestive heart failure. This is further divided into mild (P:F 200–300), moderate (P:F 100–200) and severe (P:F<100). ARDS is observed in about 6% of adult and pediatric sepsis patients.

What Is the Ventilatory Strategy for Patients with ARDS?

The ventilatory strategy for ARDS is to increase the level of positive end-expiratory pressure (PEEP) and adjust the FiO_2 to maintain SaO_2 >90%. The target FiO_2 is below 60%. An ARDSNet study published in 2000 demonstrated lung protection with low tidal volumes around 6 mL/kg compared to 12 mL/kg. Permissive hypercapnia with pH>7.25 is usually the goal to minimize barotrauma and volutrauma. Once mean airway pressure increases beyond 20 cm H_2O, consideration of advanced modes of ventilation such as oscillation is usually warranted. Nitric oxide also has a role in treating severe hypoxemia and high FiO_2, though there is a rare association with renal failure with this treatment. This can assist in ventilation/oxygenation matching and can also alleviate pulmonary hypertension, which can complicate cardiac function.

What Are Other End-Organ Manifestations of Severe Sepsis?

Renal dysfunction is another common comorbidity with severe sepsis. Fluid overload is a common manifestation following volume resuscitation and if the renal system cannot compensate for the volume, continuous renal replacement therapy (CRRT) may be warranted. CRRT is also indicated in severe refractory acidosis, uremia, or hyperkalemia. All of these can result from tumor lysis syndrome in leukemia patients such as the one discussed in the vignette. This syndrome occurs when patients with a high tumor burden have many of their tumor cells lyse at the same time, possibly secondary to treatment or severe stress. Unfortunately, the use of CRRT can be limited secondary to hemodynamic instability secondary to the fluid shifts necessary to complete dialysis.

Patients with severe sepsis also will occasionally present with disseminated intravascular coagulation. This is a syndrome secondary to release of tissue factor from endothelia and inflammatory cells, which leads to activation of the clotting cascade and consumption of intravascular endogenous anticoagulants. The lack of these endogenous anticoagulants leads to uncontrolled micro-thrombi formation, causing intravascular and intra-organ clots along with a predisposition to bleeding due to consumption of pro-coagulant factors and platelets. This is an important consideration prior to surgical intervention as many septic patients will require correction of coagulopathy represented by abnormal prothrombin and partial thromboplastin times and abnormal fibrinogen levels with fresh frozen plasma and cryoprecipitate.

Thrombocytopenia should be corrected prior to surgery. Anemia may be present, secondary to intravascular lysis secondary to DIC or hemodilution, and this should also be corrected prior to operation as it will lead to improvement in hemodynamics and oxygenation. Transfusion is indicated for hemoglobin level <7 mg/dL though some guidelines recommend transfusion when <10 mg/dL.

What Are the Anesthetic Considerations for Sepsis Patients?

The goal in choosing anesthetic induction agents is to provide pharmacologic agents with the least hemodynamic perturbation possible. Patients in septic shock are at high risk for cardiac arrest with secdation and initiation of positive pressure ventilation. Ketamine tends to slightly increase blood pressure through release of endogenous catecholamines, though in septic patients, these catecholamines can be depleted and can lead to a decrease in blood pressure, as well as a secondary myocardial depression effect of the agent. Fentanyl and midazolam have good analgesic and hypnotic properties, but can cause some decrease in myocardial output, though the amount of decrease seen with this can be minimal. Propofol tends to provide excellent intubating conditions quickly but can cause hemodynamic instability. Etomidate has a black-box warning in pediatrics due to adrenal suppression and increased mortality in septic patients and should not be used in pediatric sepsis patients.

Many of these procedures are emergent and a modified rapid sequence induction technique should be strongly considered. The likelihood of aspiration may also be higher due to a stress-induced ileus in severe sepsis. The choice of paralytic between succinylcholine and rocuronium likely depends on comorbidities including pre-existing renal dysfunction, hyperkalemia, or liver injury. Careful monitoring of induction should be used as end-organ dysfunction including hepatic and renal dysfunction may lead to significantly less need for drug dosing than commonly used. Remifentanil is a good choice as a primary agent for analgesia. Dexmedetomidine can blunt the tachycardic response desirable for pediatric patients and may cause hemodynamic instability. The effect of heart rate on cardiac output in pediatrics is important to consider given the smaller stroke volume from a smaller heart. Inhaled anesthetics cause significant peripheral vasodilation and will cause worsened hemodynamic instability.

Other anesthetic considerations for pediatric patients include a higher risk for hypothermia, which will worsen hemodynamic instability and can worsen coagulopathy. Hypoglycemia must also be avoided and severe stress associated with sepsis may lead to a requirement for a higher glucose infusion rate than usually needed. Preparation for all of these issues should be considered prior to taking a patient with sepsis to the operating room. Regular arterial blood gases, coagulation testing, lactate levels, and glucose testing are necessary. Blood counts and electrolyte levels should also be closely monitored.

What Types of Surgical Procedures Are Often Required in Patients with Septic Shock?

Septic pediatric patients may require surgical debridement of abscesses or necrotic wounds. Empyemas may require drainage following a severe pneumonia. Though many of these may occur in stable patients, there is the possibility that drainage could release bacterial products into the bloodstream and lead to a transient bacteremia and SIRS. Trauma patients can suffer infectious processes and require surgical intervention for foreign body removal or repair of intraabdominal injury or long bone fracture. Occasionally, septic shock patients will develop significant fluid overload with abdominal compartment syndrome requiring surgical decompression. Infected tunneled central lines also will require removal if the infection cannot be cleared.

What Are Common Postoperative Considerations in Sepsis Patients?

Any patient with significant ventilatory requirement or hemodynamic instability during operative procedures should be monitored in a pediatric intensive care unit until the hemodynamic instability has resolved. These patients require continued monitoring for end-organ dysfunction and intervention if necessary. Antibiotic therapy must be continued and monitored for toxicity. Nutrition should be started, though there has been some recent controversy as to the appropriate timing for this. Glycemic control should be initiated with insulin if levels are continually high, though the true benefit of this is still unknown and studies are ongoing. Children are at higher risk for hypoglycemia and this must be avoided. Patients recovering from severe illness are also at increased risk for secondary infection, which can lead to significant mortality, and this also must be monitored with indwelling central lines and catheters.

What Is Propofol Infusion Syndrome (PIS)?

While commonly used for sedation in adult ICUs, propofol for continuous sedation in pediatric patients has been issued a black-box warning by the Food & Drug Administration (FDA) after numerous reports of patient deaths. These deaths were directly attributed to the PIS in children. PIS is a complex, multifactorial constellation of symptoms. The exact etiology of PIS is unknown but postulated to result from impaired fatty acid metabolism in mitochondria.

Symptoms of PIS include acidosis, bradyarrhythmia, and rhabdomyolysis of cardiac and skeletal muscle leading to multi organ failure. In patients with PIS, a high incidence of lipemia, hypertriglyceridemia, and fatty liver changes has been noted.

Patients with prolonged infusion of propofol greater than 4 mg/kg/h or 67 mcg/kg/min are highest risk for development of PIS. Treatment requires stopping the propofol infusion and initiation of supportive therapies.

Suggested Reading

Bray RJ. Propofol infusion syndrome in children. *Paediatr Anaesth.* 1998;8(6):491–9 PMID: 9836214.

Brower RG, Matthay MA, Morris A, et al. Ventilation with lower tidal volumes as compared with traditional tidal volumes for acute lung injury and the acute respiratory distress syndrome. *N Engl J Med.* 2000;342(18):1301–8. PMID: 10793162.

Ferreira FL, Bota DP, Bross A, Mélot C, Vincent JL. Serial evaluation of the SOFA score to predict outcome in critically ill patients. *JAMA.* 2001;286(14):1754–8.

Giuliano JS Jr, Markovitz BP, Brierley J, et al. Comparison of pediatric severe sepsis managed in U.S. and European ICUs. *Pediatr Crit Care Med.* 2016;17(6):522–30. PMID: 27124566.

Goldstein B, Giroir B, Randolph A; International Consensus Conference on Pediatric Sepsis. International pediatric sepsis consensus conference: definitions for sepsis and organ dysfunction in pediatrics. *Pediatr Crit Care Med.* 2005;6(1):2–8. PMID: 15636651.

Jones AE, Trzeciak S, Kline JA. The Sequential Organ Failure Assessment score for predicting outcome in patients with severe sepsis and evidence of hypoperfusion at the time of emergency department presentation. *Crit Care Med.* 2009 May;37(5):1649–54. PMID: 19325482.

Singer M, Deutschman CS, Seymour CW, et al. The third international consensus definitions for sepsis and septic shock (Sepsis-3). *JAMA.* 2016;315(8):801–10. PMID: 26903338.

Vincent JL, de Mendonça A, Cantraine F, et al. Use of the SOFA score to assess the incidence of organ dysfunction/failure in intensive care units: results of a multicenter, prospective study. Working group on “sepsis-related problems” of the European Society of Intensive Care Medicine. *Crit Care Med.* 1998;26 (11):1793–800. PMID: 9824069.

Weiss SL, Fitzgerald JC, Pappachan J, et al. Global epidemiology of pediatric severe sepsis: the sepsis prevalence, outcomes, and therapies study. *Am J Respir Crit Care Med.* 2015;191(10):1147–57. PMID: 25734408.

Chapter 12

Malignant Hyperthermia

Giselle Torres

> A three-year-old, 18 kg male presents for tonsillectomy and adenoidectomy. No other pertinent past medical history or family history was reported. Inhalational induction and intubation without muscle relaxation was safely performed. Fifteen minutes after intubation and initiation of adequate controlled ventilation, generalized muscle rigidity is noted. Vital signs at that time include: $EtCO_2$ 110 mmHg, BP 140/80, HR 160 bpm, and T 38°C.

How Will You Approach This Constellation of Clinical Findings?

The most likely diagnosis for increased end tidal carbon dioxide, fever, and muscle rigidity in this age group is malignant hyperthermia (MH). Other possible diagnoses that are usually considered include serotonin syndrome, sepsis, pheochromocytoma, neuroleptic malignant syndrome, thyroid storm, and adverse drug reactions, but none of these alternatives have been reported in this type of patient and should not be considered.

MH is a hypermetabolic response to inhalational anesthetics or succinylcholine. Acute signs include hypercarbia, tachycardia, master muscle or generalized muscle rigidity, arrhythmia resulting from hyperkalemia, or hyperthermia as an early or later sign. A rapid elevation of temperature is associated with increased severity of disease. Arterial blood gas sampling demonstrates a respiratory acidosis and possibly metabolic acidosis. Complications from MH include disseminated intravascular coagulation (DIC) from prolonged severe hyperthermia, rhabdomyolysis and myoglobinuria, end-stage organ failure, cardiopulmonary collapse, and death.

How Is MH Diagnosed?

Acute MH is diagnosed only by clinical characteristics and index of suspicion. After the event, a diagnosis of MH susceptibility can be confirmed by a positive result of a caffeine-halothane contracture test (CHCT) from a skeletal muscle biopsy, or finding a known MH-causative mutation on genetic screening. However, only a negative CHCT can rule out MH susceptibility; a negative mutation analysis is not sufficient to rule out MH susceptibility. Most MH-causative mutations are located on the gene that encodes for the skeletal muscle ryanodine receptor (RYR1), and rarely on the *CACNA1S* gene that encodes for the dihydropyridine receptor. In very rare cases, MH has been associated with a mutation in the *STAC3* gene, which also contributes to the excitation-contraction complex in skeletal muscle.

What Is the Incidence of MH?

The approximate incidence of acute MH during general anesthesia with triggering agents has been estimated to be between 1/10,000 and 1/25,000 cases. The estimated prevalence of MH susceptibility is thought to be between 1/3,000 and 1/8,500 people. Historically, half of the diagnosed cases of MH have been found in the pediatric population. However, in recent years, studies have found that only 17–18% of patients diagnosed with MH in the United States are under the age of 18. This may be due to better detection of MH susceptibility and anesthetic preparation for MH susceptible patients by anesthesiologists. Male sex is also predominant in pediatric patients diagnosed with MH.

What Diseases Are Associated with MH Susceptibility?

Diseases that are associated with or caused by mutations in *RYR1*, *CACNA1S*, or *STAC3* should be presumed to be associated with MH susceptibility. They are summarized in Table 12.1.

What Is the Treatment for Acute MH?

Once the anesthesia provider suspects MH, the inhalational agent should be discontinued and dantrolene administered. The initial dose of dantrolene is 2.5 mg/kg and it should be continued until signs of MH begin to abate. In some reported cases, doses up to 10 mg/kg have been required. Hyperventilation with 100% oxygen is helpful to counteract rising blood CO_2 levels. The surgical procedure should be aborted or finished rapidly, and total intravenous anesthesia administered until the patient's condition has stabilized.

Table 12.1 Mutations associated with malignant hyperthermia

RYR1	*CACNA1S*	*STAC3*
Normal phenotype	Normal phenotype	Native American myopathy
Central core disease	Multiminicore disease	
Multiminicore disease	Congenital fiber type disproportion	
King–Denborough syndrome	Potassium-related periodic paralysis	
Congenital myopathy with cores and rods		
Centronuclear myopathy		
Congenital fiber type disproportion		
Potassium-related periodic paralysis		
Idiopathic hyperkalemia		

Additional priorities include treatment of hyperkalemia with calcium, bicarbonate, or glucose/insulin, and aggressive lowering of hyperthermia to maintain core body temperature below 38.5 °C. The effects of rhabdomyolysis may be minimized by increasing crystalloid administration. An indwelling urinary catheter may be necessary to monitor urine output postoperatively. After the clinical signs of MH have abated, the patient may be weaned off intravenous anesthesia, and the endotracheal tube removed. Dantrolene 1 mg/kg every 6 hours should be continued for at least 24 hours past the point that MH signs have abated and the creatine kinase is trending down.

How Would You Approach the Anesthetic Management of a Patient with a Personal or Family History of MH?

For such patients, premedication with dantrolene is not indicated; however, it should be easily available for the operative procedure. Total intravenous anesthesia (TIVA) and/or regional anesthesia should be used, avoiding inhalation agents and succinylcholine. The anesthesia machine can be prepared by replacing the CO_2 absorbent, removing or taping over the vaporizers, removing succinylcholine from the work area, and replacing the anesthesia breathing circuit. The anesthesia machine and circuit should be flushed free of residual anesthetic vapors. The use of charcoal filters will greatly shorten and facilitate this process (Figure 12.1). Although there is no known safe

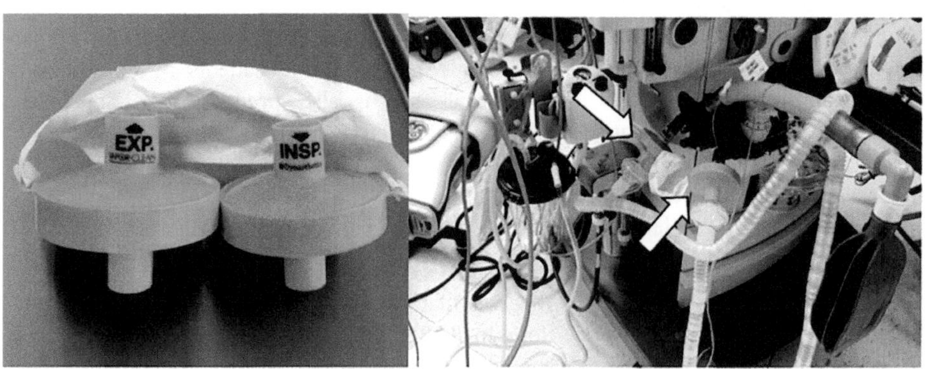

Figure 12.1 Charcoal filters in situ on the anesthesia machine circuit.

exposure level for MH-susceptible patients, the goal of these measures is to decrease the amount of inhalation anesthetic exposure to less than 5 ppm.

Patients with a history of malignant hyperthermia can be treated safely in an ambulatory care setting where dantrolene is easily accessible.

Suggested Reading

Birgenheier N, Stoker R, Westenskow D, et al. Activated charcoal effectively removes inhaled anesthetics from modern anesthesia machines. *Anesth Analg.* 2011;112 (6):1363–70. PMID: 21543783.

Kim TW, Nemergut ME. Preparation of modern anesthesia workstations for malignant hyperthermia-susceptible patients: a review of past and present practice. *Anesthesiology.* 2011;114(1):205–12. PMID: 21169802.

Larach MG, Gronert GA, Allen GC, et al. Clinical presentation, treatment, and complications of malignant hyperthermia in North America from 1987 to 2006. *Anesth Analg.* 2010 Feb 1;110(2):498–507. PMID: 20081135.

Nelson P, Litman RS. Malignant hyperthermia in children: an analysis of the North American malignant hyperthermia registry. *Anesth Analg.* 2014;118(2):369–74. PMID: 24299931.

Rosero EB, Adesanya AO, Timaran CH, et al. Trends and outcomes of malignant hyperthermia in the United States, 2000 to 2005. *Anesthesiology.* 2009;110(1):89–94. PMID: 19104175.

Salazar JH, Yang J, Shen L, et al. Pediatric malignant hyperthermia: risk factors, morbidity, and mortality identified from the Nationwide Inpatient Sample and Kids' Inpatient Database. *Paediatr Anaesth.* 2014;24(12):1212–6. PMID: 24974921.

Wappler F. Anesthesia for patients with a history of malignant hyperthermia. *Curr Opin Anaesthesiol.* 2010;23(3):417–22. PMID: 20173632.

Chapter

13 Cystic Fibrosis

Jamie W. Sinton

A nine-year-old girl with cystic fibrosis and recurrent pulmonary infections is scheduled to undergo repair of an umbilical hernia. Her home treatment regimen includes chest physiotherapy, albuterol, tobramycin, and nighttime humidified continuous positive airway pressure (CPAP), 8 mmHg.

Preoperatively her vital signs include: blood pressure 105/68; heart rate 86, respiratory rate 20; temperature 36.8°C SpO_2 97% on room air. Physical exam revealed a very thin young girl, cooperative with history and physical. Her respiratory effort is normal without the use of accessory muscles or retractions. She had coarse breath sounds bilaterally on auscultation. Airway exam was unremarkable.

What Genetic Factors Are Associated with Cystic Fibrosis?

Cystic fibrosis is caused by a mutation in the gene that encodes for the cystic fibrosis transmembrane regulator (CFTR) protein. This is a chloride channel that is found at the apical border of epithelial cells lining most exocrine glands. The mutation is the most lethal inherited disorder and displays an autosomal recessive pattern of inheritance.

What Are the Pulmonary Manifestations of Cystic Fibrosis?

Cystic fibrosis affects numerous organ systems although the primary cause of morbidity and mortality is related to pulmonary manifestations. Copious and thick secretions combined with mucociliary dysfunction lead to airway inflammation, atelectasis, and bacterial trapping. Bacterial overgrowth and inflammation cause biofilm formation and recurrent infection. With disease progression, airway obstruction from secretions causes further air trapping resulting in bronchiectasis. Patients are plagued by recurrent exacerbations leading to progressively reduced lung function, cor pulmonale, and hypercarbic, hypoxemic respiratory failure.

What Are the Nonpulmonary Clinical Manifestations of Cystic Fibrosis?

Common organ systems affected include: gastrointestinal, and genitourinary, endocrine, bone, skin, and reproductive systems (Table 13.1).

This Patient Is Scheduled for a First Case Start. However, the Patient's Pulmonologist Insists That the Patient Be Scheduled Later in the Morning. What Is the Basis for This Concern?

The timing of surgery is important as cystic fibrosis patients have very structured time-intensive treatment regimens that they adhere to in the morning. This often includes chest percussion, nebulized medication, postural drainage, and other pulmonary toileting strategies. A first start case may result in suboptimal preoperative preparation by the patient and their family on the morning of surgery.

What Are the Important Preoperative Studies in Patients with Cystic Fibrosis?

Pulmonary function studies may be useful in determining severity of disease. Cystic fibrosis patients tend to have obstructive disease with increased functional residual capacity (FRC), decreased forced expiratory volume (1 second) (FEV1), and decreased vital capacity. X-ray imaging of the chest may demonstrate air trapping as demonstrated by a flattened diaphragm. In some cases, emphysematous changes and upper lobe pulmonary blebs can also be identified on chest radiography.

Table 13.1 Pathologic and clinical manifestations in cystic fibrosis by organ system

Organ system	Pathology	Clinical manifestation
Upper respiratory tract	Copious nasal secretions	Chronic sinusitis, nasal polyps
Lower respiratory tract	Mucoid secretions, mucociliary dysfunction	Recurrent infections, bronchiectasis, chronic hypoxemia
Cardiac	Cor pulmonale	Right ventricular hypertrophy
Hepatobiliary	Bile duct obstruction	Biliary cirrhosis, portal hypertension
Gastrointestinal	Intestinal secretions	Neonatal meconium ileus, recurrent intestinal obstruction, malabsorption (vitamins A,D,E,K)
Endocrine	Obstruction and fibrosis of pancreatic ducts	Impaired pancreatic exocrine function and induced diabetes
Reproductive	Abnormal cervical secretions (females) Absence of vas deferens (males)	Decreased fertility (females and males)
Integumentary	Increased chloride levels in skin	Impaired thermoregulation
Bone	Impaired calcium, vitamin D absorption, increased bone catabolism	Early onset osteoporosis

Liver studies, complete blood count (CBC), and coagulation screen may also be indicated. Malabsorption of vitamin K from the gastrointestinal tract alongside hepatobiliary disease can lead to inadequate synthesis of vitamin K dependent factors, which places patients at risk for hemorrhage. Intraoperative hemorrhage in the setting of a concurrent malabsorptive iron deficiency anemia increases the risk of an adverse event following moderate blood loss.

Serum electrolyte levels may reveal a hypochloremic, hyponatremic, metabolic alkalosis and dehydration. Pancreatic dysfunction may lead to glucose intolerance, necessitating blood glucose checks.

Finally, CO_2 retention becomes worse with disease progression. Hypercarbia and chronic hypoxia are predisposed to the development of secondary pulmonary hypertension, and in severe cases, cor pulmonale. An arterial blood gas may be necessary to evaluate baseline respiratory status. In advanced disease, cardiac evaluation may include ECG and echocardiography.

Is Premedication Indicated in This Patient?

Premedication with the patient's usual regime of inhaled medications should be confirmed with the parents. It is crucial that the patient receive bronchodilator. Anxiolysis with midazolam benefits most children as it improves compliance with anesthetic induction.

How Would You Induce Anesthesia in This Patient?

Either inhalational or intravenous induction may be considered. Inhalational induction in this patient cohort may be somewhat delayed, due to their increased FRC, small tidal volumes and V/Q mismatch resulting in a slow uptake of volatile anesthetics. Nitrous oxide should be avoided as it can expand pulmonary blebs and lead to bleb-rupture pneumothorax.

Intravenous induction with propofol, while rapid, abolishes spontaneous ventilation and may be associated with significant obstruction due to sudden loss of airway tone. This may necessitate positive pressure ventilation, placing the patient at risk for bleb-rupture pneumothorax. Addition of intravenous dexmedetomidine may help preserve spontaneous ventilation. Regardless of induction strategy, patients should be deeply anesthetized prior to airway manipulation as cystic fibrosis is associated with high airway reactivity and a potential to provoke bronchospasm.

What Is the Optimal Anesthetic Maintenance Strategy for CF Patients?

The optimal maintenance strategy for CF patients involves maintenance of spontaneous ventilation, use of bronchodilator therapy and minimization of postoperative respiratory depression. Inhaled agents allow for maintenance of spontaneous ventilation while simultaneously serving as a bronchodilator. If positive pressure ventilation is required, employing the lowest appropriate tidal volumes with moderate positive end-expiratory pressure (PEEP) while maintaining low airway pressures is most appropriate. This serves to minimize variations in the mean airway pressure, reducing the risk of bleb rupture.

Analgesia should be provided with a multimodal approach. Opiates increase the risk of postoperative respiratory depression. Adjunctive nonsteroidal anti-inflammatories are advised. Neuraxial and regional anesthesia should be employed when possible. Ketamine, while possessing analgesic properties due to NMDA antagonism, increases airway secretions and should be used with caution.

What Special Intraoperative Concerns Exist for This Population?

Cystic fibrosis patients often have nasal polyps, combined with a possible vitamin K deficiency; this may be associated with severe bleeding with nasal instrumentation.

These patients are at risk for dehydration with a hypochloremic, hyponatremic alkalosis. Adequate intraoperative hydration is important to correct electrolyte abnormalities and reduce the viscosity of airway secretions.

Due to chronic malabsorption, cystic fibrosis patients are often thin and vulnerable to heat loss. Postoperative shivering leads to increased oxygen consumption which combined with impaired ventilation may be a dangerous stressor to the patient.

How Would You Extubate This Patient?

During the case and immediately prior to extubation, suctioning is crucial to clear the airway of secretions. Early extubation is preferred to minimize the risk of hospital acquired ventilator associated pneumonia. The use of albuterol on emergence may be indicated. Recruitment maneuvers, with low inspiratory pressures, should be used to minimize atelectasis. Finally, extubation should not take place until the patient establishes spontaneous ventilation consistent with pre-induction tidal volumes. Use of CPAP should be considered, especially in patients on home CPAP therapy.

Early reinstatement of pulmonary physiotherapy is crucial for optimal recovery.

What Are the Risk Factors for Postoperative Mechanical Ventilation?

While few studies exist, a preoperative FEV1 of <1 L and hypoxemia are risk factors for postoperative intubation. Cor pulmonale suggests elevated pulmonary arterial pressures and advanced pulmonary disease. Open abdominal incisions significantly reduce FEV1 and empiric postoperative mechanical ventilation should be considered.

Should Paralysis Be Used in This Patient Cohort?

Paralysis should be avoided in cystic fibrosis patients when possible. It is important to minimize any agents that may cause postoperative respiratory compromise. Patients with CF have progressive loss of cartilaginous airway support and must rely on muscle tone to maintain airway patency. Neuromuscular blockade may lead to increased flow obstruction. If paralysis is used then twitch monitoring is essential. Antibiotic suppression therapy including tobramycin, an aminoglycoside, will prolong the effects of neuromuscular agents. Full reversal from blockade is necessary prior to extubation, however the cholinergic effects of neostigmine may be problematic. Sugammadex, if available, may be an appropriate alternative to acetylcholinesterase inhibitors. However, in patients requiring bronchoscopy and or biopsy, use of neuromuscular blockade may be warranted as paralysis reduces the risk of pneumothoraces, especially in post lung transplantation patients.

Suggested Reading

Fitzgerald M, Ryan D. Cystic fibrosis and anaesthesia. *Continuing Education in Anaesthesia Critical Care & Pain*. 2011;11(6):204–9. https://doi.org/10.1093/bjaceaccp/mkr038.

Huffmyer JL, Littlewood KE, Nemergut EC. Perioperative management of the adult with cystic fibrosis. *Anesth Analg*. 2009;109(6):1949–61. PMID: 19923526.

Walsh TS, Young CH. Anaesthesia and cystic fibrosis. *Anaesthesia*. 1995;50(7):614–22. PMID: 7653761.

Chapter 14

Muscular Dystrophy

Jamie W. Sinton

A 16-year-old male with muscular dystrophy presents to the operating room for laparoscopic gastrostomy tube. He uses a wheelchair and undergoes physical therapy four times weekly.

The mother has brought his continuous positive airway pressure (CPAP) machine used nightly at 7 cm H_2O.

Current medications include: prednisone, albuterol, vitamin D, and calcium supplementation.

His baseline saturation is 96% on room air.

DIAGNOSIS

What Are the Important Diagnoses to Consider?

Patients undergoing muscle biopsy present with a wide range of symptoms and no definitive diagnosis. Shapiro et al. has described a classification system for these patients based on presumptive preoperative diagnosis: myopathy or muscular dystrophy (MD), neuropathy or neuronal degeneration, metabolic or mitochondrial myopathy, seizures, cardiomyopathy, dermatomyositis. Patients with suspected diagnosis categories of myopathy or muscular dystrophy as well as metabolic or mitochondrial myopathy often have diseases that will alter anesthetic management. Special consideration to management of patients in these subsets is warranted.

PREOPERATIVE EVALUATION

How Is the Diagnosis of Muscular Dystrophy Made?

Muscle biopsy is the gold standard for diagnosis of many muscular disorders. The muscle to be biopsied is chosen based on the distribution of muscle weakness on physical exam. If weakness is generalized, often the quadriceps, specifically vastus lateralis, is chosen.

What Historical and Clinical Exam Findings Are Consistent with Muscular Dystrophy?

Muscular dystrophies are quite a heterogeneous group of disorders; however, most children present under the age of 4 years for muscle biopsy. Children with more severe forms of muscular diseases will present earlier in life.

Muscular dystrophy is characterized by painless muscle degeneration and atrophy. Any exam findings of muscular tenderness make MD less likely. Assessment of muscle bulk may be of some utility as myotonias often present early in life with muscle hypertrophy while other muscular disorders present with muscle wasting and atrophy.

What Testing Is Prudent to Narrow the Differential Diagnosis and Optimize the Patient's Medical Condition Preoperatively?

Discussion with the referring physician and surgeon may be exceedingly helpful to ascertain likely diagnostic possibilities for each patient.

Muscular disorders may be suggested based on elevations of creatine phosphokinase (CK), creatine kinase of muscle (ckMB), blood urea nitrogen (BUN), aldolase, pyruvate, and lactic acid. More recently, genetic studies have become available for many disorders. For selected patients, hematologic studies and electromyography (EMG) can be suggestive of several diagnoses.

Medical optimization prior to biopsy includes determination of cardiopulmonary involvement. Tests such as chest roentgenogram, electrocardiogram, or echocardiogram may be indicated based on history, physical exam findings, and known comorbid associations with the presumptive diagnosis.

Table 14.1 Muscular disorders associated with cardiac disease

Muscular disorder	Cardiac findings
Duchenne muscular dystrophy	ECG: sinus tachycardia with short PR interval, tall R waves in V1, and deep Q waves in limb leads Echo: Dilated cardiomyopathy, papillary muscle dysfunction leading to mitral regurgitation
Nemaline rod muscular dystrophy	Echo: dilated cardiomyopathy

Muscular disorders associated with cardiac disease are shown in Table 14.1.

Are Airway Abnormalities Associated with Neuromuscular Disease?

Structural airway abnormalities, while uncommon, do occur in muscular disease. Scoliosis with relative rigidity of the spinal column may pose positioning and airway management challenges. Chondrodysplastic myotonia (Schwartz–Jampel Syndrome) is associated with micrognathia. Functional airway abnormalities, however, are quite common and are discussed below.

Cough clearance may be impaired due to neuromuscular weakness. The five phases of cough include irritation, inspiratory phase, glottic closure, compressive phase, and expulsive phase. Each of these phases may be affected by neuromuscular disease. Diaphragmatic (or other inspiratory muscle weakness) may impair inspiratory phase. Alternatively, glottic closure is affected by bulbar involvement as seen in motor neuron disease such as Duchenne muscular dystrophy. Similar to inspiratory phase compromise, expiratory phase compromise is related to weakness of the expiratory muscles. While expiration is usually passive, during coughing, expiration is facilitated by the rectus abdominis, abdominal obliques, and internal intercostal muscles.

Mucociliary airway clearance may be impaired in patients with chronic aspiration. Chronic deposition of mucus in the tracheobronchial tree prohibits proper clearance of new secretions.

Obstructive sleep apnea occurs with disease progression due to pharyngeal muscle weakness. Sleep study results should be reviewed if available.

INTRAOPERATIVE MANAGEMENT

What Anesthetic Options Are Available for This Patient?

Local, regional, and general anesthetics have been used. In a one-year-old patient, local anesthesia is unlikely to be tolerated. Regional anesthetics may selectively block innervation to the muscle to be biopsied. Spinal, epidural (including caudal), femoral, fascial iliaca blocks may provide anesthesia to the vastus lateralis. These may be used alone or in combination with sedation.

General anesthesia with dexmedetomidine and ketamine has been studied by Kako et al., who concluded that sedation with ketamine 1 mg/kg IV with dexmedetomidine 0.5 mcg/kg IV bolus over 10 min plus continuous infusion at that rate was safe and effective with limited cardiovascular effects.

For Which Patients Should a Non-MH Triggering Anesthetic Probably Be Chosen?

Non-MH triggering anesthetics are chosen for those patients whose preoperative suspected diagnosis makes them susceptible to malignant hyperthermia (MH). These patients often present with a creatine kinase level greater than 2 times normal (for age). Modern anesthesia machines should be prepared according to manufacturer instructions and recommendations from the Malignant Hyperthermia Association of the United States (MHAUS). Additionally, activated charcoal filters could be considered for use. Muscular conditions which have definite or likely association with malignant hyperthermia include chondrodysplastic myotonia (Schwartz–Jampel Syndrome), King-Denborough syndrome, central core disease, multiminicore disease, and Brody myopathy.

Less clear recommendations can be made for those with diseases associated with adverse muscular or metabolic reaction to anesthesia (AMRA), or anesthesia-induced rhabdomyolysis (AIR). See below for discussion.

For Patients Receiving a Non-MH Triggering Anesthetic, How Should Temperature Be Measured, and Why?

Core temperature should be measured because temperature measurement location is significantly associated with death if an episode of malignant hyperthermia occurs. In a retrospective study of malignant hyperthermia patients, the risk of dying from the event was 13.8 times greater with no temperature monitoring than with core temperature monitoring. Similarly, monitoring skin temperature conferred a 9.7 fold increased risk of death once a malignant hyperthermia episode occurred.

Is Succinylcholine Safe to Use for Patients with Suspected Neuromuscular Disease?

Generally, succinylcholine should be avoided in patients with suspected neuromuscular disease. Certainly, succinylcholine is not safe for patients with suspected muscle disorders that are associated with malignant hyperthermia susceptibility. Additionally, those with Duchennes or Beckers muscular dystrophy reliably develop hyperkalemia following succinylcholine. Patients with hyperkalemic periodic paralysis will experience the usual potassium release following a dose of succinylcholine; however, the rise in plasma potassium may be significant and cause delayed hyperkalemic muscle weakness.

Will the Use of Nondepolarizing Muscle Relaxants Impact the Tissue Diagnosis of the Biopsy Specimen? Are They Safe to Use in This Patient Population?

Nondepolarizing neuromuscular blockers do not impact the diagnostic yield of the muscle biopsy. Some muscle disorders, however, place the patient at risk of extreme sensitivity to such agents and prolonged weakness may ensue.

Many primary or secondary muscular disorders, (myasthenia gravis), may display significant sensitivity to these agents. Additionally, patients with myotonias may experience sustained muscular contractions following reversal of neuromuscular blockade.

POSTOPERATIVE CONSIDERATIONS

How Can Adverse Muscular or Metabolic Reaction to Anesthesia (AMRA) Be Detected Postoperatively?

Adverse reactions include any unexplained hyperkalemia with ECG changes or cardiac arrest. Muscular manifestations include myoglobinuria, and a hypermetabolic state. Pre- and intraoperative level of suspicion for AMRA based on preoperative presumptive diagnosis may guide monitoring plans.

When Is Hospital Discharge Safe?

No definitive guidelines exist regarding management and discharge timing for these patients. If no adverse muscular or metabolic reaction to anesthesia is present and airway status returns to baseline, outpatient procedures are appropriate.

Parental counseling is advised for outpatients, as the patients must return to the hospital emergently if tachypnea, dark urine, muscle pains, or elevation in temperature should occur.

Special Considerations in Duchenne Muscular Dystrophy

Duchenne muscular dystrophy (DMD) occurs in approximately 1 in 5000 live (male) births. It results from a paucity of the protein dystrophin. Dystrophin is located adjacent to the sarcolemmal membrane in myocytes and connects the extracellular matrix with the intracellular contractile apparatus. Muscle biopsy demonstrates lack of dystrophin immunostaining. Genetic mutation analysis may also be diagnostic. Affected patients (males) develop muscular weakness by age two to three years. Nearly all patients are symptomatic by age five years.

Adult patients with advanced disease may continue to present to pediatric hospitals throughout their lives, although the Muscular Dystrophy Association (MDA) center offers help to transition pediatric patients into adult care.

What Preoperative Cardiac Considerations Are Necessary in Patients with Duchenne Muscular Dystrophy?

Sedentary lifestyle and inability to gather historical information on exercise tolerance warrants cardiac evaluation prior to elective anesthetics. Further, wheelchair user status puts little stress on the heart; consequently, even those with dilated cardiomyopathy may be asymptomatic. The incidence of cardiomyopathy is 25% by age six and 59% by age ten. By age 30, 90% have cardiac involvement.

ECG changes listed in Table 14.1 are often present regardless of cardiomyopathy status (Thrush 2009). Additionally, in this study, patients' ages ranged from 3 to 27 years. Interpretation and interplay of QT and QTc varies over heart rate range and actual QT diverges from QTc with increasing heart rate. This suggests a possible small margin of safety for young children whose heart rates are faster at baseline. Dilated cardiomyopathy is common and treated with afterload reduction. Use of angiotensin converting enzyme inhibitors may predispose to post-induction hypotension. One fourth of these patients take chronic steroid therapy (even after full time wheelchair use), so adrenal suppression should be suspected (Wagner 2007).

Volatile anesthetic use. Boys with Duchenne or Becker MD are at risk for life-threatening hyperkalemia and rhabdomyolysis under general anesthesia. Although the reaction is not specifically MH, it can be equally lethal. Names for this type of reaction to inhaled anesthetics include Anesthesia Induced Rhabdomyolysis (AIR) and Adverse Muscular or Metabolic Reaction to Anesthesia (AMRA).

Previously, patients with DMD or Becker MD were often found to have positive caffeine-halothane contracture tests. For this reason, non-triggering anesthetics were recommended. Later, data from Europe suggested that dystrophin deficiency did not predispose to development of MH and that the caffeine-halothane contracture tests are unreliable in these patients. Presently, it is recognized that the genetic basis for either of DMD or Becker MD is x-linked while genetic predisposition to MH is autosomal (chromosome 19), making a genetic association between the two less likely.

In a recent retrospective chart review of 117 anesthetic exposures, the authors of the study concluded that although symptoms of leakage of muscle cell contents and resulting hyperkalemia or acidosis may be associated with volatile anesthetic exposure, severe intraoperative events also co-existed in each case. For example, one patient in the series developed metabolic acidosis but had also had 2.5 liter blood loss. As volatile anesthetic agents had not been implicated in these adverse events, the authors cannot definitively recommend against the use of volatile agents in children with Duchenne or Becker MD.

Suggested Reading

Kako H, Corridore M, Kean J, et al. Dexmedetomidine and ketamine for sedation for muscle biopsies in patients with Duchenne muscular dystrophy. *Paediatr Anaesth.* 2014;24(8):851–6. PMID: 24646124.

Larach MG, Brandom BW, Allen GC, et al. Malignant hyperthermia deaths related to inadequate temperature monitoring, 2007-2012: A report from the North American Malignant Hyperthermia Registry of the Malignant Hyperthermia Association of the United States. *Anesth Analg.* 2014;119(6):1359–66. PMID: 25268394.

Nigro G, Comi LI, Politano CL, et al. The incidence and evolution of cardiomyopathy in Duchenne muscular dystrophy. *Int J Cardiol.* 1990;26:271–7. PMID: 2312196.

Shapiro F, Athiraman U, Clendenin DJ, et al. Anesthetic management of 877 pediatric patients undergoing muscle biopsy for neuromuscular disorders: a 20 year review. *Paediatr Anaesth.* 2016;26(7):710–21. PMID: 27111691.

Thrush PT, Allen HD, Viollet L, et al. Re-examination of the electrocardiogram in boys with Duchenne muscular dystrophy and correlation with its dilated cardiomyopathy. *Am J Cardiol.* 2009;103(2):262–5. PMID: 19121448.

Chapter 15

Spinal Muscular Atrophy

Jamie W. Sinton and William D. Ryan

A three-year-old with spinal muscular atrophy presents for intrathecal administration of nusinersen (Spinraza).

What Is Spinal Muscular Atrophy?

Spinal muscular atrophy (SMA) is a motor weakness disease caused by a mutation in the survival motor neuron (SMN) gene on chromosome 5. In over 95% of cases, the defect is a homozygous deletion of exon 7 resulting in a lack of SMN protein. The SMN protein is essential for normal functioning of the motor neuron, including the neuromuscular junction. The protein is involved in transport of mRNA along axons and local RNA processing. This deletion leads to loss of anterior horn cells of the spinal cord despite the presence of normal numbers of motor neurons. Its incidence is approximately 1 in 6,000–10,000 live births, and it is inherited in an autosomal recessive fashion. Sensation is generally intact. This disorder is heterogeneous in clinical presentation and has therefore been subcategorized for prognostic utility. Muscle weakness affects most major muscle groups as well as the intercostal muscles, but the diaphragm is spared.

What Are the Different Types of SMA?

SMA type 1 (Werdnig–Hoffmann) has onset at birth or shortly thereafter. Without ventilatory support, 90% of these infants will succumb to respiratory failure before 1 year of age, and none will survive to two years. Noninvasive artificial ventilation (e.g., CPAP) may lead to survival past five years of age, and invasive ventilation via tracheostomy may increase lifespan into adulthood.

Often, the infant has no spontaneous movements of extremities except tremor of the fingers and tongue fasciculations. Intercostal muscles are so weak that diaphragmatic breathing is required.

SMA type 2 (juvenile spinal muscular atrophy) usually presents between 6–18 months of age. While infants are weak, motor milestones such as sitting unassisted are often achieved but walking is never achieved. In less severe cases, spirometry may be unaffected. If untreated, about 70% will reach adulthood, but modern medical care improves the situation considerably.

SMA type 3 (Wohlfart–Kugelberg–Welander syndrome) usually presents after two years of age with abnormal gait. Most of these children will eventually be able to walk, and survival into adulthood is not unusual.

Electromyography shows denervation with fibrillation potentials and muscle biopsy often shows neurogenic atrophy, but diagnosis of SMA is confirmed by genetic testing for the SMN mutation.

What Is Nusinersen (Spinraza)?

Nusinersen is an SMN2-directed antisense oligonucleotide indicated for the treatment of SMA in pediatric and adult patients. Nusinersen binds to a specific sequence in the intron downstream of exon 7 of the SMN2 transcript. The administration of antisense oligonucleotides should increase production of full length SMN2 proteins. Treatment begins with four loading doses. The first three loading doses should be administered at 14-day intervals. The fourth loading dose is given 30 days after the third. Patients will then receive maintenance doses every four months. Patients with SMA who require lumbar puncture and administration of nusinersen will often need sedation or general anesthesia for immobility due to the high cost of the drug and the risk of failed administration.

What Are the Important Anesthetic Considerations in Patients with SMA?

The anesthetic considerations posing the most risk to SMA patients are related to possible difficult intubation (from atrophy of the masseter muscle and ankylosis of the mandibular joint) and postoperative respiratory failure caused by global motor weakness. For minimally invasive procedures, such as the one described above, a facemask or supraglottic airway is sufficient. Infants with SMA Type I usually need postoperative respiratory support, while SMA Type II and III may not, depending upon their individual clinical condition. SMA patients tend to exhibit increased sensitivity to and prolonged effect of nondepolarizing neuromuscular blockers. Succinylcholine is usually avoided because of possible exaggerated release of potassium. Preoperative pulmonary evaluation and consultation are recommended.

How Will You Induce and Maintain Anesthesia for This Procedure?

There are no contraindications to the use of inhalational or intravenous anesthetic agents in patients with SMA. In our practice, most children with SMA receive inhalational anesthesia by facemask or tracheostomy followed by IV catheter insertion. Some practitioners prefer insertion of a supraglottic airway during the lumbar puncture procedure in the lateral position. Opioids and other respiratory depressant agents are avoided.

Suggested Reading

Graham RJ, Athiraman U, Laubach AE, et al. Anesthesia and perioperative medical management of children with spinal muscular atrophy. *Paediatr Anaesth.* 2009 Nov;19(11):1054–63. PMID: 19558636.

Islander G. Anesthesia and spinal muscle atrophy. *Paediatr Anaesth.* 2013;23(9):804–16. PMID: 23601145.

Mesfin A, Sponseller PD, Leet AI. Spinal muscular atrophy: manifestations and management. *J Am Acad Orthop Surg.* 2012;20 (6):393–401. PMID: 22661569.

Chapter 16

Burns Management

Aysha Hasan, William D. Ryan, and Arvind Chandrakantan

A healthy six-month-old female presents to the OR for treatment of burns on the right side of her body. Her grandmother laid her down onto their apartment heater for approximately 30 minutes. The child's right side of the face, neck, shoulder, arm, hand, abdomen, leg, and foot are burned. Her lung fields are clear. Her first set of vital signs are: HR: 174, BP: 76/37; SpO_2: 100% on room air.

How Do Pediatric Burns Usually Occur?

Burns are a leading cause of in-home harm to children. Infants who are not yet walking are often burned when they are placed in contact with hot surfaces, or as a result of a hot liquid spill. Mobile toddlers are able to pull a cup containing hot liquid off a table, chew on an electrical cord, or accidentally step on a hot surface. Adolescent burns may involve gasoline and fire. Overall, 70% of pediatric burns are associated with hot liquids.

What Are the Different Classifications of Burns?

Initial classification is based on the type of burn:

- **Thermal burns:** the depth of the skin injury is related to contact temperature, duration of contact, and thickness of the skin involved. There may be airway damage from hot smoke inhalation;
- **Cold exposure burns** such as frostbite occur when bodily tissues are frozen;
- **Chemical burns** cause caustic reactions, alteration of the pH, disruption of cell membranes, and/or toxic effects on metabolic processes. Acid burns cause tissue coagulation whereas alkali burns cause liquefaction necrosis;
- **Electric current burns** are transformed into thermal injury as the current passes through poorly conducting tissues. They may cause severe fractures, hematomas, visceral injury, and skeletal and cardiac muscle injury which can lead to pain, myoglobinuria, and dysrhythmias or other ECG abnormalities;
- **Inhalation burns** are typically caused by steam or fire;
- **Radiation burns** result from radiofrequency energy or ionizing radiation that causes damage to skin and tissues (e.g., sunburn).

Burns are further classified based on their penetrating depth:

- **Superficial (first-degree) burns** involve only the epidermal layer of the skin. These burns do not blister but are painful, dry, and blanch with pressure. These injuries are self-healing and require about one week to heal.
- **Partial thickness (second-degree) burns** can be classified as either superficial or deep. Superficial partial thickness burns are painful, red, weeping and also blanch with pressure. They blister within 24 hours, and do not typically scar, although skin pigmentation may change. Deep partial thickness burns extend deeper into the dermis and include damage to the hair follicles and glandular tissues. They are painful only to pressure and almost always blister. They are wet or waxy dry and have a mottled discoloration to them. They do not blanch with pressure. Without skin graft or infection, they heal in three to nine weeks.
- **Full thickness (third-degree) burns** destroy all the layers of the dermis and injure underlying subcutaneous tissue. Burn eschar typically remains intact. If the eschar is circumferential, it can compromise the area it is surrounding. These burns are usually painless. The skin appears along the spectrum of waxy white to charred black. The skin is dry, inelastic, and does not blanch with pressure. Blisters do not develop. Without

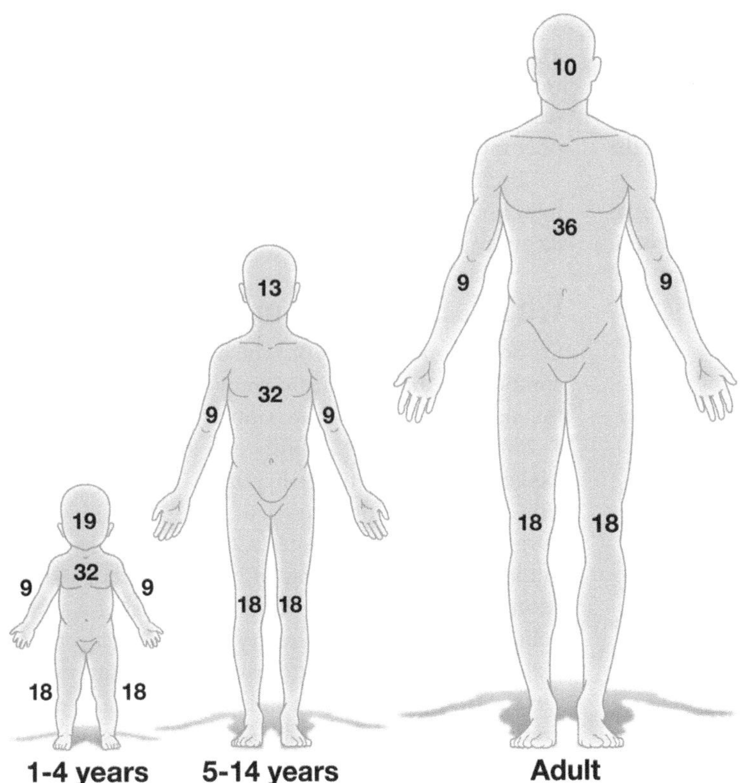

Figure 16.1 Schematic representation of body surface area (BSA) variability between children and adults. Reproduced with permission from: Litman RS, *Basics of Pediatric Anesthesia*, Philadelphia, 2014. Illustration by Rob Fedirko.

surgery, these burns heal with contractures. These burns scar severely with contractures. Surgery is required for this healing process.

- **Fourth-degree burns** are deep and potentially life-threatening burns that extend from the skin down to the fascia, muscle, and/or bone.

What Is the Estimated Percent Total Body Surface Area Burned on This Patient?

Burns can be classified according to the percentage body surface area (BSA) involved. The total percentage BSA derives from the "Rule of Nines," which is different in children than in adults since the pediatric head accounts for a larger percentage of BSA (Figure 16.1).

A *major burn* is defined as: (1) a second-degree burn with greater than 10% BSA or second-degree burn for children over 10 years old with greater than 20% BSA; (2) a third-degree burn with greater than 5% BSA; or (3) a second- or third-degree burn of the hands, feet, perineum, or major joints, electrical or chemical burns, inhalational injury, or burns in patients with preexisting medical conditions. The American Burn Association recommends that patients suffering from a major burn should be referred to a certified burn center.

Morbidity and mortality increase with increasing size and depth of the burn. Inhalational smoke injury and early shock are associated with greater mortality. The risk of mortality increases when the burn extends to greater than 60% BSA; yet there have been patients who have survived with a 90% burn. Severely burned patients may survive the initial insult, only to succumb to a secondary complication (e.g. infection). The age of the burned child is important for his or her survival, because of better prognosis with increasing age.

What Are Your Initial Anesthetic Concerns?

The initial anesthetic management of the pediatric burn patient should focus on airway evaluation and management, provision of adequate oxygenation and ventilation, as well as restoring circulatory volume. Burn patients will have difficulty regulating body temperature, so heat lamps and blankets should be used to maintain euthermia. There are pharmacokinetic implications after third-degree burns because of the upregulation of postsynaptic receptors, which can lead to acute hyperkalemia with succinylcholine administration. Wound care is usually deferred until after the acute resuscitation phase.

IV access can be difficult in cases of severe burns covering large surface areas necessitating central access. Intraosseous access can be an important tool in these patients and should be used when appropriate to avoid delay in resuscitation.

What Are the Implications for Airway Management?

Prior to tracheal intubation, the highest possible concentration of oxygen by face mask should be used. Tracheal intubation is indicated if there is evidence of inadequate ventilation, singed nasal hair, facial or upper airway edema, hoarseness, or stridor. Patients with stridor or other signs of upper airway obstruction should have tracheal intubation performed prior to the development of facial and upper airway edema, which can impede future tracheal intubation. In adults and older children, awake fiberoptic intubation is preferred if upper airway edema or injury is suspected; the extent of airway injury can be examined at the same time. Uncooperative young children will require tracheal intubation following induction of general anesthesia. Low levels of PEEP may help avoid pulmonary edema.

Respiratory failure and asphyxia may result from inhalation of toxic fumes, chemical injury from smoke, upper airway edema and, in the later stages, eschar formation on the chest wall. Inhalation of toxic chemicals can cause increased airway secretions, irritability, capillary leaking, and pulmonary edema. Clinical manifestations include hypoxia, hypercapnia, dyspnea, bronchospasm, cough, and stridor. Circumferential burns of the chest wall can cause restrictive respiratory failure for which an escharotomy may be required.

Postintubation complications may include increased secretions, bronchospasm, atelectasis, airway edema, and bronchopneumonia.

Why Are Severe Burns of the Neck and Chest Important to the Anesthesia Care Provider?

Patients with neck and chest burns are at risk for airway compromise as the eschars can become severely restrictive. Escharotomies are performed to avoid airway compression in the case of neck burns or restriction of the thoracic cavity in the case of circumferential chest burns which may result in atelectasis, pneumonia, or respiratory insufficiency.

Escharotomies may be required in the limbs as tight eschars may cause vascular compromise and loss of distal pulses.

What Is Carbon Monoxide Toxicity?

Carbon monoxide (CO), which is a byproduct of combustion and present in smoke, is responsible for the majority of deaths from smoke inhalation. CO has a 200 times greater affinity for hemoglobin than oxygen, leading to tissue hypoxia. CO will shift the oxygen dissociation curve to the left, impairing oxygen offloading to tissues. CO also interferes with mitochondrial uncoupling of oxidative phosphorylation and reduces ATP production, causing a metabolic acidosis. Pulse oximetry will not reflect CO toxicity and it will show normal oxygen saturation. Thus, carboxyhemoglobin must be specifically measured as a component of a blood gas analysis. Clinical symptoms are directly proportional to CO levels.

Low CO levels cause mild CNS symptoms and high CO levels can cause coma. The four-hour half-life of CO can be decreased to 40 minutes with 100% oxygen therapy. Severe CO intoxication can be treated with hyperbaric oxygen therapy; however, there is little evidence that it prevents permanent neurological deficits.

What Is Cyanide Toxicity?

Cyanide toxicity is commonly seen in victims who inhale or absorb combustible synthetic materials, like burning of plastic materials with elevated nitrogen content. Cyanide binds to cytochrome oxidase and impairs tissue oxygenation by converting intracellular aerobic metabolism to anaerobic metabolism. An elevated venous oxygen level and a lactic acidosis that does not improve with oxygen administration are suggestive of cyanide toxicity. Often, the patient will present with high lactic acidosis without a major burn. Blood cyanide level greater than 0.2 mg/L is toxic (lethal at about 1 mg/mL). Cyanide toxicity is measured by using a spectrophotometric assay using methemoglobin. Children who sustain cyanide poisoning as a result of inhalational injury may succumb from asphyxiation and should be treated with sodium thiosulfate or sodium nitrite if seizures, cardiopulmonary failure, or persistent lactic acidosis occurs.

How Will You Manage This Patient's Body Temperature?

Paradoxically, many patients seem adequately warm on presentation due to the nature of the injury. However, these patients can rapidly become hypothermic due to large exposed surface areas and lack of intact skin. Hypothermia can cause arrhythmias, coagulopathy, and decreased wound healing. Hypothermia in these patients is a major source of morbidity and mortality. Therefore, the clinician should treat the normothermic patient as if they are hypothermic.

Steps of therapy include room warming, blankets to unaffected areas (including the head in young children), warmed intravenous fluids, and underbody warmers whenever available.

How Will You Manage This Patient's Fluid Status?

During the acute phase of a burn, patients have a transiently decreased cardiac output due to depressed myocardial function, increased blood viscosity, and increased systemic vascular resistance from the release of vasoactive substances. Burn shock can occur due to hypovolemia from the translocation of intravascular volume to extravascular space. During the hypermetabolic phase, tissue and organ blood flow are increased due to increased cardiac output and decreased systemic vascular resistance.

Administration of IV fluids is indicated when the burn is >10% BSA. Several formulas have been proposed to estimate fluid requirements in children. The Parkland formula describes use of Lactated Ringer's solution, which is administered at the child's maintenance rate plus 4 mL/kg per 1% BSA burn for the initial 24 hours. At some institutions, half the total fluid is given over the first 8 hours with the other half given over the next 16 hours. Fluid requirements are greatest during the first 24 hours after injury.

Established formulae should be used as guides only; fluid administration should be based on parameters of adequate tissue perfusion. The rate of urine output should be maintained at a minimum of 0.5–1.0 mL/kg/h. Oliguria in burned patients is usually the result of inadequate fluid resuscitation and not renal insufficiency.

After the first day, fluid losses occur by evaporation through denuded skin and as a component of the burn exudate. Maximum weight gain due to edema occurs on the second or third day and is followed by a diuresis and return to normal weight by day 14. Protein loss through the burn exudate occurs until all wounds are grafted and healed. During graft harvesting, the surgeon may infuse crystalloid solution under the donor skin to facilitate harvesting. The amount infused can sometimes be large and should be accounted for in the total volume of fluids given. The use of colloids as a component of fluid resuscitation is controversial. In children, albumin administration increases the serum albumin level, but no data exist to support its routine administration.

What Are the Pharmacological Implications of Administering Anesthesia Drugs to Burn Patients?

Any IV induction agent is acceptable, although if significant hypovolemia is suspected, ketamine or etomidate may preserve blood pressure the best. The choice of neuromuscular blocker depends on the time since the burn. Following the initial 24-hour post-burn period, administration of succinylcholine can cause symptomatic hyperkalemia secondary to up-regulation of extrajunctional acetylcholine receptors on injured or burned muscle. This risk peaks between five days and three months and may persist for up to two years after the initial injury or until the patient has regained adequate muscle function. Burn patients may demonstrate resistance to the nondepolarizing neuromuscular blockers up to 1–2 months after the initial burn; thus, relatively larger doses are required to achieve relaxation, especially in patients with major burns. This resistance is thought to be due to changes in post-junctional acetylcholine receptors. Maintenance of general anesthesia can be accomplished using a balanced technique with an inhalational anesthetic agent. Burn patients have greater requirements for opioids due to both pharmacokinetic changes and development of tolerance. Because of the pharmacologic changes with burn injury, all drugs should be titrated to clinical effect and appropriate hemodynamic and oxygenation monitoring are required to detect opioid-induced respiratory depression. Large opioid needs during the intraoperative and postoperative periods are common.

How Much Blood Loss Is Expected during Burn Debridement?

Burn debridement commonly results in large blood losses because of the relatively large surface area of exposed skin from donor and graft sites. Once the burn eschar is excised and the large capillary bed is exposed, bandages soaked in epinephrine are often placed over the wound to decrease bleeding; this often manifests as tachycardia and hypertension. Consequently, since blood loss may be underestimated, early transfusion is often warranted during these procedures to avoid sudden hypovolemia.

Red blood cell transfusion is indicated when oxygen-carrying capacity is inadequate to meet cellular metabolic demands. The maximum allowable blood loss is determined using the estimated blood volume (EBV) of the child, which varies with age. There is no absolute hematocrit below which all patients require blood transfusion; most previously healthy children tolerate a hematocrit lower than 30% without adverse sequelae. In the trauma setting, the hematocrit is often unknown and estimates of EBV, blood loss, and blood needs are empiric. In life-threatening emergencies, immediate transfusion with type O blood is warranted. Administration of large amounts of blood to small children entails risks that include hyperkalemia from lysis of stored red cells, hypocalcemia from citrate toxicity, hypothermia, and coagulopathy that results from dilution of platelets and clotting factors.

What Are the Unique Considerations for Monitoring Children with Burns?

Standard monitoring can be challenging in the burned child. Blood pressure cuffs may have to be placed over a burned area, and needle electrodes may have to be used for the ECG. Pulse oximetry readings may not be reliable with extensive burn injury, low blood pressure, or hypothermia. In this case, pulse oximetry probes may be placed on the ear lobe, buccal mucosa, or tongue. Children that require major burn surgery will require invasive arterial blood pressure monitoring, and possibly central venous pressure monitoring to accurately track volume status acutely. Temperature measurement and maintenance of normothermia is essential since burned children are susceptible to hypothermia. The operating room and IV fluids should be warmed, inspired gases should be heated and humidified, and all exposed body surfaces covered.

What Organ System Changes Occur after a Burn?

During the acute phase of injury, the glomerular filtration rate is decreased due to decreased cardiac output and increased vascular tone from circulating catecholamines, vasopressin, and activation of the renin-angiotensin-aldosterone system. The child with a major burn is at higher risk of renal failure secondary to rhabdomyolysis, myoglobinuria, and hypotension. Neurologic dysfunction can result from hypoxia, hyperthermia, electrolyte imbalance, carbon monoxide, and hypertension. Hematologic abnormalities may include anemia from red cell hemolysis and decreased red cell survival, and thrombocytopenia due to platelet aggregation at wound sites and at damaged microvasculature. A hypercoagulable state with possible DIC can develop from increasing clotting factor production. The burned child is susceptible to development of sepsis secondary to the loss of skin and intestinal mucosal barriers, and an impaired immune response. Early enteral nutrition minimizes the intestinal mucosal barrier damage and decreases endotoxemia. Liberal application of topical antibiotic ointment has decreased the mortality from infection. Children with major burns are at risk of hypothermia from evaporative losses through large areas of exposed skin. Duodenal and gastric stress ulcers may cause chronic occult bleeding; therefore, H_2-antagonists are routinely administered. Nearly all patients will develop an ileus and will require gastric decompression with a nasogastric tube.

Children with approximately 30% BSA burn or more will demonstrate a hypermetabolic response that consists of release of stress hormones, including catecholamines, antidiuretic hormone, renin, angiotensin, aldosterone, glucagon, and cortisol. This hypermetabolic state lasts until all wounds are healed (possibly many months), and generally declines during the first 9–12 months post-injury. The degree of hypermetabolism depends on the severity of the burn. The mechanisms involved in this response are complex and may include increased adrenergic output, gut-induced endotoxemia, and endogenous resetting of energy production. The hypermetabolic state manifests as increased catabolism, nitrogen wasting, hyperthermia, hyperglycemia, increased

CO_2 production, and increased oxygen utilization. Approximately eight hours after the burn, the hypothalamic-pituitary thermoregulatory set point resets to a higher than normal body temperature. During the hypermetabolic phase, high caloric nutritional support will help prevent protein breakdown and promote wound healing. Since hypermetabolism increases oxygen consumption and CO_2 production, minute ventilation should be increased, and a warm ambient temperature ($\geq 30°C$) should be maintained to help prevent catabolism due to hypothermia.

How Is Pain Management Accomplished in the Burned Child?

Pain is a major problem in burned children. In the acute period, pain can be categorized as background pain, procedural pain, and postoperative pain. Background pain is proportional to the size of the burn and the mainstay of therapy is with oral or IV opioids. Because of rapidly developing tolerance, opioid doses need to be adjusted daily. Adjuvant analgesics such as acetaminophen, ketamine and clonidine should also be included. Procedural pain is controlled with regional anesthesia when possible, as well as opioids, benzodiazepines (for procedure-related anxiolysis), and ketamine.

What Are the Analgesic and Sedative Options for Postoperative Wound Care?

The adequate provision of anxiolysis and analgesia for daily wound care can be very challenging for providers, patients, and families. Opioid-based techniques are most commonly used, and the route of administration depends on the availability of IV access and the expected number of dressing changes over time, as well as the child's level of anxiety. Inhaled nitrous oxide is often effective for mildly painful procedures. More painful procedures may be amenable to oral or IV ketamine, in conjunction with a benzodiazepine and a topical local anesthetic. Epidural analgesia is useful for repeated wound care of the perineum or lower extremities. In some cases, administration of general anesthesia (by facemask or supraglottic device) may be required. Non-pharmacologic techniques such as hypnosis and distraction therapy have proven very useful in some children. Child-life specialists should be intimately involved with the patient and their family. Using the same medical and nursing personnel in a familiar environment with expectant management for repeated wound care lessens patient and family stress and improves provider conditions.

Suggested Reading

Battle CE, Evans V, James K, et al. Epidemiology of burns and scalds in children presenting to the emergency department of a regional burns unit: a 7-year retrospective study. *Burns Trauma*. 2016;4:19. PMID: 27574688.

Fuzaylov G, Fidkowski CW. Anesthetic considerations for major burn injury in pediatric patients. *Paediatr Anaesth*. 2009;19(3):202–11. PMID: 19187044.

Hoffman HG, Chambers GT, Meyer WJ, III, Arceneaux LL, Russell WJ, Seibel EJ, et al. Virtual reality as an adjunctive non-pharmacologic analgesic for acute burn pain during medical procedures. *Ann Behav Med*. 2011;41(2):183–91. PMID: 21264690.

Chapter 17

Pediatric Trauma

Karla E.K. Wyatt

> You are called to assist in the evaluation and care of a seven-year-old boy who will be arriving to your emergency department following a head-on motor vehicle collision. The child was an unrestrained passenger in the backseat of an automobile. The first responders report positive loss of consciousness at the scene, with two failed attempts at intubation. There is adequate bag-mask ventilation. There is no additional medical or surgical history available, as the child's parents were injured in the accident and taken to the nearest adult trauma center.
>
> His current vital signs are: blood pressure 75/32 mmHg; heart rate 140/min; temperature 35.2°C; SpO_2 92% with bag-mask ventilation.

What Are the Demographics of Pediatric Trauma?

According to the Centers for Disease Control and Prevention, unintentional injury, suicide, and homicide comprise the top three causes of morbidity and mortality in children between the ages of 1–14 years. Unintentional injuries are the leading cause of childhood death, with motor vehicle collisions reported as the most common, followed by drowning, fires/burns, and accidental suffocation. Traumatic brain injury and thoracic trauma are the leading causes of death due to motor vehicle collisions in children.

Accidental suffocation is the leading cause of *injury-related* death in children under one year, while the overall leading cause of death in children under one year is secondary to congenital anomalies.

How Is Pediatric Trauma Care Organized?

In the United States, adult and pediatric trauma centers undergo a state and local designation as well as the American College of Surgeons (ACS) verification process. The ACS designates standardized criteria for hospital entities to ensure uniform resource capability. Pediatric trauma patients are typically routed to level I or level II trauma centers. A level I facility has the means to sustain the adult and/or pediatric patient, encompassing all aspects of injury-related care including but not limited to the vast emergency, perioperative, operative, intensive care, and rehabilitation settings. Both Level I and Level II pediatric centers require the presence of trauma and subspecialty surgeons, emergency medicine, radiology, anesthesiology, and critical care personnel (24-h *in-house* for level I and 24-h *immediately available* for level II).

What Is the Initial Evaluation and Classification of the Pediatric Trauma Patient?

Evaluating the pediatric trauma patient involves a stepwise continuum of information processing including the prehospital encounter, primary survey, resuscitation, secondary survey, resuscitation, re-evaluation, and anticipatory care. The Advanced Trauma Life Support guidelines recommend a primary and secondary survey be performed on all trauma patients.

What Are the Elements of the Primary Survey?

The primary survey is a systematic approach used to identify and treat life-threatening injuries. This evaluation often includes multiple medical personnel simultaneously assessing the trauma patient. The mnemonic *ABCDE* can be used to guide the primary survey.

A. Airway. The airway is evaluated for patency, obstruction, and secretions. In the pediatric population, careful inspection should be given to oral and facial anomalies that may alert the

Table 17.1 Glasgow coma scale (GCS) in pediatric patients

	Adult and verbal children	Infants and nonverbal children	Score
Eye opening	Spontaneous	Spontaneous	4
	To speech	To speech	3
	To pain	To pain	2
	None	None	1
Verbal	Appropriate speech	Coos, babbles	5
	Confused speech	Irritable, cries but consolable	4
	Inappropriate words	Cries, inconsolable	3
	Incomprehensible words	Moans to pain, grunts	2
	None	None	1
Motor	Follows commands	Spontaneous movement	6
	Localizes pain	Withdraws to touch	5
	Withdraws to pain	Withdraws to pain	4
	Decorticate posture to pain	Decorticate posture to pain	3
	Decerebrate posture to pain	Decerebrate posture to pain	2
	None	None	1

provider to the potential difficult airway associated with an underlying syndrome. Providers should quickly determine the patient's level of consciousness and the ability to talk and/or protect the airway. Jaw-thrust, chin-lift, and airway adjuncts may assist in eliminating obstruction. Endotracheal intubation should be performed in those who cannot protect their airway. It is important to maintain cervical spine instability precautions with any head and neck manipulations during this assessment.

B. Breathing. Visual inspection of the oropharynx, neck, and chest for injuries and deviations, followed by an assessment of respiratory quality, auscultation, and palpation of the thorax should be accompanied with intervention if appropriate.

C. Circulation. During acute blood loss, children can compensate their blood pressure for a longer period of time when compared to adults. Tachycardia is often manifested as an initial sign of poor perfusion. Assessment of adequate perfusion in the pediatric patient should include palpation of the brachial and femoral pulses, capillary refill, and turgor. Two large bore intravenous catheters should be placed in the upper extremities if possible, to maintain resuscitation should the inferior vena cava be compromised. If intravenous access is difficult, pending no contraindications, intraosseous lines can also be placed. In children, hypotension becomes apparent when ~25% of the patients' blood volume is depleted. If there is evidence of poor perfusion, resuscitation with 20–30 mL/kg of a balanced salt solution should be administered. If obvious hemorrhage is occurring, direct pressure should be applied, and type O negative blood can be administered.

D. Disability. Assessment of the patients' neurological status includes the Glasgow coma scale (GCS) (Table 17.1). The pediatric modified GCS can be used in infants and nonverbal children. A GCS score $\leq$8 signals severe brain injury and endotracheal intubation with in-line stabilization is highly recommended. A GCS of 9–12 is classified as moderate, and a GCS $\geq$13 is considered minor brain injury. The next course of action in the management of a patient with a GCS in the mild to moderate range will depend on the nature of overall injury and the stability of their current clinical status.

E. Exposure. Removal of all patient clothing and accessories followed by careful inspection for further injury. During this evaluation, it is imperative to maintain patient normothermia.

What Are the Elements of the Secondary Survey?

Once the initial primary survey and resuscitation is complete and all life-threatening injuries have been addressed or ruled out, the secondary survey can take place. The secondary survey is a head-to-toe examination for any injuries that may have been overlooked during the primary survey. During this assessment radiologic, ultrasound, and laboratory data is gathered. When caregivers are available, this is the time to collect the patient's past medical history, allergies, medications, and any additional information pertinent to acute care. If clinical deterioration occurs during the secondary survey, the primary survey should promptly be re-evaluated.

What Are the Common Mechanisms of Injury?

Pediatric patients have a higher incidence of blunt traumatic injuries, with abdominal injuries occurring more often than thoracic injuries, likely secondary to the common causes of injury (i.e., falls, motor vehicle collisions, sports injuries). Adults are more likely to present with penetrating traumatic injuries, with many localized to the thorax. Thoracic trauma is the second leading cause of death due to trauma in children. However, due to the cartilaginous nature of a child's thorax, it is uncommon for them to sustain rib fractures. As a result, internal and mediastinal injury may not be immediately apparent. Furthermore, when tension and/or hemopneumothoraces occur in children, the shifting of structures within the mediastinum can lead to more pronounced hemodynamic instability. For these reasons, when such injury is suspected, consideration of needle decompression and/or chest tube placement is recommended prior to the initiation of positive pressure ventilation to avoid further hemodynamic compromise.

How Is the Traumatic Airway Assessed?

Significant respiratory distress; GCS ≤8; blunt and/or penetrating trauma to the face, neck, thorax, or abdomen; cardiovascular decompensation or direct injury; severe hemorrhage; and significant fire/burn trauma are all indicative of patients who will likely require intubation. Examination of the pediatric airway trauma should include assessment of mouth opening, consideration for restricted neck movement, debris/secretions/blood in the oropharynx, potential airway distortion, dysmorphic facies, congenital syndromes, the nature of any head and neck injuries, and consideration of the consequences of intubation with positive pressure ventilation with respect to thoracic and abdominal injury.

The approach to the airway will depend on the patient's overall clinical status. Fiberoptic airway management is ideal in the nonemergent trauma patient with a suspected difficult airway. All trauma patients should be considered to have a full stomach. Hence, there are aspiration risks associated with this approach, as it is rare for children to accommodate an awake fiberoptic technique. In emergent situations where there is no concern for a difficult airway or cervical spine instability, rapid sequence intubation with in-line stabilization of the cervical spine is preferred. Careful consideration of anesthetic induction agents that maintain hemodynamic stability and/or spontaneous ventilation is advised. In the event of a difficult airway the pediatric difficult airway algorithm should be employed.

Airway assessment should address:

- Patient cooperation
- Potential difficulty of mask ventilation
- Potential difficulty of supraglottic airway placement
- Difficulty of laryngoscopy
- Difficulty of intubation
- Difficulty of surgical airway
- Craniofacial trauma
- Head and neck trauma

What Is the Best Approach to Vascular Access?

Large bore intravenous access should be obtained as soon as possible to aid resuscitative measures. If abdominal injury is suspected, it is recommended to place lines above the diaphragm in the event that large vessels below the diaphragm are injured. Attempts should be made to avoid placing lines in injured extremities. If the head or neck has sustained a substantial injury, placement of access below the diaphragm will ensure delivery of fluids, products, and medications should there be significant vascular compromise above. It is imperative that peripheral access is obtained quickly to guide therapeutic intervention, as such large bore access should not be delayed for advanced access (central lines).

In children, intraosseous lines (IO) are often utilized when peripheral access cannot be obtained. Providers should quickly move to intraosseous line placement when peripheral IV attempts have failed to avoid undue delays in treatment and resuscitation. IO lines can aid fluid resuscitation until peripheral and or central lines can be placed. Typically, IO lines are placed in the proximal humerus or tibia. Detailed instruction and a video on placing IO lines is provided by the manufacturer (www.teleflex.com/en/usa/ezioeducation/index.html).

Contraindications to intraosseous access include fracture of the extremity, underlying bony disease, previous attempt at the same site, infection at the site, and the inability to identify landmarks. Central and arterial line placement is usually performed after the acute phase access and resuscitation has begun. The patient's clinical status and the location of their injuries often preclude initiation of early advanced monitoring.

Why Is Maintaining Normothermia Important in Trauma Patients?

Hypothermia contributes to altered mental status, left shift in the oxygen-hemoglobin dissociation curve with decreased oxygen delivery to the tissues, shivering with increased metabolic oxygen consumption, and platelet dysfunction leading to coagulopathy. These effects can lead to further deterioration of hemodynamically unstable trauma patients. Various techniques may be used to warm the patient, increasing ambient temperature, fluid warmers, forced air warming devices, and warming blankets.

In certain situations (cardiac arrest and neurotrauma), deliberate hypothermia may be employed for functional preservation. In patients returning to the operating room undergoing active cooling, decision to continue this therapy should be discussed with the critical care team. In many situations, the cooling is continued perioperatively understanding that it may result in coagulopathy.

What Are the Anesthetic Implications of Cervical Spine Injury?

Cervical spine injuries occur less commonly in children as compared to adults due to the cartilaginous nature of the spine and incomplete calcification of the vertebrae. However, pseudo-subluxation of the cervical spine, the anterior displacement of C2 on C3, is common in children. Differentiating pseudo-subluxation from a true spinal injury requires cervical manipulation and should not be attempted until potential spinal injury is discussed with a surgeon. When the mechanism of trauma involves acceleration, deceleration, or forceful impact, or neurologic deficits are present, the anesthesiologist should assume cervical instability and institute cervical immobilization with a backboard and cervical collar. A neurosurgical consultation should be obtained.

What Are the Intraoperative Anesthetic Implications of Intraoperative Management?

Intraoperative management of pediatric trauma patients is dynamic and involves all of the operating room personnel. The trauma operating room should be prepared with a warm ambient temperature, crystalloid fluids, airway adjuncts and devices, suction, fluid warmers, central venous and arterial monitoring capability, rapid transfusing devices, emergency vasoactive medications, access to an institution approved defibrillator, and commonly used anesthetic medications. If massive blood loss is anticipated, patient type specific or type O negative blood product should be readily available. This often involves close communication with blood bank personnel. Administration of red blood cells, fresh frozen plasma, and platelets in a 6:6:1 ratio has not been validated in the pediatric population. Calculation of the patient's estimated blood volume and maximal allowable blood loss, in conjunction with assessment of ongoing blood loss and laboratory data, will help guide therapy. Continuous analysis of vital signs, laboratory data, urine output, ventilator changes, and surgical interventions are variables that should be frequently reassessed.

What Are the Postoperative Anesthetic Implications?

Intensive care and enhanced monitored floor units are required postoperatively for many pediatric trauma patients. Maintaining normothermia, adequate oxygenation and ventilation, and cardiovascular stability is paramount as care transitions from the operating room to the intensive care unit. Children with large volume resuscitation are at increased risk for postoperative pulmonary edema, fluid overload, respiratory complications, hypothermia, infections, coagulopathy, and thrombosis. The decision to remain intubated should be based on the extent of the injury, degree of resuscitation, and the potential for ongoing hemodynamic instability and the need for continued resuscitation. Careful communication among anesthesia, surgery, nursing, and the receiving patient care team is paramount.

How Is Pain Managed in the Trauma Patient?

Pain is expected in trauma patients. Pain is managed using nurse or patient controlled analgesia of opioids or by continuous infusion. Understanding of the effects of narcotic medications on the patients' hemodynamic goals will help titrate pain control and maintain adequate perfusion. Pain requirements should be considered when deciding on extubation. Additionally, opioid side effects should be considered such as constipation and ileus with preventative strategies empirically started. It is prudent to avoid analgesic medications that can worsen renal function/injury and liver insult, and excessively sedate patients with fluctuating neurological status. Standardized pediatric pain scales for both verbal and nonverbal patients can be utilized for frequent assessment of pain and the adequacy of analgesia.

Is There a Role for Regional Anesthesia in the Pediatric Trauma Patient?

Prehospital and disaster medicine teams have reported the utilization of regional anesthesia for patients undergoing amputations and wound debridement during mass casualty and extreme conditions. Similar intervention has been reported in the adult military prehospital population. Epidural and peripheral nerve catheters have been used successfully with management of minor trauma in the pediatric population. However, the role for regional anesthesia has not yet been evaluated in a large-scale pediatric population. The decision to employ regional anesthesia in the polytrauma patient is often more complicated given the risk of coagulopathy, compartment syndrome, nerve injury, and labile hemodynamics. Ongoing research may enhance understanding of this in the future.

Suggested Reading

Apfelbaum JL, Hagberg CA, Caplan RA. Practice guidelines for management of the difficult airway: an updated report by the American Society of Anesthesiologists Task Force on Management of the Difficult Airway. *Anesthesiology*. 2013;118(2):251–70.

Avarello JT, Cantor RM. Pediatric major trauma: an approach to evaluation and management. *Emerg Med Clin North Am*. 2007;25 (3):803–36.

Densmore JC, Lim HJ, Oldham KT, et al. Outcomes and delivery of care in pediatric injury. *J Pediatr Surg*. 2006;41:92–8.

Myers SR, Branas CC, French B, Nance ML, Carr BG. A National Analysis of Pediatric Trauma Care Utilization and Outcomes in the United States. *Pediatric Emergency Care* 2019; 35(1):1–7.

Sperka J, Hanson S, Hoffmann R, Dasgupta M, Meyer MT. The effects of pediatric advanced life support guidelines on pediatric trauma airway management. *Pediatric Emergency Care*. 2016;32 (8):499–503.

Chapter 18

Infant Hernia Repair and Prevention of Postoperative Apnea

William D. Ryan, Adam C. Adler, and Ronald S. Litman

> A two-month-old, 6 kg male infant is scheduled for inguinal hernia repair. The patient was born at 32 weeks of gestation and is currently breast-fed.

What Is an Inguinal Hernia?

An inguinal hernia is a protrusion of a portion of fatty tissue or intestine through the inguinal canal, a tubular passage in the lower abdominal wall. It occurs in 1–5% of all newborns but its prevalence is higher in infants born prematurely and in boys. It is most common in boys because the spermatic cord and testicles descend through the inguinal canal during development.

An *incarcerated* inguinal hernia occurs when the protruding tissue cannot be massaged back into the abdomen. It can lead to strangulation, in which blood supply to the protruding tissue becomes jeopardized. Strangulated hernias require immediate surgical intervention.

Inguinal hernia repair is one of the most commonly performed surgical procedures in children. A unilateral hernia is usually diagnosed on routine physical exam in healthy school aged children. Bilateral hernias occur more commonly in premature infants and, because of the potential risk of incarceration, will usually be repaired before the child is discharged from the hospital. Therefore, these children will present with all of the usual medical problems associated with prematurity.

Which Anesthetic Method Will You Choose for This Procedure?

There are many ways to anesthetize children for hernia repairs. Different factors are taken into consideration when deciding on an anesthetic technique, including the health of the child, preference of the surgeon, and the skills of the anesthesiology provider. Older children with uncomplicated unilateral hernias can receive maintenance of general anesthesia by facemask or laryngeal mask with inhaled agents. When laparoscopic examination of the contralateral side is performed, endotracheal intubation and neuromuscular blockade may be indicated, depending on the surgeon's preference for abdominal wall relaxation and desired degree of intra-abdominal insufflation.

The anesthetic technique for bilateral hernia repair for the small infant is different from that of the older child. The hernias can consist of large bulging sacs (in the male) and can present a surgical challenge. For these cases we prefer general anesthesia with neuromuscular blockade and endotracheal intubation. In some cases of extreme prematurity and small size (e.g., less than 3 kg), when the infant is scheduled to return to the intensive care unit, we may choose to maintain endotracheal intubation into the postoperative period while the infant fully recovers. Caudal analgesia is performed for postoperative pain relief.

Pain relief for inguinal hernia repair is accomplished using regional analgesia. Caudal analgesia with dilute local anesthesia is often used for bilateral repair, and a peripheral nerve block is used for unilateral repair. However, in ambulatory children in whom a caudal block may cause lower extremity weakness, bilateral peripheral nerve blocks are performed. Analgesia may be supplemented with a small dose of an IV opioid and ketorolac.

Premature infants often exhibit central apnea following the administration of general anesthesia (GA). There are several anesthetic strategies designed to prevent this complication and these include the use of regional anesthesia instead of GA, and administration of caffeine in the perioperative period to boost ventilatory drive. Most reported studies investigating the use of spinal or epidural anesthesia report a lower incidence (not a complete absence) of postoperative apnea, as long as additional systemic sedative agents are avoided. When adjuvant sedatives, such as ketamine, are administered intraoperatively, the risk of postoperative apnea increases to a level similar to that of GA.

Caffeine is a respiratory stimulant which can decrease the incidence of postoperative apnea, bradycardia, and hypoxemia in susceptible infants. For NICU patients undergoing surgery, communication between the anesthesiologist and neonatologist is essential. The patient may currently be receiving caffeine and may not require a perioperative dose. Other patients may be going home soon after surgery; thus, a perioperative dose of caffeine will complicate discharge planning.

Almost all studies on the risk of postoperative apnea following GA were performed prior to the advent of short-acting anesthetic agents, such as sevoflurane, desflurane, and remifentanil. Some studies have shown that these newer agents of limited duration result in a decreased incidence of postoperative apnea. However, definitive data on the association of postoperative apnea with use of these agents is lacking.

Both retrospective and prospective studies have been performed in an attempt to delineate the types of patients at risk for postoperative apnea. Characteristics of premature infants that are more likely to develop postoperative apnea include low gestational age, low postconceptional age (PCA), preoperative apnea of prematurity, and anemia (usually defined as a hemoglobin level <10 g/dL) (Figure 18.1). The PCA at which postoperative apnea will not occur is unknown; however, there are no reports of postoperative apnea in infants aged greater than 60 weeks PCA (Figure 18.2). (These statements are based on older studies that attempted to determine PCA-based risk, but the term "postconceptional age" has been abandoned in favor of the more reliable "postmenstrual age.") The true risk for an individual patient is indeterminate and is likely a continuum based on the infant's gestational and chronological age, and coexisting medical conditions.

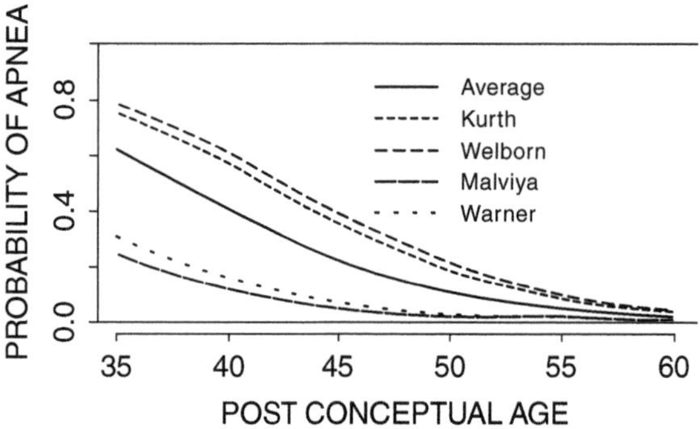

Figure 18.1 Predicted probability of apnea in recovery room and postrecovery room by weeks postconceptual age as demonstrated by review of multiple studies. Reproduced with permission from: Cote CJ, et al., *Anesthesiology* 1995;82(4):809–22. Copyright © 1995, Wolters Kluwer Health

Describe the Implications of Spinal Anesthesia in Infants

The most common use of spinal anesthesia in the pediatric population is for inguinal surgery in the preterm infant at risk for postoperative apnea following general anesthesia, especially in light of recent evidence of the possibility of neurotoxic effects of general anesthesia on the developing brain. Spinal anesthesia is most practical when the duration of the surgical procedure is less than 90 minutes. If the procedure is expected to be longer, a combined spinal-epidural or a continuous caudal-epidural anesthesia technique can be used. Contraindications to spinal anesthesia include infection at the site,

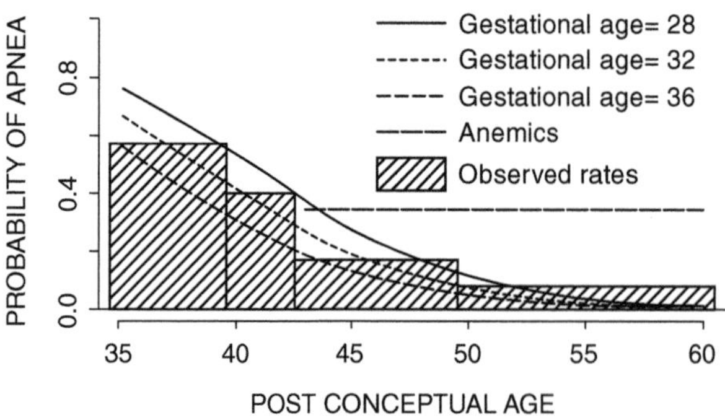

Figure 18.2 Predicted probability of apnea for all patients, by gestational age and weeks postconceptual age. Patients with anemia are shown as the horizontal hatched line. Bottom marks indicate the number of data points by postconceptual age. The risk for apnea diminishes for infants born at a later gestational age. The shaded boxes represent the overall rates of apnea for infants within that gestational age range. The probability of apnea was the same regardless of postconceptual age or gestational age for infants with anemia (horizontal hatched line). Reproduced with permission from: Cote CJ, et al. *Anesthesiology* 1995;82 (4):809–22. Copyright © 1995, Wolters Kluwer Health

increased intracranial pressure (ICP) and clinically significant hypovolemia.

Preoperative application of a topical anesthetic cream over the lumbar spine will decrease pain of the spinal injection. Some pediatric anesthesiologists prefer to obtain IV access and some administer atropine prior to performance of the block.

The choice of intrathecal local anesthetic agent will depend on the expected duration of surgery. A larger dose is required than for adults because of the relatively larger ratio of cerebrospinal fluid to bodyweight in neonates (6–10 mL/kg) compared with adults (2 mL/kg) and the resulting dilutional effect. Most reports in the literature use 1% tetracaine or 0.5–0.75% bupivacaine at doses varying from 0.3 to 1 mg/kg to provide 45–90 minutes of effective surgical anesthesia up to the T5–6 level. To prolong the duration of the spinal block, epinephrine can be added using an "epi wash" which involves drawing up epinephrine (1:1,000) into a tuberculin syringe and then ejecting it all out, thereby leaving a small amount lining the syringe and the hub of the needle prior to drawing up the local anesthetic solution.

Spinal anesthesia can be performed in either the sitting or lateral position, and is largely determined by the personal preference of the anesthesiologist. Lumbar puncture is performed at the L4–5 interspace because the spinal cord in the small infant ends at a more caudad level (L3) than in older children (L1). This landmark can be found parallel to the top of the iliac crest. With a sterile aseptic technique, a 1.5-inch, 22-gauge spinal needle is most often used and inserted approximately 1–2 cm until a light "pop" is felt as the needle penetrates the dura and subarachnoid membrane. When the stylet is removed, free flow of CSF is observed, and the syringe is firmly attached to the hub of the inserted spinal needle. (A common cause of a failed spinal block is leakage of the local anesthetic solution during injection.) The local anesthetic solution is injected over 5–10 seconds. Once the block has been performed, the infant is rapidly placed supine on the operating room table. Tape is then placed across the legs to prevent the infant from being lifted up from the table by OR staff, which may result in a high spinal block. When the electrocautery pad is placed on the infant's back, the entire infant should be lifted parallel to the table. The blood pressure cuff should be placed on a numb lower extremity to minimize stimulation of the conscious infant. Once the spinal block is completed, the anesthesiologist will know within several minutes if the block is successful when the infant's legs become limp. Conversely, if the infant's legs do not become limp within several minutes, the block was probably not successful. When this occurs we do not reattempt the spinal. Rather, we proceed with general anesthesia for the case.

With a successful spinal block, the anesthesiologist is left with a conscious infant who must be kept calm during the surgical procedure because crying or fussing increases intra-abdominal pressure, which increases the technical difficulty of inguinal surgery. Most infants will sleep during the procedure or rest quietly if offered a pacifier dipped in glucose water.

What Is the Course of Action When the Infant Is Inconsolable During the Surgical Procedure?

First, the anesthesiologist and surgeon should determine whether the surgical area is properly anesthetized. In some cases of a patchy block, the surgeon can administer local anesthesia into the wound with satisfactory results. However, if doubt remains, induction of general anesthesia is the most prudent action. If the infant is merely agitated without pain, and does not become consoled with small sugar-water feedings, the anesthesiologist's options for pharmacologic sedation are limited because the addition of sedative agents of any class will increase the risk of intra- and postoperative apnea. One exception to this is the addition of modest concentrations (<50%) of N_2O. However, N_2O does not reliably sedate all infants. If additional sedation is required to complete the surgical procedure, administration of general anesthesia is probably the best course of action.

Although cardiorespiratory effects are uncommon after spinal block in infants, complications from spinal anesthesia are not infrequent. Intra- and postoperative apnea, bradycardia, and hypoxemia may occur, necessitating immediate ventilatory assistance and possible atropine administration. A "high spinal" will cause respiratory and neurological depression with rapid onset of hypoxemia. Therefore, vigilance is required during and after the administration of the spinal anesthetic. Hypotension from a spinal anesthetic-induced sympathetic block does not usually occur in children under the age of about five to seven years. This may be due to the relatively immature sympathetic nervous system in children compared with adults, or because of the relatively

Table 18.1 Spinal vs. caudal epidural for the conscious infant. Reproduced, with permission, from "Regional anesthesia", authors Harshad Gurnaney, Andrew Costandi, James Quint, Ron Litman, Tarun Bhalla, and Joe Tobias. In: Litman RS, *Basics of Pediatric Anesthesia*, Philadelphia, 2016

	Advantages	Disadvantages
Spinal anesthesia	• Lower total dose of local anesthetic (1 mg/kg vs. 3–4 mg/kg) • Definite end-point (aspiration of CSF) • Rapid onset • Dense sensory and motor block	• Limited duration of action (60–90 minutes) • Technically difficult in small infants • Potential for high block with change in position
Caudal epidural	• High rate of success • Longer duration if catheter inserted • Minimal change in level with position	• High dose of local anesthetic agents required • Slow onset of action • Incomplete motor block

smaller intravascular volume in the lower extremities of children such that lower extremity vasodilation does not reduce preload to any appreciable extent (Table 18.1).

What Is Neonatal Apnea?

Neonatal apnea is defined as a cessation in respiratory flow of greater than 15–20 seconds or <15 seconds if accompanied by oxygen desaturation <90% and/or bradycardia of <100 beats/min. Apnea can be classified as central, obstructive, or mixed, depending upon the presence of inspiratory efforts or upper airway obstruction. Central apnea is cessation of air flow in the absence of respiratory effort. Obstructive apnea is cessation of airflow, usually at the level of the pharynx, with preserved respiratory efforts. Mixed apnea is defined as upper airway obstruction with inspiratory effort that precedes central apnea. Most neonatal apnea is central or mixed.

The prevalence of neonatal apnea is inversely related to gestational age. Apnea in term infants is uncommon and often related to other underlying medical conditions. Apnea in preterm infants is more common and is often expected in those born before 28 weeks' gestation.

What Are the Etiologies of Neonatal Apnea?

The most common cause of apnea in the neonatal intensive care unit (NICU) is related to prematurity and is thought to be a result of relative immaturity of ventilatory regulation, as well as an immature response to hypoxia and hypercarbia, and an exaggerated protective response to airway stimulation. However, there are other possible causes of apnea, such as sepsis or prenatal exposure to drugs that suppress respiration. Neurological conditions that cause apnea include intracranial hemorrhage and neonatal seizures. Cardiovascular conditions associated with apnea include pulmonary edema or congestive heart failure.

What Are Risk Factors for Neonatal Apnea?

Additional risk factors for development of neonatal apnea include airway structural anomalies, ambient temperature fluctuation, anemia, chronic lung disease, metabolic derangement, and necrotizing enterocolitis.

How Would the Discharge Criteria Differ If the Patient Was Premature or a Full-Term Infant?

The postconceptual age of the infant would determine if the patient is an appropriate candidate for discharge after recovering in the post-anesthetic care unit (PACU). Each institution has specific discharge criteria guidelines for preterm and term infants.

Some institutions have guidelines with no admission requirement for postop apnea monitoring in a term infant (greater than 37 weeks postconceptual age) for elective surgery because there is little evidence that term infants have an increased risk for apnea. Other institutions will not allow full term infants to have elective outpatient surgery until four to six weeks of age or may require that the infant be scheduled early in the day so that the infant can observed for a longer time in the PACU. If the infant exhibits a documented apnea event, then the episode will warrant an admission for observation. In studies of postoperative apnea in infants, while preterm infants have an increased incidence, the term infant does not have zero risk.

In a subanalysis of the GAS study (Davidson et al.) where general anesthesia was compared to awake regional anesthesia for inguinal hernia repair in both term and preterm infants less than 60 weeks, former premature infants had a 6.1% incidence of apnea compared to 0.3% of full-term infants.

Suggested Reading

Coté CJ, Zaslavsky A, Downes JJ, et al. Postoperative apnea in former preterm infants after inguinal herniorrhaphy. A combined analysis. *Anesthesiology.* 1995;82:809–22. PMID: 7717551.

Davidson AJ, Disma N, de Graaff JC et al. Neurodevelopmental outcome at 2 years of age after general anaesthesia and awake-regional anaesthesia in infancy (GAS): an international multicentre, randomised controlled trial. *Lancet.* 2016;387(10015):239–50. PMID: 26507180.

López T, Sánchez FJ, Garzón JC, et al. Spinal anesthesia in pediatric patients. *Minerva Anestesiol.* 2012;78:78–87. PMID: 22211775.

Sale SM, Read JA, Stoddart PA, et al. Prospective comparison of sevoflurane and desflurane in formerly premature infants undergoing inguinal herniotomy. *Br J Anaesth.* 2006;96:774–8. PMID: 16648152.

Welborn LG, Hannallah RS, Luban NL, et al. Anemia and postoperative apnea in former preterm infants. *Anesthesiology.* 1991;74:1003–6. PMID: 2042754.

Welborn LG, Rice LJ, Hannallah RS, et al. Postoperative apnea in former preterm infants: prospective comparison of spinal and general anesthesia. *Anesthesiology.* 1990;72:838–42. PMID: 2187377.

Chapter

19 Anterior Mediastinal Masses

Adam C. Adler and Sheryl Modlin

A 16-year-old female presents for a diagnostic biopsy of a cervical lymph node and central venous port placement. She had been previously healthy until several weeks prior to admission, when she was noted to have cervical and supraclavicular lymphadenopathy, facial plethora, and occasional stabbing chest pains. On examination, HR = 110 beats/min, RR = 32 breaths/min. Orthopnea is present except when her head is elevated to > 30°. Laboratory testing is significant for a WBC of 63,000 per microliter, of which 57% were blast cells. An electrocardiogram demonstrates electrical alternans. The AP chest radiograph shows an enlarged mediastinum and right pleural effusion.

What Are the Different Compartments of the Mediastinum?

The mediastinum can be divided into superior and inferior compartments, and the inferior compartment consists of the anterior, middle, and posterior sections. There is no actual anatomic separation between these compartments; however, on chest radiographs (Figure 19.1), the compartments can be delineated as:

The *superior mediastinum* is an area that is bound by the thoracic inlet superiorly, the thoracic place inferiorly, the mediastinal pleura laterally, the manubrium anteriorly and the bodies of the upper four thoracic vertebrae posteriorly;

The *inferior mediastinum* is subdivided into anterior, middle, and posterior sections:

The *anterior mediastinum* lies between the sternum and pericardium.

The *middle mediastinum* contains the pericardium, heart, ascending aorta, lower half of superior vena cava, trachea, main bronchi, pulmonary artery, pulmonary vein, and phrenic nerve.

The *posterior mediastinum* is located between the pericardium and the vertebral column.

What Is the Differential Diagnosis of an Anterior Mediastinal Mass?

While pathologies can occur in any mediastinal region and cross over to adjacent areas, it is pathology in the anterior mediastinum that is most associated with perioperative risk. Leukemias (especially T-cell) and lymphomas (Hodgkin's and non-Hodgkin's) have a predilection for the anterior mediastinum. Although thymomas and germ cell tumors with anterior mediastinal involvement may also occur in children, most anterior mediastinal masses will occur in adolescents and will likely be a type of lymphoma.

What Are the Symptoms Associated with Anterior Mediastinal Masses?

Signs and symptoms associated with anterior mediastinal masses can be divided into those related to the airway, cardiac, and vascular systems, as well as constitutional symptoms. Respiratory and cardiovascular symptoms may be dependent on the patient's position, such that lying supine may increase pressure of the mass on the trachea and cardiac structures.

Airway/Respiratory Symptoms

- Inspiratory stridor
- Dyspnea
- Nonproductive cough
- Hoarseness (due to recurrent laryngeal nerve involvement)
- Orthopnea (symptoms worsen with supine position due to tracheal compression)
- Tracheomalacia (weakened tracheal walls) caused by prolonged tumor compression
- Decreased breath sounds
- Expiratory wheeze

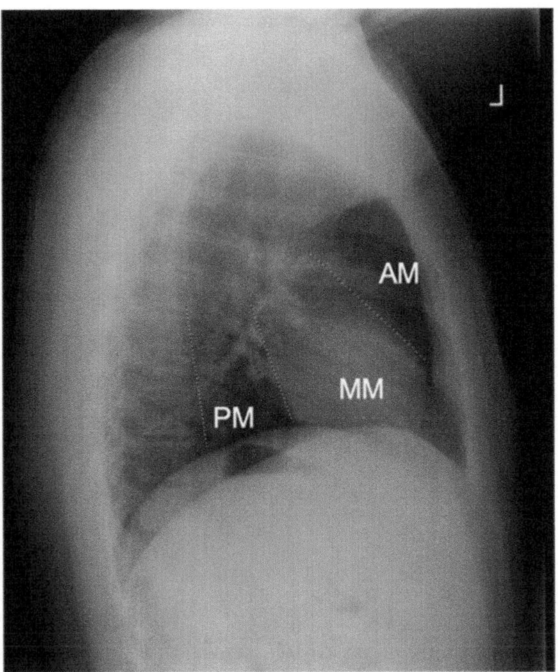

Figure 19.1 Lateral chest radiograph highlighting the anterior (AM), middle (MM), and posterior mediastinal (PM) compartments.

Cardiovascular Signs and Symptoms

- Syncope
- Tachycardia
- Plethoric facies (vascular compression): SVC syndrome
- Cyanosis
- Pleural effusion due to impaired lymphatic drainage
- Paradoxical decrease in blood pressure occurs when going from upright to supine. This is due to obstructed right ventricular filling or ejection
- Pericardial effusion
- Cardiac tamponade

Constitutional ("B Symptoms")

- Fever, chills
- Night sweats
- Weight loss

The most significant risk factors predisposing patients to anesthetic complications include:

- Orthopnea
- Upper body edema
- Great vessel compression
- Tracheal or main stem bronchus compression

What Are the Anesthetic Risks of an Anterior Mediastinal Mass?

An anterior mediastinal mass may grow so large that it causes tracheal and/or bronchial compression. Compression of the superior vena cava or right atrium may lead to obstruction of blood flow into (superior vena cava syndrome) or out of the heart. When this obstruction is severe, the negative intrathoracic pressure generated by spontaneous ventilation precariously maintains the patency of the lower airway and great vessels and is often made worse when the patient is in the supine position (i.e., orthopnea). Administration of sedatives or anesthetic agents may result in potentially life threatening airway obstruction and great vessel compression. This obstruction cannot always be overcome by administration of positive-pressure ventilation.

In one notable case from 1981, a 9-yr-old boy with a known anterior mediastinal mass developed cardiac arrest and died during inhalational induction with halothane in the sitting position despite initially breathing spontaneously. Although the child was easily intubated and ventilated, he developed asystole that was unresponsive to all resuscitative efforts. The history revealed that four days prior to the procedure, the child became cyanotic and lost consciousness while straining during a bowel movement. An autopsy revealed that a large lymphoma had enveloped the heart and pulmonary artery, but in 1981, preoperative echocardiograms were not yet standard of care for these diagnoses. If this large mass surrounding the heart had been revealed prior to the procedure, perhaps the team might have chosen a less sedating technique. This is only one of many similarly reported cases of children with anterior mediastinal masses who have succumbed during administration of general anesthesia.

What Preoperative Diagnostic Studies Should Be Performed in a Patient with an Anterior Mediastinal Mass?

Preoperative evaluation should focus on identification of risk factors associated with anesthetic complications, specifically airway collapse and cardiovascular compromise. A CT scan of the chest will delineate airway and cardiopulmonary involvement (Figure 19.2), and an ECG and echocardiogram will reveal the extent of

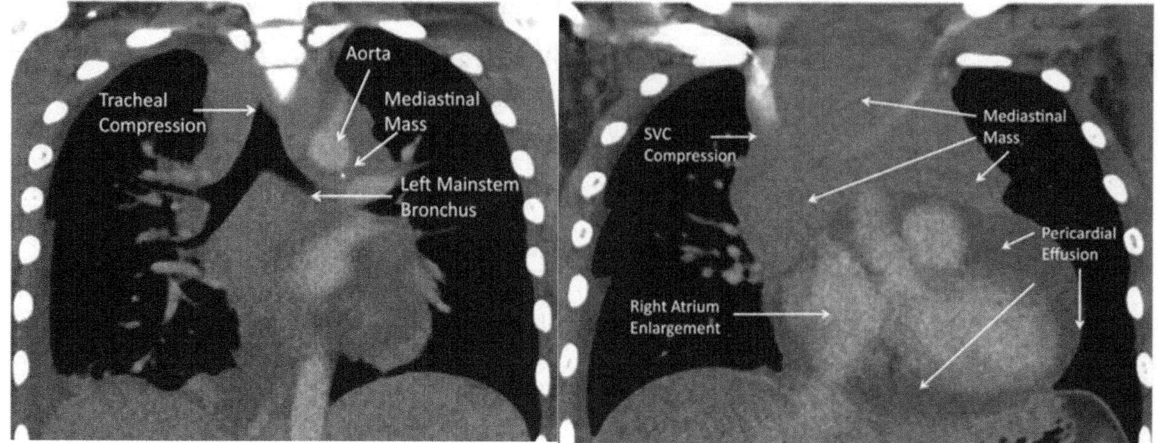

Figure 19.2 CT scan demonstrating significant tracheal compression, pericardial effusion, SVC compression, and aortic encasement. This can be compared with Figure 19.3, an AP chest X-ray from the same patient. Reproduced from: Adler AC, et al., *Anesthesiology* 2015;123(4):928 with permission. Copyright © 2015, Wolters Kluwer Health

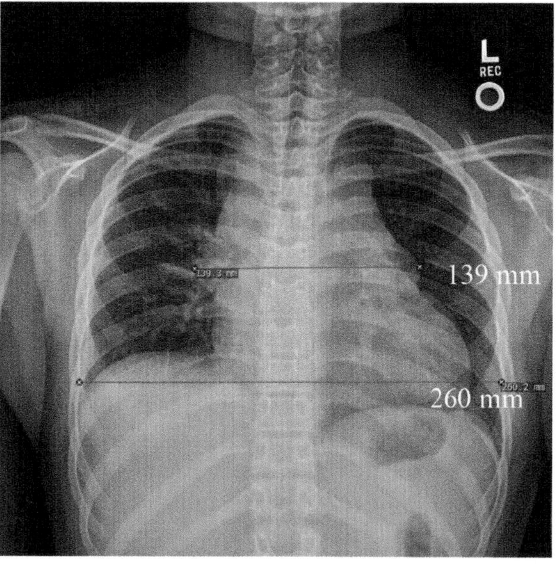

Figure 19.3 AP chest radiograph demonstrating the calculation of the mediastinal mass ratio. In this patient it is 139 mm/260 mm or 53%.

cardiovascular compression from the mass. Pulmonary function tests have not proven predictive of poor outcomes and will delay intervention, and thus, are not indicated.

The mediastinal mass ratio (MMR) and tracheal cross-sectional area (T_{CSA}) have been cited as predictors of intra-operative complications:

Mediastinal Mass Ratio (MMR)

The MMR can be calculated from an AP chest radiograph as the largest diameter of the mass divided by the largest chest diameter as measured at the level of the diaphragm (Figure 19.3). In one investigation, the risk of airway obstruction under anesthesia was 2%, 10.5%, and 33% for MMRs of <31%, 31–45%, and >45%, respectively.

Tracheal Cross-Sectional Area (T_{CSA})

The T_{CSA} is the difference between the smallest AP tracheal diameter and the largest AP tracheal diameter. A T_{CSA} <50% raises concern that airway collapse may occur during or after administration of general anesthesia, especially in children, owing to the highly compressible and cartilaginous pediatric tracheal structure.

What ECG Findings Are Suggestive of Cardiac Involvement?

- Sinus tachycardia
- Right or left axis deviation
- Electrical alternans: seen with pericardial effusion (Figure 19.4), a beat-to-beat variation in QRS axis and amplitude due to the swinging motion of the heart in the pericardial cavity

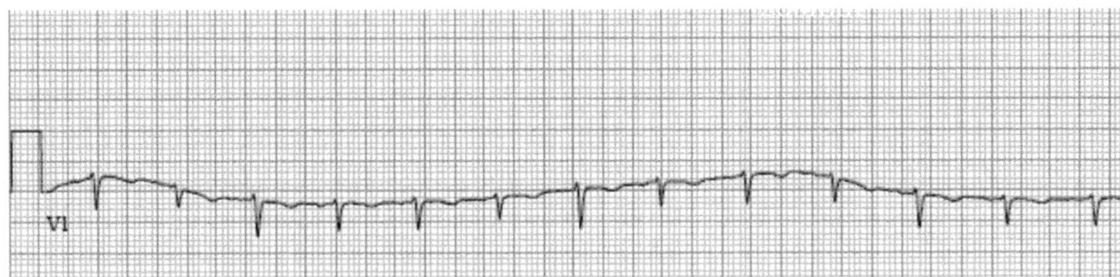

Figure 19.4 ECG strip demonstrating electrical alternans in a patient with a large pericardial effusion.

Which Echocardiographic Signs Are Concerning in Patients with Mediastinal Masses?

- Depression of right heart function may signify elevated pressures from pulmonary-tracheal compression
- Depression of left heart function may occur from direct compression or lack of preload
- Pericardial effusion
- Right atrial collapse
- Left atrial compression
- Pulmonary venous obstruction

Overall, there is no perfect algorithm for predicting the effects of general anesthesia on pulmonary or cardiovascular compromise. In general, it appears that positional dyspnea, stridor or orthopnea, presence of superior vena cava syndrome, tracheal airway compression of >50% by CT, and compression of cardiac vasculature or large pericardial effusions identified by echocardiogram all may be important indicators of further compromise during administration of general anesthesia.

In Patients with SVC Syndrome, Where Should IV Access Be Obtained?

Superior vena cava compression leads to engorgement of the veins of the head and neck and may cause thrombosis and reduce cardiac preload. IV access should be obtained in a lower extremity to ensure adequate and rapid circulation of medications. IV access should be obtained prior to induction of anesthesia in these cases.

What Are the Risks of Administering a Neuromuscular Blocking Agent to a Patient with a Mediastinal Mass?

Administration of a neuromuscular blocker will result in the loss of negative intrathoracic pressure during ventilation and may lead to life-threatening airway obstruction and great vessel compression. Unless strongly indicated by the clinical situation, paralysis should be avoided in these patients.

What Is the Preferred Anesthetic Technique in Patients with Anterior Mediastinal Masses?

The ideal anesthetic is one that maintains adequate airway tone and cardiac preload during spontaneous ventilation. Nearly all sedative or anesthetic agents can be slowly titrated to maintain spontaneous respiration. For biopsies and pericardial/pleural effusion drainage, generous use of local anesthetics will decrease the use of IV or inhaled agents. Some anesthesiologists prefer to use agents that can be reversed (i.e., opioids and benzodiazepines) and others prefer use of medications that have a history of preserving spontaneous ventilation (e.g., ketamine, dexmedetomidine) when slowly titrated. Since the mass will cause further compression in the supine position, the patient should be positioned with the head of the bed elevated during all phases of the procedure, when possible.

How Does the Ventilation Technique Affect Intrathoracic Pressure?

Patency of the airways and major vessels is best maintained during spontaneous ventilation, which preserves negative intrathoracic pressure (Table 19.1).

Describe the Possibilities for Intubation in a Patient with Airway Compromise

Patients with external airway compression pose a risk for airway collapse with induction of anesthesia. Smooth muscle supporting and maintaining airway patency relaxes with anesthesia and may result in life-threatening airway compression.

Table 19.1 Effect of ventilation on airway patency for patients with anterior mediastinal masses

	Intrathoracic pressure	Tracheal/ bronchi patency
Spontaneous ventilation (inspiration)	Decreased	Improves
Positive-pressure ventilation	Increased	Potential for complete collapse

Patients should be positioned with the back of the table upright. Awake intubation can be performed although this is generally not well tolerated in the pediatric population. Small doses of Midazolam can be helpful for amnestic purposes. Ketamine and dexmedetomidine via bolus or continuous infusion have been used for sedation while maintaining airway patency. Adequate topicalization with local anesthetic should be employed to the upper airway as well as the vocal cords.

A flexible fiberoptic scope is often used for intubation of the trachea in these situations to allow for internal assessment of airway narrowing and positioning of the endotracheal tube distal to the point of narrowing.

What Precautionary Plans Should Be Considered Prior to Sedation of These Patients?

In patients where the anesthesia provider has significant concern for airway collapse during intubation the following should be considered. A stretcher should remain in the room allowing for the patient to be flipped prone should sedation result in tracheal occlusion.

A plan of action should the patient decompensate must be discussed with the providers involved prior to sedation to avoid confusion if facing cardiopulmonary collapse.

What Is the Role of Rigid Bronchoscopy in These Patients?

Should airway collapse occur during administration of sedative or anesthetic agents, insertion of a rigid bronchoscope past the level of obstruction may be used to establish airway patency. In cases where a strong likelihood for airway obstruction exists, the bronchoscope should be opened in the OR, white-balanced, and connected to the monitor. A skilled operator, such as an ENT surgeon, should be immediately available. A separate stretcher or gurney should be kept in the OR to place the patient in the lateral or prone position in the event of ventilatory or cardiopulmonary compromise, as this may help alleviate airway compression.

Is There a Role for Extracorporeal Membrane Oxygenation (ECMO) in a Patient with an Anterior Mediastinal Mass?

If cardiopulmonary arrest results from compression of the trachea or heart, the ability to perform high quality CPR and maintain adequate cerebral perfusion is minimal. If the mass is so severe as to cause life-threatening obstruction, while the patient is conscious and prior to the administration of sedating agents, groin cannulation should occur as the time from cannulation to cardiopulmonary bypass (CPB) (5–10 minutes) generally exceeds the time in which significant morbidity and mortality will occur should cardiac arrest occur. ECMO is a theoretical rescue tool that, in reality, is unlikely to save a patient following arrest without prior preparation.

Is a Lymph Node Biopsy for Tissue Diagnosis Always Indicated in a Patient with an Anterior Mediastinal Mass?

In some cases, the risk of administration of sedating agents outweighs the need for an immediate tissue diagnosis. In patients with critical respiratory or vascular compromise, an attempt should be made to obtain tissue for diagnosis in a minimally invasive manner without heavy sedation or general anesthesia. Examples of diagnostic interventions include peripheral blood flow cytometry for leukemia; or lymph node, mediastinal mass, or bone marrow biopsy performed under local anesthetic. Chemotherapy and/or radiation can be used to decrease the size of the mediastinal mass prior to diagnostic procedures. Elective placement of central vascular lines should be postponed until the patient's symptoms have largely resolved and the anesthetic risk is minimal.

What Is Tumor Lysis Syndrome?

Tumor lysis syndrome (TLS) describes a constellation of metabolic abnormalities resulting from spontaneous or treatment-induced tumor cell death. Rapid cell death results in severe hyperphosphatemia and hyperuricemia, leading to acute kidney failure. Hyperkalemia may also occur leading to heart failure or cardiac dysrhythmias. Other symptoms may include gastrointestinal upset, lethargy, hematuria, seizures, muscle cramps, tetany, or syncope. Tumors with rapid growth rates such as T-cell leukemia and Burkitt's lymphoma are at highest risk of TLS. High WBC counts (>100,000/μL) and evidence of significant disease burden (hepatosplenomegaly or lymphadenopathy) also increase the likelihood of developing TLS. The risk for tumor lysis is greatest during the first 3–7 days after the initiation of chemotherapy. Prevention of TLS includes aggressive IV hydration with non-potassium–containing fluids and sometimes diuretic therapy with furosemide. Uric acid reduction with allopurinol can be initiated immediately. However, if the patient already has a very elevated uric acid, requires ICU level care, or is at very high risk of TLS, rasburicase is recommended for its more efficient onset. Hyperphosphatemia should be treated with oral agents such as phosphate binders. Fluid restriction of patients with renal insufficiency will worsen the crystal induced nephropathy and should be avoided. Temporary dialysis is sometimes required to manage fluid overload, metabolic abnormalities and/or renal insufficiency. Replacing potassium or calcium should be done carefully.

It is important for anesthesia personnel to recognize that administration of steroids, especially dexamethasone, may cause or exacerbate TLS. Numerous case reports exist demonstrating TLS after a single dose of an IV steroid. Dexamethasone is routinely given during the chemotherapy induction phase and is preferably given to these patients under the care of the oncology team. Steroids should be used with caution in patients with vague symptoms and lymphadenopathy and without a defined diagnosis.

Suggested Reading

Anghelescu DL, Burgoyne LL, Liu T, Li CS, Pui CH, Hudson MM, et al. Clinical and diagnostic imaging findings predict anesthetic complications in children presenting with malignant mediastinal masses. *Paediatr Anaesth.* 2007;17(11):1090–8. PMID: 17897276.

Howard SC, Jones DP, Pui CH. The tumor lysis syndrome. *N Engl J Med.* 2011;364(19):1844–54. PMID: 21561350.

King DR, Patrick LE, Ginn-Pease ME, McCoy KS, Klopfenstein K. Pulmonary function is compromised in children with mediastinal lymphoma. *J Pediatr Surg.* 1997;32(2):294–9. PMID: 16481238.

Pearson JK, Tan GM. Pediatric Anterior Mediastinal Mass: A Review Article. *Semin Cardiothorac Vasc Anesth.* 2015;19 (3):248–54. PMID: 25814524.

Shamberger RC, Holzman RS, Griscom NT, Tarbell NJ, Weinstein HJ. CT quantitation of tracheal cross-sectional area as a guide to the surgical and anesthetic management of children with anterior mediastinal masses. *J Pediatr Surg.* 1991;26(2):138–42. PMID: 2023069.

Stricker PA, Gurnaney HG, Litman RS. Anesthetic management of children with an anterior mediastinal mass. *J Clin Anesth.* 2010;22(3):159–63. PMID: 20399999.

Chapter 20

Esophageal Atresia and Tracheoesophageal Fistula

Adam C. Adler

A six-day-old male presents with excessive drooling and tachypnea with feeding. When drinking his bottle, he coughs and desaturates to the high 80s. A nasogastric tube was placed in the nursey with postplacement X-ray (Figure 20.1). He was born via spontaneous vaginal delivery at 38 weeks. There is no additional medical or surgical history.

His current vital signs are: blood pressure 60/37 mmHg; heart rate 150/min; respiratory rate 32/min; temperature 37.1°C; SpO_2 100% on room air. Weight is 3.45 kg.

How Is the Diagnosis of Esophageal Atresia Made?

Esophageal atresia (EA) often presents soon after birth with inability to eat. Children with EA often choke and become cyanotic with feeding. Food that is unable to enter the GI tract enters the trachea and lungs. Esophageal atresia may be diagnosed by failure to pass an oro/nasogastric tube (OGT/NGT). X-ray may demonstrate an OGT/NGT coiled in the chest or a blind stomach air pocket. Esophageal atresia may be full or partial and may occur in association with other congenital anomalies such as cardiac anomalies or trachea-esophageal fistulae (TEF). Prenatal ultrasound may show polyhydramnios as the infant is unable to swallow amniotic fluid.

What Is the Most Likely Age for Presentation?

Generally, the diagnosis is made shortly after birth; however, a variant (H-type fistula) exists with a small fistula between the trachea and esophagus which can result in a delayed diagnosis. These children can often present with recurrent aspiration prior to diagnosis of a fistula.

What Is the Incidence of EA?

Esophageal atresia has an incidence of 1 in 3,000–4,000. The incidence of EA/TEF is greater in patients with trisomy 21 and 18.

Idenify the Fistula Variants Presents in Patients with EA/TEF

Five main variants exist for congenital malformations of the esophagus (Figure 20.2).

In What Percentage of Patients with EA/TEF Are Other Anomalies Present?

More than 50% of patients with EA/TEF have associated congenital anomalies.

What Anomalies Are Most Commonly Associated with EA/TEF?

The most common association is that of VACTERL/VATER syndrome. VACTERL/VATER is really an association in which certain congenital anomalies are seen grouped together with a significant degree of frequency.

The following anomalies are known to be associated and therefore require diagnostic testing when a patient presents with EA/TEF.

- **V**: Vertebral
- **A**: Anal defects
- **C**: Cardiac anomalies
- **TE**: Tracheoesophageal fistulae
- **R**: Renal
- **L**: Limb deformities (often radial absence)

Additionally, numerous other associated anomalies may be present (i.e., cleft lip and palate, gastric wall defects)

What Are the Classic Vertebral Defects in VACTERL Syndrome?

Generally, the defects involve the vertebral bodies which may be absent or incompletely formed. The defects may occur anywhere but are most common in the cervical and lumbar regions. These defects can result in instability of the neck due to incompletely formed vertebral bodies. These children also have an increased incidence of scoliosis as they mature.

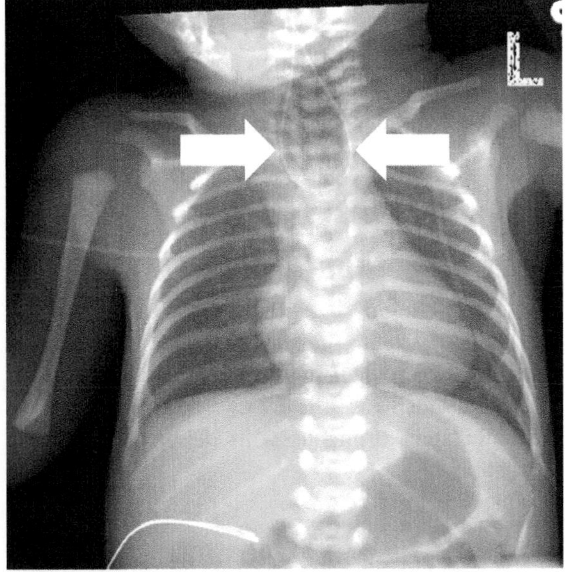

Figure 20.1 Chest X-ray of infant with tracheoesophageal fistula revealing coiling of gastric tube in the upper gastric pouch. Reproduced from: Adler AC, et al. A A *Case Rep* 2017;8(7):172–174. Copyright © 2017 International Anesthesia Research Society

What Are the Classic Anal Defects in VACTERL Syndrome?

Most commonly, these defects include anal atresia or imperforate anus. This necessitates the need for early surgical intervention generally with a multistaged procedure requiring an ostomy, recreation of an anus, and a colonic pull-through to reestablish continuity. The repair of the EA/TEF precedes the anal surgical intervention.

In What Percent of Patients with EA/TEF Is a Cardiac Defect Present?

Approximately one-third of patients with EA/TEF are found to have an associated congenital heart defect.

The most common defects are atrial and ventricular septal defects, patent ductus arteriosus, and Tetralogy of Fallot.

What Are the Classic Renal Defects in VACTERL Syndrome?

Renal defects can include hypoplasia or aplasia of the kidneys and issues related to ureteral valves. If left untreated, these unrelated valve defects can progress to hydronephrosis and/or renal failure.

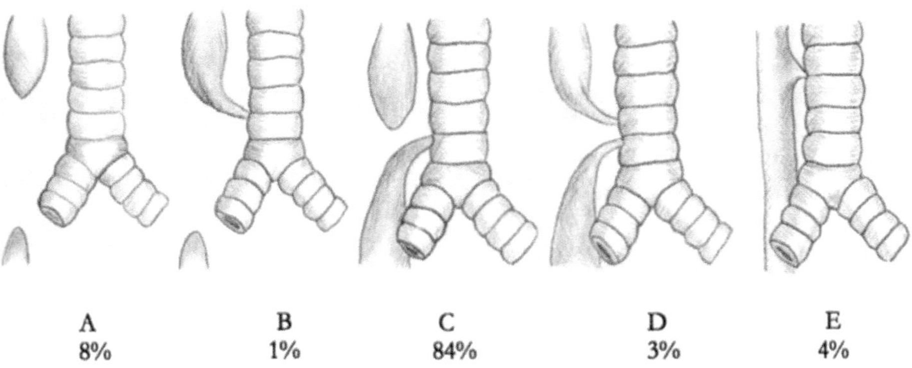

Figure 20.2 Schematic of the types of five main variants of congenital esophageal malformations and their incidences. Courtesy of Adam C. Adler, MD. Drawn by J. Daynes

What Are the Classic Limb Defects in VACTERL Syndrome?

Digital issues including: hypoplastic thumb, polydactyly, and syndactyly, as well as disorders of the forearm including absent radius. Interestingly, limb and renal defects are often ipsilateral and patients with bilateral limb deformities often have bilateral renal issues.

Is Neurocognitive Function Altered in Patients with VACTERL Syndrome?

Most patients with VACTERL have normal intelligence.

What Is the Expected Mortality in Patients with EA/TEF?

Outcomes after EA/TEF repair have been excellent in recent years with minimal mortality. Patients with cardiac defects, low birth weight (<1,500 grams) and those suffering postoperative respiratory complications have a significantly increased mortality.

Describe the Preoperative Evaluation in Patients with EA/TEF

Aside from the general evaluation of the neonate, patients with suspected EA/TEF should undergo a comprehensive work-up aimed at identifying commonly associated pathologies. In particular, a cardiac anomaly should be excluded as this both contributes to increased mortality and may have significant anesthetic considerations based on the cardiac lesion. A transthoracic echocardiogram should be performed to identify the majority of the pathologies as well as presence of a right aortic arch (2–3%) which has implications for the surgical approach.

Other evaluations include ultrasound of the kidneys for renal anomalies, and radiographs of the spine if concern for vertebral anomalies exist.

Upon diagnosis, a catheter can be placed (with fluoroscopy if needed) in the esophageal blind pouch to remove secretions. These patients are kept NPO with maintenance IV fluid and regular glucose checks.

What Is the Preferred Method of Induction in Patients with EA/TEF?

Classically, the patient is induced with inhalational agents to maintain spontaneous ventilation and avoidance of muscle relaxants prior to fistula ligation. Positive pressure ventilation should be minimized to avoid insufflation of the gastrointestinal tract.

What Is the Benefit of Performing a Bronchoscopy Prior to Intubation?

Many surgeons will perform a flexible or rigid bronchoscopy after induction to allow for confirmation of diagnosis, localization of fistula, and to exclude the presence of multiple fistulae or other pathology.

Describe the Proper Positioning of the Endotracheal Tube (ETT)

The ETT should be positioned (under vision, Figure 20.3) distal to the fistula to avoid gastric insufflation. At times, the fistulous portion may involve the carina, in which case the ETT is generally placed in the main stem bronchus with deliberate one lung ventilation.

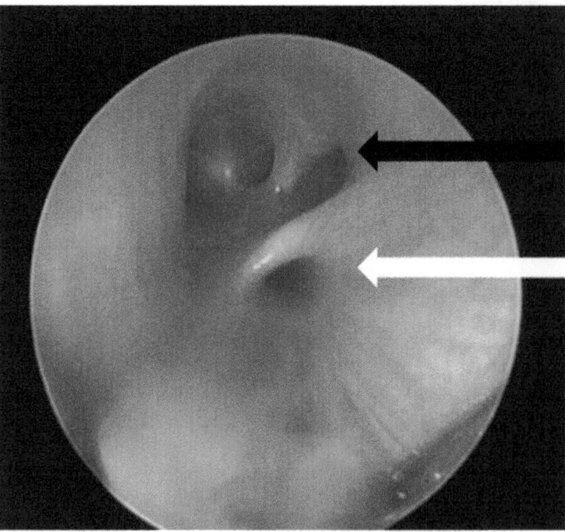

Figure 20.3 Intraoperative rigid bronchoscopic view of EA/TEF showing the fistula arising from the carina (black arrow); also present is a tracheal take-off of the right upper lobe bronchus (pig bronchus) (white arrow). Reproduced from: Adler AC, et al. A A *Case Rep* 2017;8(7):172–174. Copyright © 2017 International Anesthesia Research Society

What Is the Most Concerning Consequence of Continued Gastric Insufflation?

Continuous gastric insufflation can result in significant gastric/abdominal distension significantly impacting ventilation. Conversely, gastric insufflation, if severe, can result in gastrointestinal rupture and pneumoperitoneum. Treatment relies on early recognition and decompression.

What Is the Intraoperative Approach to EA Repair and TEF Ligation?

The approach is often via an open thoracotomy or a minimally invasive thoracoscopic approach. In cases of two lung ventilation (absent or high fistula) the ipsilateral lung can be manually retracted or is deflated by the pressure of insufflation in cases using a thoracoscopic approach.

The approach to this procedure is dictated by the type of fistula. With most being type C (blind, proximal esophageal pouch with distal tracheal/esophageal fistula), the repair includes ligation of the fistula and anastomosis of the esophageal pouches. In some cases, the distance between the proximal and distal esophageal pouches is too long to perform a primary anastomosis without placing the esophagus under tension.

Aside from standard ASA monitoring, placement of an arterial line may be considered in certain patients. IV access should be sufficient to allow for for rapid administration of blood products if significant bleeding is encountered.

What Is the Postoperative Approach to EA Repair and TEF Ligation?

This is strongly dictated by the type of fistula and presence of associated anomalies (especially cardiac anomalies). Depending on the type of TEF and difficulty of the esophageal repair, the patient may be extubated. In general, low birth weight babies, premature infants, co-existing cardiac anomalies, and those with a "tight" anastomosis should remain intubated.

What Head/Neck Maneuver Should Be Avoided in Patients Post-EA Anastomosis?

In patients following esophageal anastomosis and especially one under some degree of tension, neck extension should be avoided as this can exacerbate the degree of tension on the suture line.

What Regional Anesthetics Can Be Offered to These Patients?

Post thoracotomy patients may benefit from either a thoracic epidural or a caudally placed thoracic epidural. Paravertebral blocks (and catheters) and the newer erector spinae block can be performed as well. Intercostal blocks are usually avoided due to their high absorption, short duration of action, and concern for local anesthetic toxicity.

Suggested Reading

Choudhury SR, Ashcraft KW, Sharp RJ, Murphy JP, Snyder CL, Sigalet DL. Survival of patients with esophageal atresia: influence of birth weight, cardiac anomaly, and late respiratory complications. *J Pediatr Surg*. 1999;34(1):70–3. PMID: 10022146.

Diaz LK, Akpek EA, Dinavahi R, Andropoulos DB. Tracheoesophageal fistula and associated congenital heart disease: implications for anesthetic management and survival. *Paediatr Anaesth*. 2005;15(10):862–9. PMID: 16176315.

Okamoto T, Takamizawa S, Arai H, Bitoh Y, Nakao M, Yokoi A, Nishijima E. Esophageal atresia: prognostic classification revisited. *Surgery*. 2009;145(6):675–81. PMID: 19486772.

Chapter 21

Pyloric Stenosis

Adam C. Adler

A six-week-old male arrives to the emergency room with sudden onset of projectile vomiting, which occurs shortly after feeding. He was born via spontaneous vaginal delivery at 38 weeks. There is no additional medical or surgical history.

His current vital signs are: blood pressure 60/37 mmHg; heart rate 146/min; respiratory rate 32/min; temperature 37.1°C; SpO_2 100% on room air. Weight is 3.8 kg.

DIAGNOSIS

What Are the Important Diagnoses to Consider?

Severe reflux, esophageal atresia, and pyloric stenosis should be considered in a patient with this presentation. Intussusception may also be part of the differential but usually results in intermittent pain and vomiting.

Severe reflux is usually a medical diagnosis and common at this age. Treatment includes oral medication for gastric acid secretion such as H2 receptor blockers and/or proton pump inhibitors. Esophagogastroduodenoscopy (EGD) may be considered as well as placement of a pH probe.

Pyloric stenosis (PS) is a potentially life-threating condition in which the pyloric musculature becomes hypertrophied leading to gastric outlet obstruction. The muscle is usually normal at birth and hypertrophies in the first few weeks to months of life. Children with PS present with feeding difficulties, weight loss, significant dehydration, and electrolyte disturbances. The vomiting is usually non-bilious as the thick pylorus prevents bile regurgitation. Interestingly, the pyloric hypertrophy generally resolves if left untreated. Historically, the treatment was frequent but small feedings until spontaneous resolution and thus why PS remains a medical and not surgical emergency. With the advances in surgical treatment and technique, the preferred method after medical stabilization is via a small incision and pyloromyotomy (incising of the pyloric muscle), immediately relieving the gastric outflow obstruction.

Briefly Review the Historical Overview of Pyloric Stenosis

Reports of PS exist as early as the 15th century, however, the modern description is owed to Hirschsprung who reported clinical and autopsy findings of pyloric hypertrophy in 1887. Initially, PS was uniformly fatal in the first weeks to months, with most infants succumbing to malnutrition and dehydration. Early surgical intervention was via full thickness incision of the pyloric musculature and transverse closure. This was successful but mortality rates were still as high as 50%. In the early 20th century, Ramstedt introduced the suture-less technique of longitudinal division of the pyloric muscle while leaving the mucosa intact. This modification still serves as the basis for current operative management. Presently, advances in minimally invasive surgery make the laparoscopic approach the preferred method owing to decreased wound complications and a shorter length of stay.

What Is the Incidence of Pyloric Stenosis?

The incidence of PS is 1.8 per 1,000 births. There is a significant male predominance of 5:1 for development of pyloric stenosis.

What Is the Most Likely Age for Presentation?

Pyloric stenosis can present from infancy to around four months of age. Most patients typically present between 3 and 10 weeks.

Is There a Genetic Component to Pyloric Stenosis?

To date, five genetic loci have been identified for idiopathic infantile pyloric stenosis. Pyloric stenosis is also associated with the following congenital syndromes: trisomy 21, trisomy 18, Cornelia de Lange, Apert, Opitz FG, Marden-Walker, Smith-Lemli-Opitz, Zellweger, duplication 1q, duplication 9q, deletion 11q, ring 12, Denys–Drash, and paramyotonia congenita.

What Are the Risk Factors for Development of Pyloric Stenosis?

Risk for development of PS can be divided into maternal and infant factors.

Maternal factors include: smoking of >10 cigarettes/day in early pregnancy, erythromycin use, age <25 years, and being overweight (but not obese).

Infant factors include: Very preterm infants, delivery by cesarean section and a birth order <2.

It has been suggested that infant exposure to prostaglandins (usually for congenital heart disease) may relay an increased risk of development of PS.

Preterm infants are generally diagnosed at a later post gestational age.

PREOPERATIVE EVALUATION

The Surgeon Requests to Perform the Pyloromyotomy after His Next Case. Is This Appropriate?

The next step is a thorough examination of the infant followed by IV placement in which labs are obtained. Dehydration and electrolyte status dictates when the patient is ready for operative intervention.

How Is the Diagnosis of Pyloric Stenosis Made?

Typically, the history and physical examination are suggestive. A small (olive size) mass may be palpated in the upper abdomen and carries a 99% positive predictive value but cannot always be felt.

In the past, upper GI series was the imaging method used to diagnose PS (Figure 21.1). Widespread use and availability of ultrasound has made sonography the imaging test of choice in these patients. While the diagnosis of PS can be made clinically based on the history and physical examination, most patients will undergo ultrasound evaluation.

What Is the Appropriate Workup for Patients with Pyloric Stenosis?

Evaluation should begin with a history of presenting symptoms to assess the degree of dehydration. Hydration status at this age should include observation for skin turgor, sunken eyes, mucous membranes, fontanelle, weight change, and number of dry diapers per day (Table 21.1).

Unlike adults, children have the ability to maintain their hemodynamics until they are profoundly dehydrated. Estimation of the degree of dehydration in children can be found in Table 21.1.

Laboratory evaluation should focus on the electrolytes to assess the degree of derangement. Intravenous access should be established.

Fluid administration in the form of 0.9% saline or D5NS should be given until the electrolytes, and

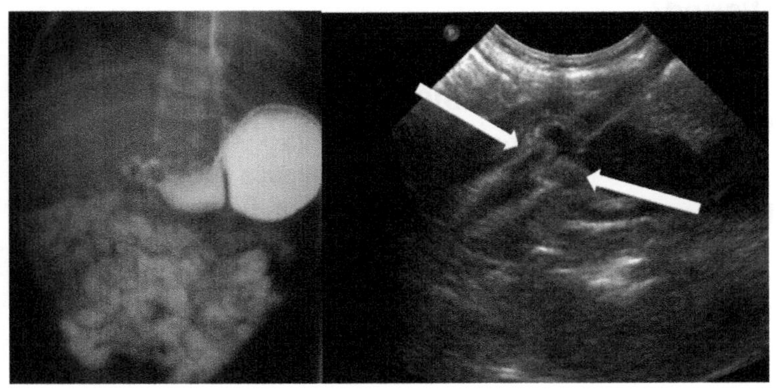

Figure 21.1 Left: Upper GI demonstrating slow emptying of barium past the pylorus. **Right**: Abdominal ultrasound

Table 21.1 Assessment of dehydration severity in children

	Mild	Moderate	Severe
Percentage of fluid loss	5	10	15–20
Fontanelle and eyes	Normal	Sunken fontanelle	Sunken eyes
Mucous membranes	Dry	Dry	Parched
Skin turgor	Normal / poor	Poor	Parched
Blood pressure	Normal	Mildly hypotensive	Severe hypotension / shock
Heart rate	Normal	Mild tachycardia / weak pulse	Significant tachycardia
Respiratory rate	Normal	Deep	Deep and rapid
Urine output	Normal / mild oliguria	Oliguria	Oliguria / anuria

especially the chloride, return to normal. Potassium is often added to fluids to avoid hypokalemia that may occur with absorption of sodium.

What Is the Expected Initial Metabolic Profile in Pyloric Stenosis?

Due to chronic emesis, sodium, chloride, and hydrochloric acid become depleted. This leads to a hyponatremic, hypokalemic, hypochloremic metabolic alkalosis.

What Is the Endpoint of Resuscitation?

The goal of fluid resuscitation is aimed at normalizing intravascular volume and repletion of electrolytes. Fluid administration should ensue with the initial goal of approximately 2 cc/kg/h of urine production.

Electrolyte correction should continue with a goal of reaching chloride values of >100 mEq/L and a bicarbonate of <28 mEq/L.

Why Is Bicarbonate Correction Important in the Preoperative Period?

Correction of the metabolic alkalosis is important in prevention of alkalosis induced postoperative apnea. Persistent alkalosis can depress the respiratory drive and preclude safe extubation.

Is the Preferred Method of Induction an Awake Intubation?

Formerly, awake intubation was considered the method of choice for securing the airway in patients with PS. Cook-Sather et al. revealed that awake suctioning of the stomach decreases the gastric volume to a safe level, allowing for induction of anesthesia and asleep intubation.

Generally, the stomach is suctioned with an OGT multiple times in the awake infant, rotating the child until minimal to no gastric contents return. This should be followed by a rapid sequence intubation to secure the airway.

POSTOPERATIVE CONSIDERATIONS

What Is the Optimal Time for Postoperative Discharge?

Patients should be able to tolerate PO feeding prior to discharge. Young infants <50 weeks post conceptual age are at risk for postoperative apnea and should be monitored. Risk of postoperative apnea is increased with opioid administration.

When Should Patients Resume a Regular Diet Postoperatively?

Numerous studies have attempted to determine the optimum time for resumption of feeding post PS repair, as there is concern for post-op vomiting. While there is no consensus as to the timeframe for feeding, a small period of NPO time appears to decrease the frequency of post-op emesis and decreases hospital length of stay.

Suggested Reading

Cook-Sather SD, Tulloch HV, Cnaan A, et al. A comparison of awake versus paralyzed tracheal intubation for infants with pyloric stenosis. *Anesth Analg.* 1998;86(5):945–51. PMID: 9585274.

Graham KA, Laituri CA, Markel TA, et al. A review of postoperative feeding regimens in infantile hypertrophic pyloric stenosis. *J Pediatr Surg.* 2013;48(10):2175–9. PMID: 24094977.

Kamata M, Cartabuke RS, Tobias JD. Perioperative care of infants with pyloric stenosis. *Paediatr Anaesth.* 2015;25(12):1193–206. PMID: 26490352.

Pandya S, Heiss K. Pyloric stenosis in pediatric surgery: an evidence-based review. *Surg Clin North Am.* 2012;92 (3):527–39. PMID: 22595707.

Ranells JD, Carver JD, Kirby RS. Infantile hypertrophic pyloric stenosis: epidemiology, genetics, and clinical update. *Adv Pediatr.* 2011;58(1):195–206. PMID: 21736982.

Sola JE, Neville HL. Laparoscopic vs open pyloromyotomy: a systematic review and meta-analysis. *J Pediatr Surg.* 2009;44(8):1631–7. PMID: 19635317.

Chapter 22

Congenital Diaphragmatic Hernia

Titilopemi A.O. Aina

An eight-day-old, ex-35-week gestation female presents for repair of a prenatally diagnosed left-sided congenital diaphragmatic hernia (CDH). The percent predicted lung volume (PPLV) was reported to be ~15–20%. Fetal echocardiogram showed no other abnormalities. She was delivered via emergency cesarean section due to nonreassuring fetal heart tracings. APGAR scores were 1 and 6, at one and five minutes respectively. CPR was initiated in the delivery room and she was transferred to the intensive care unit, intubated, and ventilated.

What Is a Congenital Diaphragmatic Hernia (CDH)?

A congenital diaphragmatic hernia (CDH) is a defect in the diaphragm occurring during embryologic development that results in herniation of the abdominal contents into the chest. This leads to the compression of the lungs and abnormal pulmonary vascular development. The diaphragm normally develops in the first trimester, with the right diaphragm closing before the left. The organs that are typically found herniated into the thoracic cavity are the stomach, intestines, spleen, and/or liver (Figure 22.1). There are two common types of diaphragmatic hernias: Bochdalek and Morgagni. The Bochdalek hernia occurs on the posterior-lateral portion of the diaphragm, and the Morgagni hernia on the anterior aspect. These hernias can be right-sided, left-sided (most common), or bilateral.

The incidence of CDH has been reported to be between 1-in-2000 and 1-in-5000 live births.

Describe the Pathophysiology of CDH

CDH results in pulmonary hypoplasia from compression of the fetal lungs during development. Pulmonary vascular hyper-reactivity, or persistent pulmonary hypertension may also occur. Hypoxia, hypercapnia, respiratory acidosis, and hypothermia contribute to worsening pulmonary hypertension and persistence of the fetal circulation. This will lead to right-to-left shunting across a patent ductus arteriosus.

How Is the Diagnosis of CDH Made?

CDH is most commonly diagnosed with prenatal ultrasound, usually in the second or third trimester. However, fetal magnetic resonance imaging may also be used. The abdominal contents can be observed in the fetal chest on imaging. Ultrasound Doppler examination of the hepatic and umbilical vessels can aid in diagnosis. Echocardiography and genetic testing may be performed to exclude co-existing anatomic anomalies and syndromic associations.

Early diagnosis allows for counseling, coordination of delivery at a specialized tertiary center, and consideration of elective termination if desired by the family.

What Is the Differential Diagnosis for CDH?

Other diagnoses to be considered in suspected CDH include diaphragm eventration, teratoma, bronchogenic or enteric cysts, and congenital cystic adenomatoid malformation.

How Is the Prognosis Determined?

Prognosis in CDH is determined by prenatal lung volume-based prognostication. The lung-to-head (LHR) ratio is most commonly used. Another method used is percent predicted lung volume (PPLV).

The presence and extent of liver herniation, or concomitant major anomalies, is indicative of poor prognosis.

Presence of liver herniation correlates with the need for extracorporeal membrane oxygenation (ECMO) support. Greater than 80% of patients with liver herniation into the thorax require ECMO

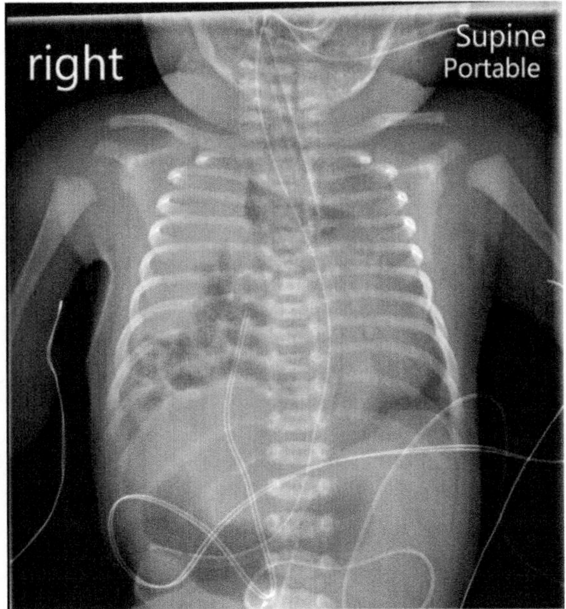

Figure 22.1 Chest X-ray demonstrating a large right-sided congenital diaphragmatic hernia with herniation of the bowel into the right hemithorax. The right lung markings are absent and the trachea is deviated leftwards. Courtesy of Adam C. Adler MD

support compared with 25% of patients without liver herniation.

What Is the Lung-to-Head Ratio (LHR)?

The LHR is calculated by measuring the lung area (on the contralateral side of the hernia) using ultrasound, and then dividing the number by the head circumference. A value less than 0.9 denotes a low rate of survival, whereas above 1.4 favors survival.

What Is Percent Predicted Lung Volume (PPLV)?

The PPLV is calculated by taking the total measured thoracic volume, and subtracting the measured mediastinal volume from this value. These measurements are based on fetal magnetic resonance imaging. A value of 15 or less denotes high risk of pulmonary morbidity and/or death.

What Is the Morbidity/Mortality Rate for CDH?

A survival rate of approximately 70% and higher has been reported in specialized tertiary care centers.

The extent of abdominal viscera herniation and presence of associated anomalies also contributes to the overall morbidity and mortality. Infants with single ventricle physiology in combination with CHD have a near 100% mortality. Patients with familial, bilateral, or syndromic CDH and those in which CDH is associated with specific genetic abnormalities are all associated with poor outcomes.

What Prenatal Interventions Are Available for CDH?

Fetal intervention has evolved in the treatment of CDH. Previously, anatomical repair of the diaphragm defect was performed in-utero; however, due to lack of improvement in overall survival, this is no longer performed. Currently, endoscopic tracheal occlusion is the most common fetal intervention for CDH. This procedure is performed between 23 and 27 weeks of gestation. A balloon in the trachea blocks the exit of lung fluid and results in large fluid-filled lungs. An Ex-Utero Intrapartum Treatment (EXIT) procedure is performed at term to remove the balloon from the trachea prior to delivery.

This approach may still result in impaired pulmonary function and is generally reserved for severe cases of CDH. Antenatal maternal steroids may be administered to improve lung maturity; however improved outcomes have not been demonstrated.

What Is the Plan for Delivery of a Fetus with CDH?

Ideally, vaginal delivery can be accomplished with induction of labor around 38 weeks of gestation. Vaginal delivery is beneficial for lung function with extrusion of lung amniotic fluid during descent. A cesarean delivery may be performed when the clinical context dictates. Regardless of the type of delivery, all infants should undergo tracheal intubation and placement of an orogastric tube at the time of birth to prevent distension of abdominal contents within the chest cavity.

What Are the Ventilator Management Options?

Gentle ventilation and permissive hypercapnia are most often used to minimize lung trauma to the hypo-plastic lung. Occasionally high-frequency oscillation and inhaled nitric oxide are required. Surgical repair is usually delayed until after the pulmonary vascular reactivity is improved. Early institution of extracorporeal membrane oxygenation (ECMO) prior to surgical repair may be necessary.

What Are Gentle Ventilation Strategies for CDH?

- Low peak inspiratory pressures, less than 25 cm H_2O
- Minimal positive end expiratory pressures, less than 5 cm H_2O
- Permissive hypercapnia
- Transitioning to high-frequency oscillation ventilation to prevent severe hypercapnia

What Type of ECMO Is Used in CDH?

Veno-arterial (VA) ECMO provides full cardiopulmonary support, with the right common carotid artery and right internal jugular vein being cannulated. Veno-venous (VV) ECMO provides only pulmonary support. In VV ECMO, a double-lumen cannula is inserted into the internal jugular vein. Both VV- and VA-ECMO are equally effective in managing CDH patients, however VA-ECMO is the most common form used.

When Should ECMO Be Instituted?

ECMO should be instituted when conventional therapy has been exhausted. The exact criteria depend on the institution. The EURO consensus criteria are:

- Inability to maintain pre-ductal saturations >85% or post-ductal saturations >70%.
- Increased $PaCO_2$ and respiratory acidosis with pH <7.15 despite optimal ventilator management.
- Peak inspiratory pressure >28 cm H_2O or mean airway pressure >17 cm H_2O is required to achieve saturation >85%.
- Inadequate oxygen delivery with metabolic acidosis as measured by elevated lactate > or = to 5 mmol/L and pH <7.15.
- Systemic hypotension, resistant to fluid or inotropic therapy, resulting in urine output <0.5 mL/kg/h for 12–24 hours.
- Oxygenation index (mean airway pressure × FiO_2 × $100/PaO_2$) > or = 40 for at least 3 hours.

How Is CDH Repaired Surgically?

Laparoscopic, thoracoscopic, or open repair closure techniques have all been reported. With smaller diaphragmatic defects, primary closure can be accomplished; for larger defects, a Gore-Tex patch is placed.

When Is a Patient Considered Ready for Surgery?

The EURO consensus surgical criteria are:

- Mean arterial blood pressure is normal for gestation age.
- Pre-ductal saturation levels of 8–95% on FiO_2 below 50%.
- Lactate below 3 mmol/L.
- Urine output more than 1 mL/kg/h.

How Can You Manage the Associated Pulmonary Hypertension?

Inhaled nitric oxide can be used in the treatment of pulmonary hypertension. Other medical therapies, such as sildenafil, have been used but have not shown consistent benefit in CDH.

What Are the Long-Term Complications of CDH?

There are a number of long-term sequelae that have been observed in patients with CDH.

These include:

- recurrent diaphragmatic hernias,
- patch infection,
- intestinal obstruction (10% of patients),
- neurological impairment (intraventricular hemorrhage/post ECMO sequelae),
- gastroesophageal reflux disease (from alterations in normal anatomic relationships),
- chronic lung disease,
- pulmonary hypertension,
- failure-to-thrive,
- sensorineural hearing loss,
- chest asymmetry (pectus excavatum or carinatum), and
- scoliosis.

Suggested Reading

Barnewolt CE, Kunisaki SM, Fauza DO, et al. Percent predicted lung volumes as measured on fetal magnetic resonance imaging: a useful biometric parameter for risk stratification in congenital diaphragmatic hernia. *J Pediatr Surg.* 2007;42(1):193–7. PMID: 17208564.

Guner YS, Khemani RG, Qureshi FG, et al. Outcome analysis of neonates with congenital diaphragmatic hernia treated with venovenous vs venoarterial extracorporeal membrane oxygenation. *J Pediatr Surg.* 2009;44:1691–1701. PMID: 19735810.

Hedrick H. Management of prenatally diagnosed congenital diaphragmatic hernia. *Semin Pediatr Surg.* 2013; 22(1):37–43. PMID: 23395144.

Haroon J, Chamberlain RS. An evidence-based review of the current treatment of congenital diaphragmatic hernia. *Clin Pediatr* 2013;52(2):115–24. PMID: 23378478.

Harrison MR, Keller RL, Hawgood SB, et al. A randomized trial of fetal endoscopic tracheal occlusion for severe fetal congenital diaphragmatic hernia. *N Engl J Med.* 2003;349(20):1916–24. PMID: 14614166.

Keijzer R, Wilschut DE, Jan Houmes R, et al. Congenital diaphragmatic hernia: to repair on or off extracorporeal membrane oxygenation? *J Pediatr Surg.* 2012; 47(4):631–6. PMID: 22498373.

Morini F, Goldman A, Pierro A. Extracorporeal membrane oxygenation in infants with congenital diaphragmatic hernia: a systematic review of the evidence. *Eur J Pediatr Surg.* 2006;16:385–91. PMID: 17211783.

Snoek KG, Reiss IKM, Greenough A, et al. Standardized postnatal management of infants with congenital diaphragmatic hernia in Europe: The CDH EURO Consortium Consensus - 2015 Update. *Neonatology.* 2016;110: 66–74. PMID: 29283134.

Chapter 23

Thoracic Surgery in Children

Kasia Rubin

> Case 1: A six-year-old with a history of osteosarcoma postchemotherapy and resection 18 months prior, presents with a new cough, shortness of breath and expiratory wheezing. The workup reveals a new mass in the right middle lobe as well as a large pleural effusion. Following CT-guided biopsy confirming metastatic disease, the surgeons plan to resect the mass via video-assisted thoracoscopic surgery (VATS).

What Is the Most Likely Cause of This Lung Mass?

Primary lung tumors are uncommon in children, with benign lung lesions being 10 times more common than malignant ones.

Secondary lung tumors are unfortunately more common with metastatic tumors comprising 80% of all lung tumors, of which 95% are malignant. In this patient, despite previous treatment, the most likely scenario of a new lung mass is recurrence of osteosarcoma with lung metastases.

In a child with no history of malignancy, the workup for new solitary lung tumors is quite different. Recommendations are to treat per symptoms, obtaining a baseline chest X-ray and labs. If symptoms persist beyond two to four weeks, a chest CT is warranted as is pulmonology consultation. If the chest CT is negative, treatment is continued for another two to four weeks prior to repeating a chest CT and bronchoscopy. If the CT reveals a lung mass, biopsy is warranted. Peripheral lung lesions are often amenable to open surgical biopsy or percutaneous biopsy in interventional radiology. Central lesions are biopsied via a bronchoscopic approach.

What Are the Differences Between VATS and Open Thoracotomy?

Video-assisted thoracoscopic surgery (VATS) was first performed in children in the mid-1970s. The contraindications to VATS include: (1) empyema with development of fibrosis obliterating obvious space between the ribs and (2) densely adherent tumor infiltrating the chest wall. The advantages of VATS over conventional thoracotomy include:

1. A reduction in postoperative pain from rib retraction during thoracotomy which occurs even if muscle sparing incisions are performed.
2. Reduction in musculoskeletal sequelae, as conventional thoracotomy leads to asymmetry of the thoracic wall from atrophy of the chest muscles as well as the development of ipsilateral scoliosis.
3. Improved recovery, with shorter hospitalizations and faster return to normal activities of daily life.

What Are the Preoperative Considerations Prior to Lung Tumor Resection?

Preoperative evaluation typically includes routine labs, chest X-ray, and CT scan of the chest. Preoperative echocardiography is necessary in settings where external cardiac compression is considered. Type- and cross-matched blood should be available. Despite plans for a thoracoscopic approach, conversion to open thoracotomy with potential for significant blood loss always remains a possibility.

What Are the Options for Lung Isolation?

The primary need for any endoscopic procedure is adequate visualization and space to work. This is achieved by collapsing the operative lung. Lung isolation in small children may prove difficult.

1. Double Lumen Tube (DLT)

   This device fuses two tubes of unequal length, with one terminating in the trachea and the other in a bronchus (right or left) allowing for ventilation of one or both lungs. The DLT also helps minimize the risk of contralateral lung contamination and allows for suction and maintenance of positive pressure as needed to either lung. Its limitation is size as the smallest DLT is a 26Fr, acceptable for ages 8–10, with an outer dimeter of 8.7 mm, comparable to a 6.5 mm internal diameter endotracheal tube, preventing its general use in younger pediatric patients.

2. Bronchial Blocker

   A balloon catheter is positioned in the proximal mainstem bronchus under fiberoptic visualization. If no true bronchial blocker is available, a Fogarty Occlusion Catheter or balloon wedge pressure catheter may be substituted. Inflation of the balloon blocks ventilation to the distal lobes or entire lung. Disadvantages include difficult placement in small children and frequent dislodgement. In situations where the balloon migrates into the trachea, full ventilatory obstruction may occur. Other issues include potential over-distension of the balloon with resultant tissue damage of the airway, inability to suction the operative lung, and an inability to apply continuous positive airway pressure to the operative lung. A bronchial blocker is often used in young children <8 years.

3. Univent Tube

   This is a tracheal tube with a bronchial blocker within a separate lumen, allowing advancement with inflation or withdrawal and deflation should double-lung ventilation be required. These tubes are available for pediatric sizes in 3.5 and 4.5 mm ID, allowing the youngest age of use to be approximately 6 years. This provides an optimal option between ages six and eight, at which point a double lumen tube is the preferred option.

4. Standard Single Lumen Endotracheal Tube with Intentional Mainstem Bronchus Intubation

   This is the preferred method for children ages zero to six months, but can be acceptable up to 18 years.
   A fiberoptic bronchoscope may be passed to confirm placement. Disadvantages include failure to provide an adequate seal, an inability to suction the operative lung, and hypoxemia due to obstruction of the right upper lobe bronchus. The inability to quickly change from one lung ventilation to two lung ventilation is the major drawback of this technique for occlusion of the operative lung.

5. Capnothorax

   In young infants, carbon dioxide insufflation into the operative hemithorax produces lung collapse. It provides adequate surgical visualization but may lead to hemodynamic effects that may not be well tolerated for long periods of time. To ameliorate these effects, low pressure insufflation is necessary, with discontinuation of insufflation should hemodynamic changes occur. Additional considerations for the anesthesiologist include hypothermia caused by a large volume of cold CO_2 in the thoracic cavity and prolonged hypercapnia in the setting of longer procedures.

Both the bronchial blocker and mainstem intubation methods of lung isolation rely on obstruction of the nonventilated bronchus for lung collapse via "absorption atelectasis." This leads to relatively slow lung deflation and reinflation. Verification of appropriate position of any device is necessary following changes in position of the patient.

How Do You Treat Resultant Hypoxemia Associated with One-Lung Ventilation?

1. If severe, switch to two-lung ventilation immediately.
2. Check position of the occluding device with fiberoptic bronchoscopy.
3. If possible, apply continuous positive airway pressure (CPAP) to the nondependent lung.
4. Apply positive end expiratory pressure (PEEP) to the dependent lung.
5. Intermittently ventilate both lungs.
6. In an emergency, the surgeon can clamp the ipsilateral pulmonary artery reducing ventilation: perfusion mismatch.

What Are the Options for Postoperative Pain Control?

Optimal analgesia is provided via a combination of regional anesthesia, opioids, and other adjuncts. Thoracic epidural blockade is achieved via placement of the epidural catheter inserted directly between T4 and T8 (depending on the level of the thoracotomy) and can be used to provide intraoperative and postoperative analgesia. Placement of a thoracic epidural catheter can safely be performed by experienced practitioners in neonates, with extremely low complication rates. Some providers prefer to approach the thoracic space using a caudally threaded epidural catheter. In this case, the caudal space is accessed and a wire reinforced catheter is advanced to the appropriate thoracic level. Often, fluoroscopy is used to confirm the epidural tip location.

Options for local anesthetics in the epidural space include bupivacaine, chloroprocaine, and ropivacaine. Adjunct agents most commonly selected are clonidine, fentanyl, or hydromorphone. Intravenous analgesia can be obtained with continuous infusions of opioid.

Intracostal nerve blocks, thoracic paravertebral blocks, or intrapleural installation of local anesthetic also aids in providing pain relief from chest tubes or incisions. Newer options such as erector spinae plane blocks and catheters have been successfully replacing thoracic epidurals. This technique affords a substantially improved safety profile, especially in small neonates.

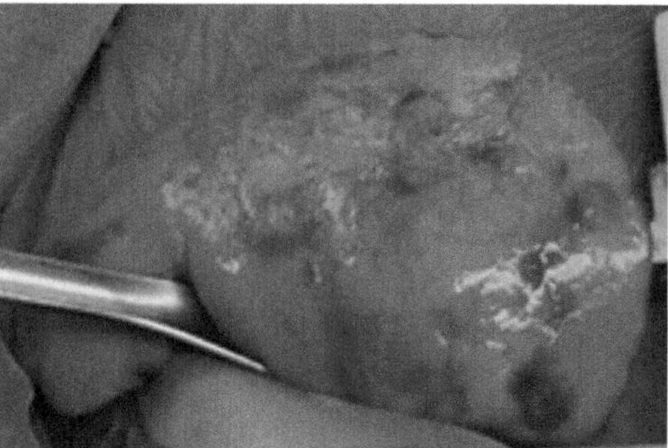

Figure 23.1 Intraoperative specimen of lung demonstrating numerous cystic malformations.

> Case 2: A five-day-old, 3.3 kg full term neonate, with no prenatal care, presents with increasing respiratory distress, tachypnea with room air oxygen saturation of 93%. Chest X-ray shows hyperinflation of the left lung; CT scan shows emphysematous hyperinflation of the left upper lobe. A diagnosis of congenital lobar emphysema is made.

What Are the Major Congenital Lung Malformations?

1. Congenital lobar emphysema (CLE) or Congenital Lobar Overinflation (CLO)

   Progressive lobar expansion leads to compression of the ipsilateral lung, due to either extrinsic airway compression or intrinsic cartilage abnormalities, leading to air trapping. This typically involves only one lobe, and is often diagnosed on prenatal ultrasound. Symptoms vary, with less severe CLE not presenting until the child is older. Approximately 10–15% of patients with CLE have associated cardiovascular anomalies. Neonates in severe distress or those with progressive decompensation will require emergent thoracotomy and resection, while elective surgery may be an option for the older child with moderate symptoms in no distress. Asymptomatic patients with small lesions may not need surgery.

2. Congenital Pulmonary Airway Malformation (CPAM) and Congenital Cystic Adenomatous Malformation (CCAM)

   This group of cystic and non-cystic lesions result from abnormalities in early airway development (Figure 23.1). They are often recognized on prenatal ultrasounds or discovered due to respiratory difficulties or recurrent infections. CPAMs are classified based on cyst size and histologic features. Symptomatic infants are treated with lobectomy or segmental resection.

3. Bronchopulmonary Sequestration

   This developmental lung lesion involves a portion of the lung that is independent of the tracheobronchial tree and has a separate systemic arterial supply, usually from the thoracic or abdominal aorta. The extra-lobar form has its own pleura and venous drainage, while the intra-lobar form shares pleura with the normal lung and drains into the pulmonary venous system. Extra-lobar lesions are usually diagnosed via prenatal ultrasound, while intra-lobar sequestration is often diagnosed in childhood or adulthood, often identified during a workup for recurrent lower lobe pneumonia. Symptomatic infants need urgent resection of the lesion. Asymptomatic patients undergo surgical resection in an elective fashion.

What Are the Management Strategies in a Symptomatic Neonate with a Congenital Lung Mass?

1. Preserve spontaneous respirations.
   a. Escalate noninvasive respiratory support as needed (blow-by oxygen, CPAP, bi-level positive airway pressure (BiPAP).
2. Intubate if in respiratory distress.
3. Ventilation after intubation.
   a. Spontaneous vs. controlled vs. high frequency oscillatory ventilation.

b. Positive pressure ventilation may lead to rapid inflation of the cystic lesion, with subsequent mediastinal shift and cardiopulmonary decompensation. Emergency decompression of hyperinflated cyst may be necessary from positive pressure ventilation.

c. High frequency oscillatory ventilation (HFOV) maybe indicated to keep constant pressures and avoid barotrauma.

4. Emergency surgery may be needed in settings of severe respiratory compromise.

Suggested Reading

Adler AC, Yim MM, Chandrakantan A. Erector spinae plane catheter for neonatal thoracotomy: a potentially safer alternative to a thoracic epidural. *Can J Anaesth.* 2019;66 (5):607–8. PMID: 30656616.

Biyyam DR, Chapman T, Ferguson MR, et al. Congenital lung abnormalities: embryologic features, prenatal diagnosis, and postnatal radiologic-pathologic correlation. *Radiographics.* 2010;30 (6):1721–38. PMID: 21071385.

Dishop MK, Kuruvilla S. Primary and metastatic lung tumors in the pediatric population: a review and 25-year experience at a large children's hospital. *Arch Pathol Lab Med.* 2008;132(7):1079–103. PMID: 18605764.

Golianu B, Hammer GB. Pediatric thoracic anesthesia and pain management for pediatric thoracic surgery. *Curr Opin Anaesthesiol.* 2005;18(1):5–11. PMID: 16534311.

Kumar K, Basker S, Jeslin L, et al. Anaesthesia for pediatric video assisted thoracoscopic surgery. *J Anaesthesiol Clin Pharmacol.* 2011;27(1):12–26. PMID: 21804698.

Patel NV, Glover C, Adler AC. Erector spinae plane catheter for postoperative analgesia after thoracotomy in a pediatric patient: A case report. *A A Pract.* 2019;12(9):299–301. PMID: 30844822.

Shah R, Reddy AS, Dhende NP. Video assisted thoracic surgery in children. *J Minim Access Surg.* 2007;3 (4):161–7. PMID: 19789677.

Chapter

24 Abdominal Masses

Neuroblastoma

Yeona Chun and Michael R. King

A 20-month-old girl presents with abdominal distension and a palpable, firm mass in her right abdomen. She is scheduled for open resection of the tumor. Vital signs include: Temp 37.6°C, BP 116/79, HR 88 bpm, SpO_2 100%. Heart and lung sounds are normal. Her CT scan is seen in Figure 24.1.

What Is the Differential Diagnosis for This Child's Abdominal Mass?

Malignancy is a serious concern with a new pediatric abdominal mass. Pediatric abdominal malignancies to consider include neuroblastoma, Wilms tumor (nephroblastoma), lymphoma, rhabdomyosarcoma, renal cell carcinoma, leiomyosarcoma, teratoma, and germ cell tumors. Other organ pathologies that may manifest as an abdominal mass include polycystic kidney disease, Meckel's diverticulum, and hepatic storage diseases. In a neonate one should also consider pyloric stenosis.

What Are the Clinical Characteristics of Neuroblastoma and Wilms Tumors?

Neuroblastoma is the most common extracranial pediatric tumor overall (with 65% of abdominal or adrenal origin), while Wilms tumor is the most common abdominal tumor in children. Both commonly present as palpable, painless abdominal masses without associated symptoms. Neuroblastomas may have associated hypertension, abdominal pain, constipation, or distension, while Wilms tumor often presents with hematuria and hypertension.

Children with localized disease may be asymptomatic other than a palpable mass, whereas those with advanced disease may appear cachectic and have constitutional symptoms (fever, weight loss). Large abdominal tumors may present with mass effect symptoms such as abdominal pain, fullness, bowel obstruction, or lower extremity edema. Mediastinal neuroblastoma can cause all of the most perilous symptoms of mediastinal masses including dyspnea from compression of the trachea or great vessels. Thoracic or cervical tumors may compress the sympathetic trunk causing Horner's syndrome, while larger thoracic tumors may cause superior vena cava syndrome. Metastatic disease can occur in the liver, bone, and skin.

What Is Neuroblastoma?

Neuroblastoma is a malignancy of the primordial neural crest cells that give rise to the sympathetic chains and adrenal glands. Their origin can stem from any part of the sympathetic nervous system, namely the adrenal glands and sympathetic chains of the abdomen, thorax, pelvis, and cervical area. As they are derived of neural crest they are capable of catecholamine secretion, although unlike pheochromocytoma they do not typically present primarily with symptoms of hypertension.

What Is the Incidence and Epidemiology of Neuroblastoma?

There are about 700 new cases of neuroblastoma annually in the United States. They account for around 10% of pediatric malignancies, though they are responsible for approximately 15% of pediatric cancer-related deaths. Most children are diagnosed before the age of 4, with a median age at diagnosis of 19 months.

How Is Neuroblastoma Diagnosed?

A definitive diagnosis of neuroblastoma requires one of the following:

(1) Tumor biopsy
(2) Evidence of bone metastasis seen on bone marrow aspirate with concomitant elevation of serum or

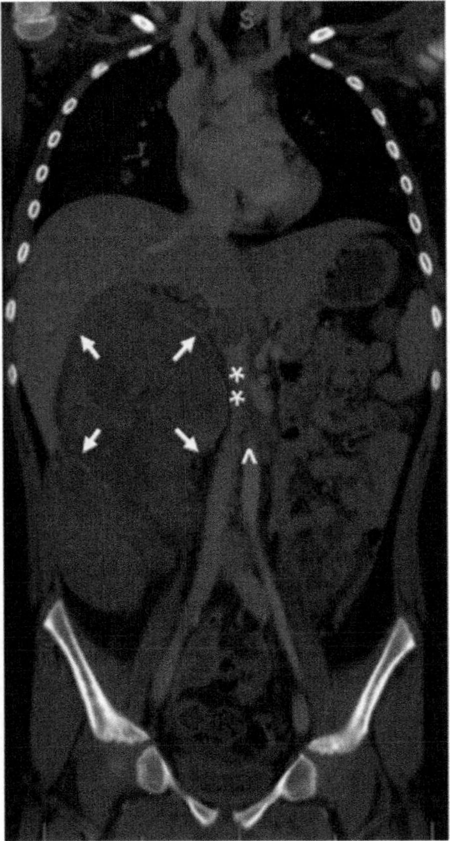

Figure 24.1 CT image of large circumferential neuroblastoma highlighted by arrows. Tumor size resulted in compression of the inferior vena cava (*) and aorta (^).

urine catecholamines/catecholamine metabolites (vanillylmandelic acid [VMA] and homovanillic acid [HVA]).

What Are the Currently Used Staging Systems for Neuroblastoma that Guide Treatment?

Ultrasound may be the initial study when an abdominal mass is discovered; however, CT or MRI is required for staging and evaluation of the extent of the mass if neuroblastoma is considered the likely diagnosis. A nuclear uptake scan is performed to evaluate for metastatic bone disease. Bone marrow biopsies should also be performed.

The International Neuroblastoma Risk Group Staging System (INRGSS) stages the patient based on radiology, clinical exam, and histology (Box 24.1). Surgical and histopathological factors are not part of the staging.

Box 24.1 International Neuroblastoma Risk Group Staging System (INRGSS)

Stage L1: Localized disease without image-defined risk factors

Stage L2: Localized disease with image-defined risk factors

Stage M: Distant metastatic disease (excluding stage MS)

Stage MS: Metastatic disease "special" in children younger than 18 months with metastases limited to liver, skin, and/or bone marrow

What Are the Commonly Used Chemotherapy Drugs and Relevant Side Effects That May Influence Your Anesthetic Management?

Chemotherapy can cause both acute side effects as well as lasting toxicities. Acute toxicities include nausea/vomiting, alopecia, myelosuppression and subsequent infection, and mucositis. Chemotherapeutic agents with well-known chronic side effects include doxorubicin (cardiotoxicity, arrhythmia), vincristine (peripheral neuropathy), and bleomycin (pulmonary fibrosis). The cardiovascular effects, specifically cardiomyopathy should be evaluated prior to anesthesia by echocardiography. Pulmonary involvement of chemotherapeutics, specifically in the presence of severe pulmonary fibrosis may warrant additional preoperative evaluation. In situations of severe end organ involvement, certain procedures may best be accomplished with regional anesthesia when appropriate (e.g., line placement).

What Major Anesthetic Concerns Do You Have for the Surgical Resection of the Tumor?

Hypertension: Hypertension may be present prior to the procedure due to catecholamine secretion from the tumor, but its absence does not necessarily mean that the tumor does not have catecholamine-secreting properties. If present preoperatively, blood pressure should be corrected with oral antihypertensive medications. As the patient may also be intravascularly volume depleted, intravenous hydration should also be used. During the procedure, hypertension may occur at any point, but has most commonly been reported at induction and with tumor manipulation. After removal, hypotension may be observed with the sudden absence of catecholamine secretion. Intravenous antihypertensive and pressor agents can be used intraoperatively, as indicated, and arterial and central venous catheters should be placed if hemodynamic lability is anticipated.

Bleeding and third space fluid losses: Neuroblastoma may surround or border large vessels. Large bore intravenous access should be obtained in the upper extremities given the potential for inferior vena cava (IVC) damage during resection or reduced IVC flow from tumor invasion. Blood products should be typed and cross-matched. Monitoring with invasive arterial blood pressure and central venous pressure should be considered.

Difficult ventilation: There may be respiratory compromise from the increased abdominal pressure caused by a large abdominal tumor. Ventilation may also become difficult during the case due to surgical retraction.

As the Surgeon Exposes and Manipulates the Tumor, the Patient Becomes Suddenly Extremely Hypertensive. What Are Your Next Steps?

Unlike pheochromocytoma, routine preoperative alpha blockade is not indicated for patients with neuroblastoma. However, intraoperative hypertension is not uncommon and may need to be treated. Case studies have reported successful use of beta blockers (labetalol, propranolol, esmolol), hydralazine, clevidipine, sodium nitroprusside, fenoldopam, and magnesium sulfate. Reported treatments for preoperative hypertension, if present, included phenoxybenzamine, enalapril, doxazosin, and labetalol.

What Other Anesthetic Strategies May Be Beneficial for This Child?

Resection of large abdominal masses often require large incisions. A caudal, lumbar, or thoracic epidural should be considered for intraoperative and postoperative pain control. Alternatively, bilateral paravertebral catheters may be considered.

Suggested Reading

Irwin MS, Park JR. Neuroblastoma: paradigm for precision medicine. *Pediatr Clin North Am.* 2015;62:225–56.

Ivani G, Suresh S, Ecoffey C, et al. The European Society of Regional Anesthesia and Pain Therapy and the American Society of Regional Anesthesia and Pain Medicine Joint Committee practice advisory on controversial topics in pediatric regional anesthesia. *Reg Anesth Pain Med.* 2015;40(5):526–32.

Przybylo HJ, Stevenson GW, Backer C, Luck SR, Webb CL, Morgan E, Hall SC. Anesthetic management of children with intracardiac extension of abdominal tumors. *Anesth Analg.* 1994;78(1):172–5.

Taenzer AH, Walker BJ, Bosenberg AT, et al. Asleep versus awake: does it matter?: Pediatric regional block complications by patient state: a report from the Pediatric Regional Anesthesia Network. *Reg Anesth Pain Med.* 2014;39(4):279–83.

Chapter 25

Abdominal Masses

Wilms Tumor

Yeona Chun and Michael R. King

A 20-month-old girl presents with abdominal distension and a palpable, firm mass in her right abdomen. Ultrasound and CT exams confirm an intra-abdominal mass, and she is scheduled for open resection. Vital signs include: Temp 37.6°C, BP 116/79, HR 88 bpm, SpO_2 100%. Heart and lung sounds are normal.

What Is the Differential Diagnosis for This Child's Abdominal Mass?

Pediatric abdominal malignancies to consider include neuroblastoma, Wilms tumor (nephroblastoma), lymphoma, rhabdomyosarcoma, renal cell carcinoma, leiomyosarcoma, teratoma, and germ cell tumors (see Chapter 24). Other organ pathologies that may present as an abdominal mass include polycystic kidney disease, Meckel's diverticulum, and hepatic storage diseases.

What Is the Incidence and Epidemiology of Wilms Tumor?

There are approximately 500 new cases of Wilms tumor annually in the United States. It is the most common renal malignancy in young children, while renal cell carcinoma is more common in adults and children older than 15 years. Most cases are diagnosed before five years of age, while nearly all are diagnosed before 10 years of age.

What Congenital Syndromes Are Associated with Wilms Tumor?

Most cases of Wilms tumor are sporadic. A minority of cases are part of congenital syndromes including WAGR (Wilms tumor, aniridia, genitourinary anomalies, intellectual disability) syndrome, Beckwith–Wiedemann syndrome, Perlman syndrome, and Sotos syndrome.

What Anesthetic Concerns Do You Have for Wilms Tumor Resection?

Neoadjuvant chemotherapy is often given before surgery and related toxicities may be present, similar to those described in neuroblastoma as discussed in Chapter 24. For those previously exposed to anthracyclines, a preoperative cardiac workup should be obtained including echocardiography. Serum creatinine and electrolytes should be checked, although most patients present with normal renal function (even with bilateral disease). Coagulation status should be evaluated as 10% of patients have an acquired von Willebrand disorder. A particularly important condition to rule out is renal vein and inferior vena cava (IVC) invasion. Intravascular tumor extension increases the risk of pulmonary tumor embolization, and presence of tumor in the IVC or cardiac chambers must be considered if obtaining central venous access. If the tumor is associated with a congenital syndrome, preparation should be made for associated anesthetic concerns, such as difficult airway due to macroglossia in Beckwith-Wiedemann and Sotos syndromes.

How Would Involvement of IVC and Intracardiac Extension of the Tumor Affect the Anesthetic Management?

Wilms tumors often have intraluminal venous extension. Renal vein involvement occurs in less than 40% of cases, with IVC extension in less than 10% and cardiac invasion in less than 1%. The patient may present with lower extremity edema if lower IVC involvement is significant. In the case of cardiac involvement, pleural effusions, hepatomegaly, ascites, or a new murmur may be present. Preoperative detection of tumor extension is thus imperative, and the IVC and right atrium should be checked for involvement by ultrasound or CT as part of the preoperative workup of patients with renal tumors. With cardiac involvement, cardiopulmonary bypass is utilized to assist in cardiac resection.

Upper extremity IV access should be secured due to the possibility of IVC compression and impairing venous return. Large bore or central access is strongly advised because of the possibility of large and rapid blood loss during resection when the IVC or aorta is involved?

How Will You Induce Anesthesia in This Child?

Intravenous and inhalational inductions are both options. If the tumor is large and there is concern for central vascular compression or displacement of abdominal contents, judicious intravenous induction with fluid and vasopressor administration may be preferred. Full stomach precautions should be taken if abdominal distension is present and there is potential for delayed gastric emptying.

How Would You Maintain General Anesthesia in This Patient?

Inhalational agent maintenance with air and oxygen is most often employed. Nitrous oxide should be avoided intraoperatively to prevent bowel distension. Analgesia can be achieved intraoperatively with epidural or opioid analgesia.

What Options for Postoperative Analgesia Would You Consider After Abdominal Mass Resection?

An abdominal incision will be painful after surgery and requires either opioid or epidural analgesia. A nurse-controlled opioid analgesic with both demand and continuous doses is appropriate given the patient's age and inability to cooperate with patient-controlled analgesia. A parent may also be given permission to deliver doses if deemed appropriate. Typical opioid choices include morphine or hydromorphone, although if the mass is renal in origin, caution should be taken when using morphine as decreased renal function may result in buildup of opioid metabolites causing toxicity. If an epidural was placed, continuous epidural infusion with or without nurse-controlled analgesia can be utilized. If an epidural was not placed, depending on the location of the incision a regional block such as a transversus abdominis plane or paravertebral block may also be useful.

Suggested Reading

Ivani G, Suresh S, Ecoffey C, et al. The European Society of Regional Anesthesia and Pain Therapy and the American Society of Regional Anesthesia and Pain Medicine Joint Committee practice advisory on controversial topics in pediatric regional anesthesia. *Reg Anesth Pain Med.* 2015;40(5):526–32. PMID: 26192549.

Przybylo HJ, Stevenson GW, Backer C, Luck SR, Webb CL, Morgan E, Hall SC. Anesthetic management of children with intracardiac extension of abdominal tumors. *Anesth & Analg.* 1994;78(1):172–5. PMID: 8267158.

Taenzer AH, Walker BJ, Bosenberg AT et al. Asleep versus awake: does it matter?: Pediatric regional block complications by patient state: a report from the Pediatric Regional Anesthesia Network. *Reg Anesth Pain Med.* 2014;39(4):279–83. PMID: 24918334.

Whyte SD, Mark Ansermino J. Anesthetic considerations in the management of Wilms' tumor. *Paediatr Anaesth.* 2006 May;16 (5):504–13. PMID: 16677259.

Chapter 26

Congenital Hyperinsulinism and Pancreatectomy

Maureen E. Scollon-McCarthy

An 18-day-old 4.3 kg female was admitted for evaluation of persistent hypoglycemia. The patient was born full term at 37 weeks 2/7 days. At one hour of life, the patient was listless and tremulous. Point of care glucose was noted to be <25 and the patient was treated and transferred to the NICU on a 20% dextrose infusion. Vital signs: Temp 37.2°C, RR 63, HR 138, BP 76/34.

What Is the Differential Diagnosis for Neonatal Hypoglycemia?

- Acquired hyperinsulinism from diabetic mother
- Beckwith–Wiedemann syndrome
- Congenital hyperinsulinism
- Fatty acid oxidation disorders
- Glycogen storage disease
- Growth hormone deficiency
- Hypopituitarism
- Inborn errors of metabolism
- Ketotic hypoglycemia
- Primary or central adrenal insufficiency
- Type 1 diabetes mellitus
- Exogenous insulin administration or other antidiabetic agents
- Administration of beta blockers

What Are the Clinical Characteristics of Neonatal Hypoglycemia?

Hypoglycemia in newborns or young infants may be characterized by lethargy, feeding difficulty, hypothermia, sweating, respiratory distress, cyanosis, or apnea. However, seizures are often the presenting symptom.

What Is Congenital Hyperinsulinism?

Congenital hyperinsulinism (HI) is the most common hypoglycemic disorder in infants. It is a heterogeneous disorder of the pancreas consisting of two main types of histologic abnormalities of pancreatic structure: focal adenomatous hyperplasia and diffuse abnormality of the islet cells.

HI results from inappropriately high insulin secretion by the pancreatic B-cells. A failure to reduce pancreatic insulin secretion in the presence of hypoglycemia (serum glucose <60 mg/dL) is caused by structural or functional molecular abnormalities in the insulin secretory mechanism or glucose-sensing mechanism.

Increased insulin levels cause hepatic and skeletal muscle glycogenesis. Glycogenesis decreases the amount of free glucose in the bloodstream causing a suppression of free fatty acids (FFA) formation resulting in hypoglycemia.

What Is the Genetic Component of HI?

The congenital pancreatic abnormalities associated with HI are caused by genetic mutations on various genes that regulate insulin secretion. Although approximately 50% of HI cases have no known genetic abnormality, 11 genes have been identified in relation to pancreatic beta cells involved in insulin secretion regulation. The most common cause of HI is inactivating mutations in ABCC8 or KCNJ11 genes of the Na^+/K^+ ATP channel.

What Are the Two Types of HI?

There are two forms of HI, diffuse and focal. In diffuse HI, beta cells throughout the pancreas are affected, with nucleomegaly seen through the pancreas. In focal HI, a distinct area of beta cell adenomatosis is seen. Focal HI involves the combination of paternally inherited ABCC8 or KCN11 mutations along with the somatic loss of the maternal tumor suppressor genes on chromosome 11p 15.

What Is the Incidence of HI?

The estimated incidence of HI is 1/50,000 live births. However, in countries with substantial consanguinity incidences may be as high as 1/25,000.

What Is the Age of Presentation?

HI can present between birth and 18 months of age, with most cases diagnosed shortly after birth. Although rare, adult-onset cases have been documented.

What Is the Presentation of HI?

Patients present with hypoglycemia ranging from asymptomatic hypoglycemia noted on routine blood glucose monitoring, to life-threatening hypoglycemic coma or status epilepticus. Many are diagnosed by routine blood work, while others are diagnosed later when they present with hypoglycemia symptoms. The risk of severe hypoglycemia causing seizures and permanent brain damage is high. Some infants may be large for gestational age.

How Is the Diagnosis of HI Made?

Diagnostic criteria for HI include blood glucose <40 mg/dL, +/− detectable insulin, decrease in beta-hydroxybutyrate, decrease in free fatty acids, decrease in IGF-BP1, and positive glucagon response.

How Is Congenital Hyperinsulinism Managed?

First-line treatment is diazoxide, a benzothiazine derivative, which activates the SUR 1 subunit of the K^+/ATP channel and opens the K/$^+$ATP channel leading to a decrease in insulin. Diazoxide dose range is 5–15 mg/kg/day given orally twice a day. Side effects include hypertrichosis and fluid retention. Many neonates require diuretic therapy along with diazoxide. Pulmonary hypertension may occur in patients without adequate diuretic therapy.

Diazoxide is given as a 5-day trial (Figure 26.1). If diazoxide is not successful in maintaining a blood glucose >70 mg/dL during a 12 hour fast, it may suggest that the patient has a defect on the K^+ ATP channel. A genetic workup should be initiated immediately.

If diazoxide is stopped, then IV dextrose with/without glucagon infusion is started to maintain blood glucose >70 mg/dL. Blood glucose, vital signs, and mental status should be assessed regularly.

A second-line agent for managing HI is the somatostatin analog octreotide, which acts on the somatostatin receptors by inhibiting the secretion of a variety of hormones including insulin. Insulin secretion is decreased through beta cell hyperpolarization and calcium channel inhibition.

Glucagon, a polypeptide hormone secreted by the alpha cells of the pancreatic islets, triggers glycogenolysis and gluconeogenesis to increase hepatic glucose output. HI patients generally have an inappropriate rise in blood glucose due to the mobilization of hepatic glycogen by glucagon. Glucagon can be used as a rescue medication for acute or severe hypoglycemia.

What If Medical Management Is Ineffective?

If the patient fails to respond to the maximum dose of diazoxide (15 mg/kg/day) after five days of treatment, a K^+ ATP channel defect is suspected as the cause of hyperinsulinism. These children are potential surgical candidates and require referral to a specialized HI center to undergo an 18–fluorol-3, 4-dihydroxphenylalanine positron emission tomography (18-F-Dopa PET) scan.

18 [F]–Dopa, an analog of L-Dopa, is a dopamine precursor and is used as a positron emitting compound. In the pancreas, normal islet cells take up a small amount of 18 F-DOPA and decarboxylate it to produce insulin. The uptake of the tracer in hyperfunctioning islets can be quite pronounced. 18 F-DOPA uptake in diffuse HI is uniform, whereas in focal HI the uptake is greater in a specific region compared to the surrounding tissue. 18 F-DOPA PET scans diagnose 75% of focal cases and are 100% accurate in identifying the location of the lesion (Figure 26.2).

What Is the Surgical Management for Congenital HI?

If medical management is ineffective a focal (partial) or diffuse (sub-total) pancreatectomy is indicated. The extent of the pancreatic resection depends on the

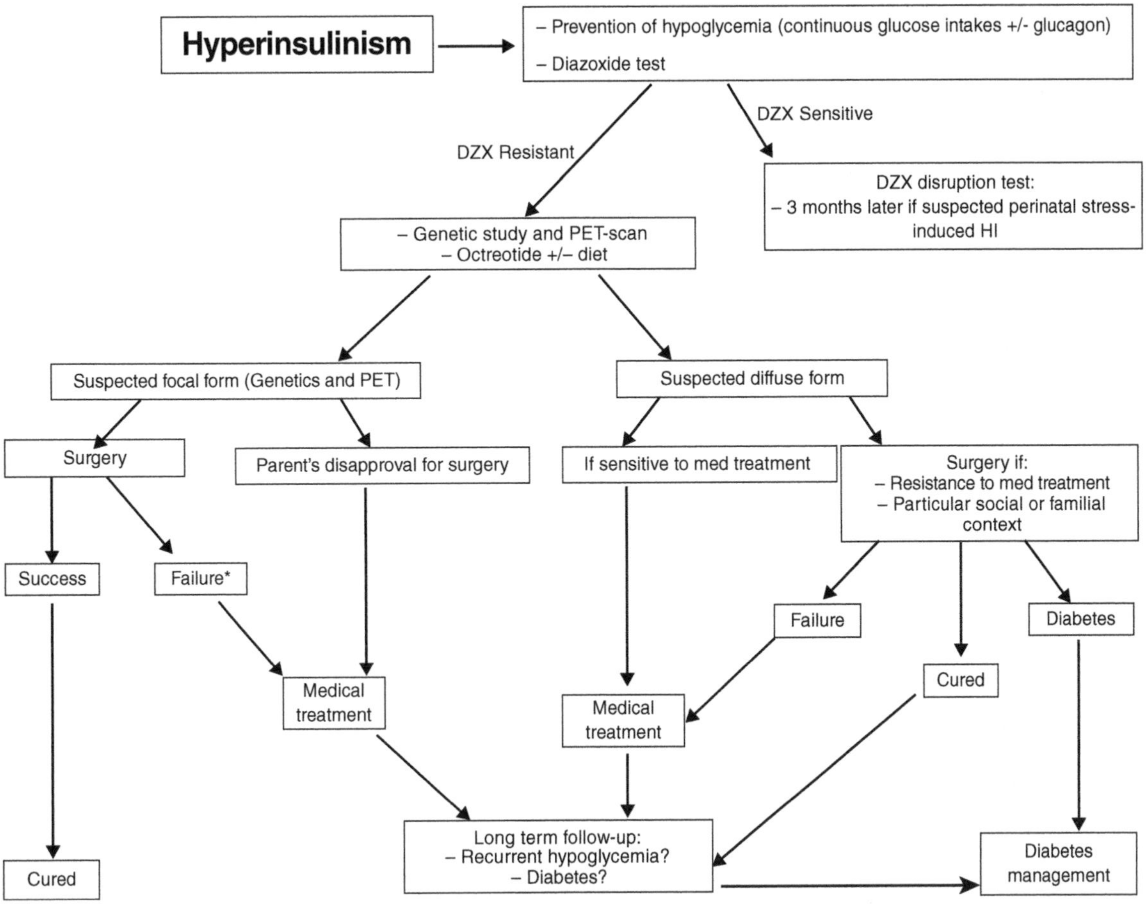

Hyperinsulinism

– Prevention of hypoglycemia (continuous glucose intakes +/- glucagon)
– Diazoxide test

DZX Resistant

– Genetic study and PET-scan
– Octreotide +/– diet

DZX Sensitive

DZX disruption test:
– 3 months later if suspected perinatal stress-induced HI

Suspected focal form (Genetics and PET)

Surgery

Success

Cured

Failure*

Medical treatment

Parent's disapproval for surgery

Suspected diffuse form

If sensitive to med treatment

Medical treatment

Surgery if:
– Resistance to med treatment
– Particular social or familial context

Failure

Cured

Diabetes

Long term follow-up:
– Recurrent hypoglycemia?
– Diabetes?

Diabetes management

Figure 26.1 Diagnostic and management schematic for patients with suspected hyperinsulinism. DZX, diazoxide. Adapted from (open access copyright) Arnoux JB, et al. Congenital hyperinsulinism: current trends in diagnosis and therapy. *Orphanet Journal of Rare Diseases* 2011;6:63

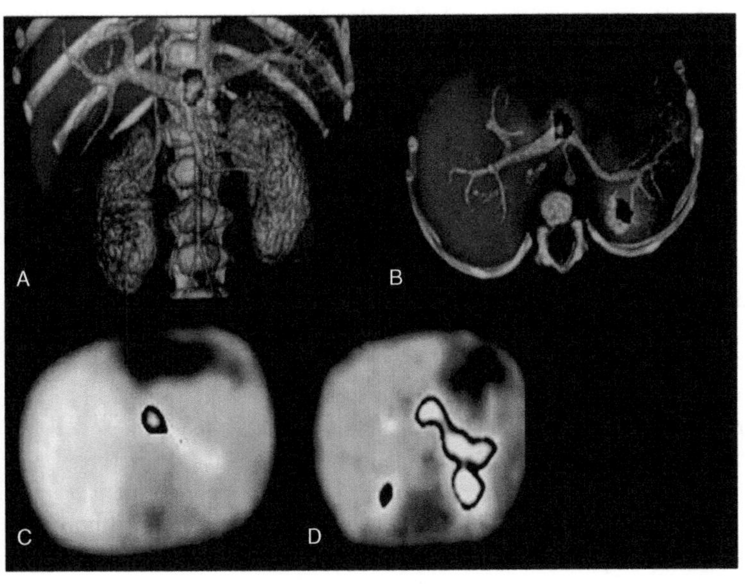

Figure 26.2 18 F-fluoro-L-DOPA PET-scan imaging in patients with HI. Focal form (A, B, C): PET-scan localizes accurately the focal lesion. A, B: 3D CT-scan reconstruction fused with PET imaging showing pancreatic uptake of the radiotracer to be almost exclusively located at the head of the pancreas. C: Transversal PET imaging in a suspected focal form. D: Transversal PET imaging in a suspected diffuse form showing uptake of the radiotracer appears in the whole pancreas. Adapted from (open access copyright) Arnoux JB, et al. Congenital hyperinsulinism: current trends in diagnosis and therapy. *Orphanet Journal of Rare Diseases* 2011;6:63

Table 26.1 Postoperative management of glucose post pancreatectomy. GIR, glucose infusion rate; BG, blood glucose; TPN, total parenteral nutrition

POD 0	POD 1
IV D30W @ 2xGIR with 0.45NaCl titrated to 80–100 mL/kg/day	IV D30W infusion is increased to provide GIRx5, TPN is ordered to provide a GIR=8
Hourly BG measurement targeting 80–180 mg/dL	GIR remains at 8 until feeds started
BG >250 is tolerated for 6–8 h. postoperatively prior to starting insulin. For BG >250 within the 6–8 h. Post-op, urine should be checked for presence of ketones.	Sepsis evaluation considered for persistent hyper C or hypoglycemia following the immediately postoperative period
If BG >250 consistently, insulin infusion should be started at 0.005 Units/kg/h GIR is not reduced when starting insulin infusion	Consider residual lesions for patients with persistent hypoglycemia requiring GIR>8
	Monitor BG every 1–2 h
	Do not wean GIR if insulin infusion required

results of the PET scan. All open procedures are performed via a transverse supra-umbilical laparotomy.

A partial pancreatectomy is performed for those patients with a focal lesion, which may necessitate a longer OR time. If a focal lesion is not identified, intraoperative biopsies are taken and immediately analyzed by frozen section from the head, body, and tail of the pancreas. Patients with diffuse HI undergo near total pancreatectomy (removal of >95% of tissue). In these cases, a small portion of pancreatic tissue is left between the common bile duct and duodenum. In patients undergoing partial resection, a Roux-en Y pancreatojejunostomy may be necessary to ensure adequate pancreatic duct drainage, if the head of the pancreas is resected. These patients usually do not need to have a G-tube placed and are less likely to require insulin. For those patients who have a diffuse disease a near-total pancreatectomy is indicated. These patients require G-tube placement and will most likely require insulin.

What Are the Anesthetic Considerations for Congenital HI?

For patients undergoing a pancreatectomy, room set up should include all standard considerations for neonates.

Point of care glucometer must be readily available.

At minimum, a type and screen should be performed preoperatively, however, consideration should be given to have cross-matched blood available in the operating room.

Intra and postoperative pain control may be augmented with a caudally threaded epidural catheter which may be placed using the assistance of fluoroscopy and a radiopaque catheter.

Glucose homeostasis may be extremely challenging in these patients. The patient will present to the OR on concentrated IV dextrose solutions. The dextrose concentration should be maintained at the level at which the patient is best managed to avoid hypoglycemia (i.e., if using 20% dextrose, 20% should be maintained). General anesthesia will cause a hyperglycemic response. The blood glucose level may rise as the abnormal pancreatic tissue is excised and the surplus insulin secretin tissue is removed. Glucose monitoring should be performed approximately every 30 minutes during the procedure.

Prior to anesthetic induction, the glucose maintenance solution should be decreased to one-half to two-thirds of the original rate. Hypoglycemia and hyperglycemia should be corrected. At the end of the procedure, the target is 2xGIR as provided below:

$$\textbf{Glucose infusion rate (mg/kg/min)} = \frac{\%\textbf{Dextrose} \times IV\ \textbf{rate} \times 0.167}{\textbf{Weight in kg}}$$

Postoperative Care

A sample template for glucose management for the first 48 h postoperatively is seen in Table 26.1.

Adequate analgesia is vital, as poor pain management may result in hyperglycemia. Therefore, when an epidural is present, the pain management team is consulted to manage. Epidural infusion of chloroprocaine is used in patients less than 12 months old. If patients are older than 12 months, an epidural infusion of ropivacaine with/without adjuncts such as fentanyl or clonidine is given. Morphine and nalbuphine rescues of 0.05 mg/kg per dose can be given every 3–4 hours as needed for pain. However, if pain is not controlled with epidural and rescue medications, a continuous opioid infusion may be required to augment analgesia.

On Post Op Day #1

Ketorolac 0.5 mg/kg per dose every 6 hours maybe considered if creatinine and platelets are normal.

On Post Op Day #2

Consider removing the epidural. The epidural is usually maintained for 48–72 hours post-op.

Considerations for Care

Throughout the postoperative course, it is essential to monitor the blood glucose and maintain adequate hydration and nutrition by adjusting the IV fluid rate. All medications should be ordered in normal saline. Any persistent hyperglycemia or hypoglycemia will warrant a sepsis evaluation including blood and urine cultures.

A feeding regimen may commence once the bowel function has returned, usually five to seven days post-op. Infants with extensive duodenal manipulation or Roux-en-Y pancreaticojejunostomy may have duodenal edema necessitating longer NPO durations (one to two weeks).

Symptoms of bilious emesis and retractable pain could indicate bowel obstruction or intussusception. These patients commonly need antireflux medication and a small amount of emesis is expected when advancing feeds.

Outcomes

The outcomes are based on the presence of focal vs. diffuse disease. The cure rate without medication management for focal disease approaches 95%. For patients with diffuse disease, approximately 15% are controlled without medication, 50% require ongoing management with insulin, and 35% require ongoing management for control of hypoglycemia.

Suggested Reading

Adzick NS, Thornton PS, Stanley CA, et al. A multidisciplinary approach to the focal form of congenital hyperinsulinism leads to successful treatment by partial pancreatectomy. *J Pediatr Surg.* 2004;39(3):270–5. PMID: 15017536.

Arnoux JB, Verkarre V, Saint-Martin C, et al. Congenital hyperinsulinism: current trends in diagnosis and therapy. *Orphanet J Rare Dis.* 2011;6:63. PMID: 21967988.

Hardy O, Hernandez-Pampaloni M, Saffer JR, et al. Diagnosis and localization of focal congenital hyperinsulinism by 18F-fluorodopa PET scan. *J Pediatr.* 2007;150 (2):140–5. PMID: 17236890.

Hardy O, Litman, RL. Congenital hyperinsulinism: a review of the disorder and a discussion of the anesthesia management. *Pediatr Anesth.* 2007;17(7):616–21.

Laje P, Stanley CA, Palladino AA, et al. Pancreatic head resection and Roux-en-Y pancreaticojejunostomy for the treatment of the focal form of congenital hyperinsulinism. *J Pediatr Surg.* 2012;47(1):130–5. PMID: 22244405.

Nanni C, Fanti S, Rubello D. 18F-DOPA PET and PET/CT. *J Nucl Med.* 2007;48(10):1577–9. PMID: 17909255.

Yorifuji T. Congenital hyperinsulinism: current status and future perspectives. *Ann Pediatr Endocrinol Metab.* 2014;19 (2):57–68. PMID: 25077087.

Chapter 27

Hepatic Portoenterostomy; Kasai Procedure

Rahul G. Baijal and Nihar V. Patel*

A nine-month-old male recently adopted from abroad with a past medical history significant for biliary atresia, arrives for preoperative evaluation for the Kasai procedure.

He was recently admitted for hematemesis requiring transfusion, followed by esophagogastroduodenoscopy with sclerotherapy and variceal band ligation. His oxygen saturation is 88% on room air. Physical examination is consistent with nail bed clubbing, scleral icterus, and a distended abdomen from ascites. He has scratch marks on his skin, some with scabbing and some appearing infected.

The preoperative clinic asks for guidance in performing a preoperative evaluation.

What Is Biliary Atresia?

Biliary atresia, with an incidence between 1 in 8,000 and 1 in 18,000 live births, is the most common cause of neonatal cholestasis and the most frequent indication for liver transplantation in children. Biliary atresia is a progressive fibro-inflammatory cholangiopathy leading to a complete obliteration of the extra-hepatic bile ducts. There is a slight female predominance with a female to male ratio of 1.7:1.

What Is the Natural History of Biliary Atresia?

Biliary atresia presents as neonatal jaundice. Neonatal jaundice beyond the first two weeks of life should raise suspicion for biliary atresia as morbidity and mortality depend on the timing of surgical intervention. Biliary cirrhosis, portal hypertension, and end-stage liver disease will occur in about 50% of children by two years of age with no surgical intervention. Clinical findings may include a conjugated hyperbilirubinemia, elevated gamma-glutamyl transferase, and elevated serum liver transaminases.

Neonatal jaundice progresses to hepatic fibrosis at four to six weeks of age. From two to six months, chronic hepatic fibrosis/cirrhosis results in the changes noted later in the chapter. If untreated, end-stage liver disease requiring liver transplantation occurs.

Associated congenital anomalies include polysplenia, situs inversus, absent vena cava, malrotation, and cardiac anomalies.

What Are the Associated Pathophysiologic Issues Related to Chronic Biliary Atresia?

- Biliary obstruction leads to hepatic fibrosis and eventually cirrhosis.
- Hepatic failure (usually after a few months of life) results in:
  - Anemia secondary to liver disease
  - Ascites (hypoalbuminemia)
  - Coagulopathy: intrahepatic factor production and inability to absorb vitamin K due to lack of bile salts
  - Hypoxemia: reduced functional residual capacity secondary to large volume ascites
  - Jaundice: acholic stool and dark urine
  - Malnutrition: malabsorption
  - Portal hypertension and esophageal varices
  - Secondary splenomegaly
  - Recurrent cholangitis/sepsis

* Drs. Baijal and Patel have contributed equally to this chapter to constitute first authorship.

What Is a Kasai Procedure (Hepatic Portoenterostomy)?

The Kasai procedure, or a hepatic portoenterostomy, involves:

(1) Mobilization of the liver to identify the porta hepatis
(2) Excision of all extrahepatic fibrous biliary remnants at the point where the portal vein enters the hepatic parenchyma.
(3) Creation of a Roux-en-Y loop of the proximal jejunum.
(4) Anastamosis of the Roux-en-Y loop of the jejunum to the porta hepatis.

The result is a conduit for biliary drainage to exit the liver.

What Is the Timing of and Prognosis for the Kasai Procedure?

The timing of the surgical intervention affects the morbidity and mortality of children with biliary atresia. Early intervention (8–12 weeks) affords the best prognosis.

Approximately one-third of children who have undergone a Kasai procedure will require no further surgical intervention whereas the other two-thirds of children will require a liver transplantation with development of portal hypertension, ascites, malnutrition, poor growth, and recurrent cholangitis.

What Is the Cause of Hematemesis in This Case?

Portal hypertension is an elevated portal venous pressure above 10–20 mmHg causing increased resistance to portal venous inflow. The increased resistance occurs not only because of hepatic fibrosis but also because of nitric oxide deficient vasoconstriction. Esophageal variceal bleeding is the most common presentation of portal hypertension with increasing blood flow from inadequate forward portal venous inflow, causing variceal expansion and rupture.

Why Is the Patient Hypoxemic?

Hypoxemia with impaired respiratory function occurs secondary to mechanical impairment from ascites and hepatosplenomegaly with reduced functional residual capacity. Pulmonary edema and pleural effusions, often reaccumulate despite drainage, due to hypoalbuminemia and reduced oncotic pressure. These changes combine to reduce functional residual capacity and increased work of breathing.

What Is Hepatopulmonary Syndrome (HPS)?

Hepatopulmonary syndrome (HPS) may also cause hypoxemia with right to left shunting secondary to intrapulmonary arteriovenous shunting and intrapulmonary vasodilation. HPS is diagnosed clinically with a PaO_2 <70 mmHg or an alveolar-arterial gradient greater than 20 mmHg on room air.

Technetium-99 radiolabeled microalbumin may also be used to diagnose HPS; normally, 95% of the microalbumin is taken up in the lungs, whereas in HPS secondary to intrapulmonary right to left shunting, the microalbumin is taken up in the systemic capillary beds. Additionally, a bubble study with a transthoracic echocardiogram may also be used to assess right-to-left shunting in the pulmonary vasculature bed with appearance of bubbles in the left atrium. Supplemental oxygen is used as supportive therapy. Hepatopulmonary syndrome is reversible following a liver transplantation.

What Is Hepatorenal Syndrome (HRS)?

Hepatorenal syndrome may be acute (type 1) or chronic (type 2). HRS is characterized by renal insufficiency in the setting of portal hypertension, presumably caused by prerenal azotemia or acute tubular necrosis. Children with metabolic disorders are prone to renal insufficiency and may be on renal replacement therapy preoperatively. Type I is characterized by rapid progression of renal failure with 100% rise in creatinine in 2 weeks, whereas type 2 progresses over several weeks to months. Liver transplantation is the definitive therapy for HRS.

What Other Major Organ Systems Are Affected by End-Stage Liver Disease?

End-stage liver disease is a multisystem disorder.

Circulatory. The cardiovascular system undergoes significant changes with end-stage liver disease. End-stage liver disease is associated with a hyperdynamic circulation with an increased cardiac output and systemic vasodilation. The pathophysiology of this condition has been attributed to sympathetic nervous system hyperactivity, inadequate clearance of vasoactive substances, arteriovenous (A-V) shunting, and tissue hypoxemia. The hyperdynamic circulation decreases sensitivity to catecholamines and vasoconstrictors, exaggerating the vasodilatory effects of most anesthetics.

Pulmonary Vasculature. Portopulmonary hypertension (PPHN) is defined as a mean pulmonary artery pressure greater than 25 mmHg with a normal pulmonary capillary wedge pressure in the presence of portal hypertension.

PPHN may present with a new-onset murmur with a loud P2 sound, dyspnea, and syncope. PPHN may be diagnosed by echocardiography or catheterization. Patients with a mean pulmonary artery pressure (mPAP) <35 mmHg do not have increased mortality during liver transplantation whereas those with a mPAP between 35 and 45 mmHg have a mortality of approximately 50%, and those with a mPAP > 50 mmHg have a 100% mortality.

Gastrointestinal. Gastrointestinal complications of portal hypertension include ascites and gastrointestinal bleeding from esophageal and gastric varices.

Coagulation. Hepatic synthetic dysfunction reduces plasma concentrations of albumin, plasma cholinesterases, and coagulation proteins. Hypoalbuminemia reduces serum oncotic pressure predisposing to intravascular hypovolemia, ascites, pulmonary edema, and pleural effusions. Decreased plasma cholinesterase concentrations only mildly prolong neuromuscular blockade after succinylcholine administration since this enzyme is produced in excess even in children with end-stage liver disease.

What Is Hepatic Encephalopathy?

Hepatic encephalopathy is graded by the severity of the altered mental status as defined by West Haven (Table 27.1). The etiology of hepatic encephalopathy is multifactorial, including electrolyte disturbances such as hyponatremia, hypoglycemia, hyperammonia, and coagulopathy. Low blood urea nitrogen with elevated ammonia is present in children with end-stage liver disease. Furthermore, gastrointestinal hemorrhage may produce hyperammonia from bacterial deamination of intestinal blood.

Table 27.1 West Haven criteria for hepatic encephalopathy

Grade	Clinical presentation
0	Minimal: no detectable changes in personality or behavior, no asterixis
1	Lack of awareness, shortened attention span, sleep disturbance, altered mood, and slowing of the ability to perform mental tasks; asterixis may be present
2	Lethargy or apathy, disorientation to time, amnesia of recent events, impaired computations, inappropriate behavior, and slurred speech; asterixis present
3	Somnolence, confusion, disorientation to place, bizarre behavior, clonus, nystagmus, and positive Babinski sign; asterixis absent
4	Coma, lack of verbal, eye, and oral response

Ammonia crosses the blood brain barrier, resulting in cerebral edema. Ammonia levels greater than 200 μg/mL have been associated with cerebral herniation and death. Lactulose is prescribed to produce an osmotic diuresis and acidify the gut lumen to trap ammonia and minimize absorption, yet has not been shown to improve survival.

Children with grade 3–5 hepatic encephalopathy require endotracheal intubation to protect airway reflexes and therapeutic measures to reduce increased intracranial pressure, including elevation of the head of the bed, sedation, acute hyperventilation, osmolar diuretics, and hypertonic saline.

What Are the Anesthetic Implications of the Kasai Procedure?

Preoperative Considerations

Blood products should be prepared prior to surgery (especially in the setting of past transfusion and potential for antibody presence).

Blood should be irradiated as these patients should always be considered for future transplantation potential. Blood prior to transfusion undergoes brief irradiation to reduce donor lymphocytes. The aim is to prevent graft vs. host disease in a newly immune suppressed patient.

The patient has severe itch due to build up of bile salts; secondary infection should be treated.

Laboratory examinations should include: CBC, coagulation studies, electrolyte, glucose, albumin, blood urea nitrogen (BUN)/Cr, and liver function tests.

A chest X-ray to evaluate for fluid overload and an echocardiogram to evaluate for PPHN are also important preoperatively especially given this patient's late presentation.

Intraoperative Considerations

- In the absence of large ascites, inhalation induction is appropriate.
- Large IV access should be obtained, specifically in the upper extremities.
- Central line (internal jugular vein or subclavian) if inadequate access, pressor support or TPN considered.
- Blood should be in the operating room.
- Arterial access should be obtained for hemodynamic monitoring and frequent laboratory examination.
- Temperature maintenance should be carefully monitored, especially in the setting of coagulopathy.
- Frequent monitoring of electrolytes, glucose, and lactate is needed.
- Transfusion of blood products as required for bleeding (especially in small neonates undergoing procedure).
- Fluid homeostasis is vital with third spacing and evaporative losses during long intra-abdominal procedure.
- Vasopressors should be immediately available.

Postoperative Considerations

Depending on the preoperative severity of illness and the intra-operative course these children may be suitable for extubation at the end of the procedure.

Analgesia is critical with the large intra-abdominal incision. In the absence of coagulopathy, thoracic epidural (direct vs. caudally threaded epidural is appropriate). The epidural may be used to reduce intra- and postoperative opioids and associated complications.

Suggested Reading

Bromley P, Bennett J. Anesthesia for children with liver disease. *Cont Educ Anaesth.* 2014:14(5):207–12.

Green DW, Howard ER, Davenport M. Anaesthesia, perioperative management and outcome of correction of extrahepatic biliary atresia in the infant: a review of 50 cases in the King's College Hospital series. *Paediatr Anaesth.* 2000;10(6):581–9. PMID: 11119190.

Chapter

28 Liver Transplantation

Rahul G. Baijal and Nihar V. Patel*

Three years following his Kasai procedure, a four-year-old male with biliary atresia (see Chapter 27) is posted for orthotopic liver transplantation for end-stage liver disease. He is currently intubated in the Pediatric ICU on dopamine and epinephrine infusions to maintain his blood pressure. Total parenteral nutrition and intralipids are infusing through a right subclavian line. Oxygen saturation on room air is 91%. His international normalized ratio (INR) is 5.6 and has required multiple transfusions of Elsewhere in book this is written as PRBCs. Make consistent to PRBCs, fresh frozen plasma (FFP), and platelets.

Hemoglobin: 8.0, Hematocrit: 23.8, Platelets: 60,000, PT: 49.6, INR: 5.6, PTT 88.3

Na: 129, K: 3.1, Cl: 105, HCO_3: 19, BUN: 30, Cr: 2.3, Glucose 65, Ca: 0.85, Mg: 1.9

Albumin: 2.5, Total Bilirubin 3.9.

What Are the Indications for and Underlying Diagnoses Associated with Pediatric Liver Transplantation?

The primary indications for liver transplantation are acute fulminant hepatic failure, chronic end-stage liver disease, and progressive primary liver disease refractory to maximal medical management and metabolic disease. Table 28.1 lists the common underlying diagnoses associated with liver transplantation.

What Is the PELD Score and How Is It Used in Pediatric Liver Transplantation?

The Pediatric End-Stage Liver Disease (PELD) score was implemented in 2002 to prioritize organ allocation to the sickest patients, rather than those who had been waiting the longest. It is used for children 12 years and younger. PELD uses the patient's values for serum bilirubin, serum albumin, the international normalized ratio for prothrombin time (INR), whether the patient is less than 1 year old, and whether the patient has growth failure (<2 standard deviation) to predict survival. It is calculated according to the following formula:

PELD = 4.80[Ln serum bilirubin (mg/dL)] + 18.57[Ln INR] − 6.87[Ln albumin (g/dL)] + 4.36(<1 year old) + 6.67(growth failure)

The PELD score is used to calculate a numerical value that is an accurate predictor of three-month mortality, independent of portal hypertension and etiology of the liver disease. A higher score correlates with a more critical condition. Thus, liver donations are usually allocated by United Network for Organ Sharing (UNOS) according to the PELD score to maximize the life-saving capability of each donated liver.

What Are the Common Pathophysiologic Derangements of End-Stage Liver Failure?

The pathophysiologic derangements common in patients undergoing liver transplantation are summarized in Table 28.2.

What Preoperative Workup Is Needed for Pediatric Liver Transplantation?

A liver transplant preoperative evaluation should include a standard history and physical exam to identify the primary cause of liver failure and identify the specific anatomic and physiologic derangements that need to be addressed. Standard preoperative workup includes past medical and surgical history, medication list, drug allergies, and NPO interval. Additional considerations include treating active infections, optimizing preexisting cardiac conditions, and completing the patient's immunization schedule.

* Drs. Baijal and Patel have contributed equally to this chapter to constitute first authorship.

Table 28.1 Relative frequency of the primary indications for liver transplantation in children. Data from Cote and Lerman, eds. *A Practice of Anesthesia for Infants and Children.* 5th Ed. Elsevier 2013

Diagnosis	Frequency (%)
Cholestatic liver disease	54
Biliary atresia	
Alagille syndrome	
Primary sclerosing cholangitis	
Intrahepatic cholestasis	
Biliary cirrhosis	
Fulminant hepatic failure	14
Acute liver failure	
Cirrhosis	
Autoimmune hepatitis	
Neonatal hepatitis cirrhosis	
Metabolic disease	14
Alpha 1 antitrypsin deficiency	
Urea cycle defects	
Cystic fibrosis	
Wilson's disease	
Tyrosinemia	
Primary hyperoxaluria	
Crigler-Najjar syndrome	
Glycogen storage disease	
Primary hepatic malignancy	6
Hepatoblastoma	
Other	
Other	6
Congenital hepatic fibrosis	
Budd–Chiari syndrome	

Based on the organ systems affected in liver disease, specific tests should be considered (Table 28.3).

How Can Liver Failure Be Treated Prior to Transplantation?

It is not uncommon for liver failure patients to wait months for a suitable organ to transplant. It is then

Table 28.2 Pathophysiologic derangements common in patients undergoing liver transplantation

Organ system	Common findings
Cardiovascular	Hyperdynamic circulation: ↑cardiac output, ↓systemic vascular resistance (SVR)
	Pericardial effusions
	Arteriovenous (AV) shunting Long term: cardiomyopathy, high output heart failure
Pulmonary	Hypoxemia due to V/Q mismatch
	Impaired hypoxic pulmonary vasoconstriction
	Intrapulmonary shunting
	↓ functional residual capacity (FRC) due to ascites
	Pulmonary hypertension
	Hepatopulmonary syndrome Pleural effusions
CNS	Encephalopathy
	Cerebral edema
Renal	Prerenal azotemia
	Hepatorenal syndrome
GI	Hepatic dysfunction: synthetic, metabolic and excretory
	Portal hypertension
	Delayed gastric emptying
Hematologic	Thrombocytopenia
	Coagulopathy
	Anemia
	Hypofibrinogenemia, dysfibrinogenemia Disseminated intravascular coagulopathy
Laboratory/ electrolyte anomalies	Metabolic acidosis
	Hypokalemia Hyponatremia
	Intravascular volume depletion

Table 28.3 Specific preoperative evaluation tests for consideration prior to liver transplantation

Organ system	Exam	Rationale
CV	Echocardiography	Identify cardiomyopathy or congenital defects
	ECG	Identify arrhythmias and prolonged QT
Pulmonary	CXR	Identify pleural effusions
	ABG	Hepatopulmonary syndrome
Renal	Chemistry panel	BUN and creatinine levels for ARF
Hematologic	CBC	Assess anemia and thrombocytopenia
	PT/PTT/INR	Coagulopathy
	TEG	Coagulopathy
	Type and cross	Blood products needed for surgery
Laboratory/electrolyte anomalies	Chemistry panel	Hyponatremia, hypokalemia, hypocalcemia, glucose
	Liver panel	Albumin, AST, ALT

necessary to reduce the severity of the complications from liver failure. In a trans-jugular intrahepatic portosystemic shunt (TIPS), a stent connects the portal vein to the hepatic veins to bypass and decompress the hepatic circulation. The aim is to reduce portal hypertension and its sequelae, ascites, and esophageal varices.

Molecular adsorbent recirculating system (MARS) therapy is a liver dialysis of sorts. Similar to dialysis, it uses albumin with and without a traditional hemodialysis machine to cleanse the blood of toxins that would otherwise be cleared by the liver. While traditional hemodialysis removes water-soluble toxins, albumin is used to remove lipophilic toxins. MARS therapy is usually reserved as a short-term treatment for fulminant liver failure and as a bridge to transplantation. MARS requires insertion of a central hemodialysis catheter. It is associated with hypocalcemia, thrombocytopenia, and hypotension that must be treated aggressively. The patient described above, with two vasopressor therapy, would be the prototypical end-stage liver disease (ESLD) patient on MARS therapy as a bridge to transplant.

What Is the Etiology of the Hematologic Abnormalities of Liver Failure?

Hematologic abnormalities include decreased synthesis of coagulation factors, including fibrinogen and factors II, V, VII, IX, and X. In addition, decreased absorption of vitamin K results from decreased bile acid secretion, and leads to elevation of prothrombin time (PT) and partial thromboplastin time (PTT). Thromobocytopenia occurs secondary to hypersplenism. Production of the procoagulant factors, proteins S and C, and antithrombin III, are also decreased.

What Is the Etiology of the Electrolyte Abnormalities? How Will These Results Modify Your Perioperative Management?

Preoperative renal insufficiency exacerbates acid-base and electrolyte abnormalities whereas diuretic therapy may also cause electrolyte disturbances, such as hyponatremia, hypokalemia, and hypocalcemia. Hypoglycemia may also occur secondary to impaired gluconeogenesis and glycogenolysis with reduced glycogen stores.

What Monitors Are Needed for the Case?

In addition to standard ASA monitors, it is necessary to have an arterial line to help draw frequent labs needed throughout the case, and to guide strict control of blood pressure. A central venous line facilitates infusion of vasopressors and rapid administration of blood products. In addition, one to two large-bore peripheral IVs are placed in the upper extremity because the inferior vena cava (IVC) is clamped for a significant portion of the procedure. Fluid warmers, external warmers, and heat/moisture exchangers are used as well to keep the patient warm as hypothermia can exacerbate coagulopathy and alter drug metabolism.

How Does Liver Failure Affect Your Choice of Medications?

Since the liver is the primary organ for drug metabolism and plays a central role in both drug pharmacodynamics and pharmacokinetics, end-stage liver disease alters the expected pharmacokinetics and pharmacodynamics of drug administration. In the absence of dose alteration, one can expect to see extended drug duration of action and possible toxic levels for hepatically metabolized medications. This occurs due to impaired protein synthesis involving alpha-1-glycoprotein and albumin increasing the free fraction of drugs (i.e., opioids), potentially exaggerating their effects. Second, the biotransformation of drugs via cytochrome P450 is decreased, allowing the drug to persist far longer than expected. However, end-stage liver disease also affects volume of distribution, hepatic extraction and metabolism, and renal excretion, making broad recommendations for drug administration difficult.

As a result of this alteration in drug effect, medications should be titrated to effect. Long-acting medications need to be carefully selected as their duration of action may outlast their desired effects. In the case of muscle paralysis, it may not be an issue if extubation is not intended and pancuronium is administered. However, in the event of administration of morphine or vecuronium with the intent of extubation at the conclusion of the procedure, there might be accumulation of drug and residual narcosis and paralysis, respectively.

How Will You Proceed with Induction of Anesthesia?

There is no established standard induction for liver transplantation. If ascites is present, or there is recent food ingestion or delayed gastric emptying, a rapid sequence induction is indicated. Succinylcholine can be used in the absence of hyperkalemia associated with hepatorenal syndrome. Rocuronium, 1–1.2 mg/kg, provides muscle relaxation in a timeframe sufficient for rapid sequence induction. Fentanyl will not accumulate with renal disease and has minimal histamine release.

During the Preanhepatic Phase of Liver Transplantation, What Major Surgical Steps Occur and What Management Options Are Available?

The preanhepatic phase starts with induction of anesthesia and concludes with placement of clamp on the hepatic artery to effectively isolate the native liver. The superior vena cava (SVC), IVC, and portal vein are all clamped as well, and the bile duct is divided. The key issues encountered during this phase are hypotension secondary to any bleeding related to a preexisting coagulopathy, especially in patients who have had a prior Kasai procedure. Fresh frozen plasma and packed red blood cells are given to correct coagulopathy and bleeding respectively. Hypotension will occur when a large amount of ascites is drained on incision. Albumin is used to quickly expand the intravascular volume in anticipation of loss of venous return that accompanies the placement of the vena caval clamps. With the piggyback technique, only a partial cross clamp of the IVC is necessary which decreases the loss of cardiac preload. Metabolic issues with hyperkalemia, hypocalcemia, and acidosis can occur and need to be corrected. A previous Kasai procedure may make dissection of the native liver difficult secondary to scarring and adhesions as well as increase the risk for major bleeding.

A hemoglobin between 9 and 10 g/dL and an INR of 1.5 are appropriate if there is no hemodynamic instability. Thromboelastography (TEG) has been used successfully in pediatric liver transplantation, providing an indicator of clotting factor activity, platelet function, and fibrinolysis (see Chapter 9).

During the Anhepatic Phase of Liver Transplantation, What Major Surgical Steps Occur and What Management Options Are Available?

The anhepatic phase begins with en-bloc resection of the native, diseased liver and ends with release of the clamps and reperfusion of the new liver. Any hypotension resulting from the loss of preload with caval clamping should be treated with volume expansion and vasopressors to maintain blood pressure. However, aggressive fluid therapy can cause hepatic venous congestion after reperfusion. Dopamine and/or epinephrine may be needed to maintain mean arterial pressure

(MAP) during this stage. In the absence of a functioning liver, anesthetic adjustments will be necessary as drug metabolism can be profoundly depressed. Excessive fluid administration should be avoided to prevent elevated right atrial pressure at reperfusion, which can cause graft congestion following reperfusion. Children often have normal urine output during this stage because of collateral vessels; therefore, urine output should not be used as a guide to fluid administration during the anhepatic phase. Because the portal vein is clamped during the anhepatic stage, portal venous hypertension develops with fluid translocation and bowel edema. Colloid administration may theoretically reduce the amount of bowel edema and potentially facilitate easier abdominal closure at the end of the procedure.

Metabolic abnormalities may occur following cross-clamping. Ionized calcium may decrease because the liver does not metabolize citrate, and metabolic acidosis may worsen because the liver does not metabolize lactate to bicarbonate. Metabolic acidosis also occurs secondary to impaired tissue perfusion. Hypoglycemia is further exacerbated with loss of gluconeogenesis and glycogenolysis. An infusion of 0.25–0.5 g/kg of glucose and 0.2 units/kg regular insulin may also be administered to reduce the serum K^+ concentration.

Monitoring and correction of pH, electrolytes, calcium, and glucose are necessary. Calcium chloride and calcium gluconate are equally efficacious in improving ionized calcium concentrations. As a result of these metabolic challenges, serial ABGs are drawn to ensure correction of electrolyte and acid base disturbances.

Intraoperative administration of blood products, particularly fresh frozen plasma, further decreases ionized calcium and magnesium because citrate-based anticoagulant solutions used in blood collection and storage bind these ions. Significant bleeding may still occur from collateral vessels and previous scar tissue. An underbody forced air warmer should be used as patients become hypothermic when the new liver (previously on ice) is inserted. Body temperature should be increased to 36–37°C prior to reperfusion.

During the Reperfusion Phase of Liver Transplantation, What Major Surgical Steps Occur and What Management Options Are Available?

The reperfusion stage (also known as neohepatic phase) starts with release of all clamps with blood flow established to the new liver.

Reperfusion begins with the release of the suprahepatic IVC clamp followed by removal of the portal vein and infrahepatic IVC clamps. Inadequate fluid resuscitation, insufficient flushing of the cold preservative solution, and release of vasoactive substances into the central circulation may cause hemodynamic instability from elevated pulmonary vascular resistance, decreased cardiac output, and decreased systemic vascular resistance. The cold solution may directly decrease cardiac output, necessitating warm irrigating solution in the surgical field. Aggressive fluid resuscitation (central venous pressure (CVP) >10 mmHg) may cause graft engorgement and cause areas of the graft to become ischemic during this phase. Volume resuscitation should occur prior to clamp removal.

Within One Minute After the Vascular Clamps Are Removed, a Prolonged QT Interval, Peaked T Waves, Bradycardia, and Hypotension Occur. What Is This Reaction and How Is It Treated?

ECG changes are often caused by the rapid intravenous infusion of effluent from the transplanted liver. The transplant preservative fluid has a low pH and temperature and is high in potassium. In addition, infusion of air and/or microthrombi into the heart may precipitate acute pulmonary hypertensive crisis. Vigorous flushing of the liver (by the surgeon) with colloid solution followed by retrograde flushing with the recipient's blood prior to reperfusion reduces the potassium concentration and acid content of the effluent as the preservation fluid is very high in potassium (125 mmol/L in University of Wisconsin solution (UWS) solution). Preemptive treatment with sodium bicarbonate, calcium chloride as well as inotropic support can help maintain stability during this phase. At this point, any coagulopathy that needs correction will be treated, as well as restoration of circulating intravascular volume to maintain urine output and MAP sufficient to perfuse the liver. In addition, the biliary drainage system is constructed with either a Roux-en-Y in the case of biliary atresia or a direct biliary anastomosis.

Hepatic artery thrombosis may result from coagulation and hematologic disorders and/or technical factors during hepatic artery anastomosis. Intraoperative and postoperative Doppler ultrasound may be used to assess anastomosis patency. Hemoglobin concentrations should be maintained between 8 and 10 mg/dL to decrease blood viscosity while maintaining oxygen delivery. Aggressive fresh frozen plasma and platelet administration may also increase blood viscosity, increasing the risk of hepatic artery thrombosis. PT and PTT should be maintained no less than 1.5 times prolonged, and platelet counts of 50,000–100,000 are acceptable, if there are no signs of microvascular bleeding and hemodynamic instability. Furthermore, children are hypercoagulable following liver transplantation secondary to decreased protein C and antithrombin III, additionally increasing the risk of hepatic artery thrombosis.

What Intraoperative Clinical Findings Indicate a Well Functioning Graft?

Reduction in calcium supplementation requirements are consistent with adequate hepatic allograft function secondary to improved citrate metabolism. The development of metabolic alkalosis is also an indicator of adequate graft function secondary to lactate metabolism to bicarbonate. Hyperglycemia post reperfusion is an additional marker of adequate graft function with the restoration of gluconeogenesis and glycogenolysis.

What Are Immediate Postoperative Considerations?

It is common practice to leave patients intubated for the first 24–48 hours after liver transplant and transport to the ICU although early extubation is appropriate in uneventful and hemodynamically stable transplantations. Given the large subcostal incision, the child should be comfortable enough to adequately oxygenate and minimize atelectasis. If the patient remains intubated, PEEP is used to minimize atelectasis during positive pressure ventilation as ascites, pulmonary edema, and pleural effusions may occur. Third-spacing and blood loss will continue and may manifest as hypotension. IVF and albumin along with any necessary blood products should be considered in an effort to maintain euvolemia. Hepatic artery thrombosis is a very common vascular complication that occurs in pediatric liver transplantation. Some surgeons may request anticoagulation in the immediate postoperative period if risk of thrombosis is high. Bowel perforation is less likely, but also known to occur and requires returning to the operating room for laparotomy.

> The patient is extubated in the operating room and transported to the intensive care unit, where 12 hours later the patient has worsening coagulation studies, metabolic acidosis, and hypoglycemia.

What Is the Main Etiology of Graft Failure?

Patients may be started on a heparin or dopamine infusion to maintain hepatic artery patency as hepatic artery thrombosis (HAT) is the most common etiology for graft failure. HAT is directly related to the size of the vessels and thus is most likely in the smallest pediatric recipients. HAT is a serious postoperative complication that can result in bacteremia, biliary stricture, and hepatic necrosis with resultant loss of the graft. The incidence has been found to be as high as 25%, with children younger than three years at greatest risk. Transplant recipients with HAT have a 50% survival rate (and most undergo retransplant) compared to an 80% survival rate of those without HAT. Surgical factors that may play a role include technique of anastomosis, vessel size less than 3 mm, use of grafts, and donor anatomy. Medical factors include use of procoagulants and hyperviscosity from blood product administration. Bile leaks resulting from bile duct ischemia secondary to early HAT require retransplantation.

Suggested Reading

Cladis F, et al. Organ Transplantation. In Cote and Lerman, eds. *A Practice of Anesthesia for Infants and Children*. 5th Ed. Elsevier 2013.

Chapter 29

Renal Transplantation

Miguel R. Prada

The first case in your operating room assignment is a living related donor kidney transplant. The recipient is a 16-year-old Caucasian female with chronic kidney disease (CKD) 5 due to obstructive nephropathy. She initially presented six months ago with progressive fatigue, headaches, nausea, and vomiting.

Initial workup demonstrated a serum creatinine of 7.5, BUN 105, sodium 134, potassium 5.8, bicarbonate 12, calcium 6.2, phosphorus 10.3, hemoglobin 7.2. Vital signs: heart rate 89, BP 148/89, temperature 36.5°C.

Renal ultrasound demonstrated bilateral small kidneys with loss of cortico-medullary differentiation and bilateral severely dilated collective systems. Since the initial diagnosis, she has been treated with sodium bicarbonate tablets, calcitriol, darbepoietin alfa, atenolol, and sevelamer carbonate. The related donor is her mother, a 38-year-old healthy woman with no significant past medical history.

Immediate preoperative vital signs include: blood pressure 138/86, heart rate 62, temperature 36.5°C, SpO_2 100% on room air.

What Is Chronic Kidney Disease (CKD)?

Chronic kidney disease (CKD) is defined by the National Kidney Foundation Kidney Disease and Outcome Quality Initiative (KDOQI) Group in any patient older than two years, with kidney damage lasting for at least three months with or without a decreased glomerular filtration rate (GFR), or any patient who has a GFR of less than 60 mL/min per 1.73 m^2 lasting for 3 months with or without kidney damage.

What Are the Stages of CKD?

The KDOQI Group classifies CKD into five stages based on GFR (Table 29.1).

When Are Patients with CKD Eligible for Kidney Transplantation?

Discussion for renal replacement therapy including renal transplantation starts when the patient reaches stage 4 CKD. Initial workup for renal transplantation is also initiated. Preemptive kidney transplantation is done when dialysis has not been started prior to transplant and it is the optimal treatment to avoid the four-fold increase in morbidity and mortality associated with dialysis.

What Organ Systems Are Affected in Patients with End-Stage Renal Disease (ESRD)?

Multiple systems are affected by ESRD including:

- cardiovascular
- endocrine
- hematologic
- bone and mineralization homeostasis.

What Laboratory Abnormalities Would You Expect in a Patient with ESRD?

Anemia. Anemia of CKD develops as a result of both decreased production secondary to low erythropoietin and increased red blood cell turnover due to uremic toxins in patients with shortened lifespans. It presents as moderate to severe normochromic and normocytic anemia without increased reticulocytes.

Electrolyte Abnormalities. Common electrolyte disturbances include mild hyponatremia due to volume overload and hyperkalemia due to decreased clearance of potassium and acidosis.

Impairment of tubular excretion function results in hyperphosphatemia with hypocalcemia due to

Table 29.1 Classification of chronic kidney disease (CKD) by glomerular filtration rate (GFR).

CKD Stage	Glomerular filtration rate (GFR) mL/min/1.73 m^2
Stage 1	Kidney disease with GFR greater than 90
Stage 2	60–89
Stage 3	30–59
Stage 4	15–29
Stage 5: End-stage renal disease (ESRD)	<15

secondary hyperparathyroidism and vitamin D deficiency as there is no conversion of 25-hydroxyvitamin D to 1,25 (OH)2D in renal proximal tubules.

Acid Base Disturbance. The high-anion gap metabolic acidosis is a consequence of failure of adequate excretion of acid anions (mainly ammonium but also phosphate and sulfate).

There is also a significant decrease in reabsorption and synthesis of bicarbonate which would serve as body buffer.

The deleterious consequences for metabolic derangements include renal osteodystrophy, arterial calcification, and increased risk of death.

What Are the Most Common Clinical Manifestations of ESRD?

- Neurological: Headaches, dysautonomia, uremic encephalopathy, cognitive alteration, fatigue, muscle weakness, peripheral neuropathy, increased risk of stroke, and in severe cases seizures and coma.
- Cardiovascular: Hypertension, fluid overload, left ventricular hypertrophy, arterial calcifications, early atherosclerosis, increased risk of cardiovascular disease.
- Endocrine: Vitamin D deficiency, renal osteodystrophy, short stature, growth retardation, dyslipidemia, malnourishment, sick euthyroid syndrome, delayed puberty, anovulation.
- Gastrointestinal: nausea, emesis, gastric paresis, insulin resistance.
- Hematologic: anemia, increased bleeding risk (uremia induced platelet dysfunction), immunosuppression due to T and B cell dysfunction.

What Is the Incidence of ESRD in Children?

In 2007, the reported incidence of ESRD in the United States was 1.48 per 100,000 children. As per the United States Renal Data System (USRDS) 2016 report, a total of 9,721 children were treated for ESRD by December 31, 2014.

What Are the Most Common Initial Treatment Options in Children with ESRD?

Treatment for ESRD includes renal replacement therapy and renal transplantation. Peritoneal dialysis (PD) was the most common initial ESRD treatment modality in children younger than nine years weighing less than 20 kg. Overall, the most common treatment for children with ESRD is hemodialysis (HD) at 50.4%.

What Are the Most Common Diagnoses Leading to Transplantation for Children with ESRD?

As per the 2014 annual transplant report from the North American Pediatric Renal Trials and Collaborative Studies (NAPRTCS), out of 11,186 pediatric renal transplants:

- Aplastic/hypoplastic/dysplastic kidney disease = 15.8%.
- Obstructive uropathy (15.3%) most common cause of ESRD requiring renal transplantation.
- Focal Segmental Glomerulosclerosis (FSGS) = 11.7%.
    - FSGS is the most frequent cause of ESRD in African American patients.

What Is the Age Distribution for Pediatric Renal Transplants?

Of the 718 listed pediatric renal transplants in 2015:

- Less than 1 year of age: 2 transplants (0.28%).
- 1 and 5 years old: 163 transplants (22.7%).
- 6–10 years: 145 transplants (20.2%).
- 11–17 years: 408 transplants (56.8%).

What Preoperative Workup Should You Order Before Proceeding?

A deceased donor kidney transplant (DDKT) is considered a semi-urgent procedure in an attempt to decrease the cold ischemia time. Cold ischemic time is the time between cooling of the kidney after organ procurement to the time when the kidney reaches physiological temperature during implantation into the recipient. On the other hand, a living donor kidney transplant is entirely an elective procedure. For both cases, workup should be completed prior to surgery.

Clinical workup should be focused on current vital signs and ever-changing volume status. In patients with hypertension, the blood pressure target should be below goals for stage 2 hypertension.

Hypertension. Preoperative administration of scheduled antihypertensive medications is recommended with the exception of Angiotensin-Converting Enzyme Inhibitors (ACEI) and Angiotensin II Receptor Blockers (ARBII), which are still controversial due to risk of intraoperative hypotension. Recently, Roshanov et al. demonstrated that in adults, withholding ACEI/ARBII before major non-cardiac surgery was associated with a lower risk of death and postoperative vascular events. However, no such studies exist in children undergoing renal transplantation regarding ACEI/ARBII administration. The major risk of withholding these medications is postoperative hypertension.

Volume Maintenance. Perioperative volume status is vital during renal transplant. ESRD patients managed by hemodialysis (HD) or peritoneal dialysis (PD) have a specific target weight after dialysis called estimated dry weight. Comparison of actual weight with dry weight gives the best evidence of fluid depletion or fluid overload. In scheduled kidney transplant cases, discussion with a pediatric nephrologist about lower fluid removal during HD or PD before surgery is key. Intravascular volume depletion after dialysis is a risk factor for graft acute tubular necrosis (ATN) or delayed function.

Laboratory Workup. Workup should, at minimum, include:

- Complete blood count (CBC), mainly hemoglobin and platelets
- Electrolytes/chemistry including Na^+, K^+, Ca^{2+}, Cl^-, HCO_3^-, BUN, creatinine, and glucose
- Coagulation studies: PT, PTT and INR
- Blood type and screen and/or type and cross-matching.

Imaging Studies. Yearly echocardiogram is usually obtained in patients with CKD 5 and ESRD to monitor for development of left ventricular hypertrophy, ventricular dilation, and both aortic and coronary calcifications. The leading cause of morbidity and mortality in children with ESRD in dialysis and post renal transplantation is cardiovascular disease.

What Are the Transfusion Goals for Patients Undergoing Renal Transplantation?

Most patients undergoing kidney transplant will have mild anemia. The KDIGO (Kidney Disease, Improving Global Outcomes) guidelines on anemia sets a treatment goal hemoglobin of 10–12 mg/dL with erythropoietin-stimulating agent (ESA).

If required, red blood cells should be irradiated (due to immunosuppression) and washed to decrease risk of hyperkalemia.

Are There Any Contraindications to Renal Transplantation in Children?

Children with uncontrolled extrarenal malignancies, sepsis, or multiorgan failure are usually not considered to be candidates for renal transplantation.

Improvements in immunosuppression protocols have permitted transplantation in ABO incompatibility situations but is not frequently seen in pediatrics.

Kidney transplant should be delayed for 12 months in patients with rapid progressive glomerulonephritis due to elevated levels of circulating antibodies and high risk of disease recurrence in the transplanted kidney.

What Monitors Do You Plan to Employ During the Transplant Operation?

In addition to the ASA standard monitors, providers should consider a 5 lead EKG, central venous pressure (CVP), and possible beat-to-beat invasive arterial blood pressure monitoring (IABP). The noninvasive blood pressure (NIBP) cuff should be placed on the upper extremity contralateral to the AV-fistula site. In addition to protecting the fistula, should great vessels need to be clamped, lower extremity blood pressure will not be accurate.

CVP is useful for intraoperative fluid management and can be monitored using an existing dialysis catheter or after placement of an internal jugular central line (ideally multilumen).

The IABP placement should be discussed with the Pediatric Nephrologist because of the possibility of a future need for an arterio-venous (AV) fistula. It should be considered in children less than 12 years of age, renal transplant requiring anastomosis of allograft into aorta and inferior vena cava, history of stage 2 hypertension, significant coronary and aortic calcifications, moderate to severe cardiac valvular disease, and heart failure. If IABP is needed, we recommend use of ultrasound guided placement and avoidance of brachial vessels with goal of placement one attempt, distal radial artery (in order to prevent damage) or dorsalis pedis artery.

How Would You Induce Anesthesia in This Patient?

Most patients will have intravenous access (IV) as usually they are admitted for prehydration, laboratory workup, and blood cross-match. Premedication with IV midazolam is generally safe and will alleviate anxiety in already highly medicalized patients.

Patients should be NPO except for medications including oral immunosuppression agents such as tacrolimus and mycophenolate mofetil, in addition to regular antihypertensives. Induction with opioids and propofol should commence with the goal of avoiding hypotension, followed by a short-acting non-depolarizing neuromuscular blocker (NDMR) (unless need for rapid sequence intubation) like rocuronium or ideally cisatracurium which is neither metabolized nor excreted by the kidney. Intermittent doses of NDMR should be continued to maintain 1–2 twitches for adequate relaxation during the procedure. After adequate placement of endotracheal tube if needed an arterial line should be placed and baseline arterial blood gas should be sent along with baseline hemoglobin. If the patient does not have an existing HD catheter to monitor CVP, placement of a right internal jugular catheter should be considered. As most patients typically have undergone prior IJ vascular access for HD catheters, vessels should be scanned with ultrasound for patency and to rule out thrombus presence.

What Are the Options for Intraoperative Analgesia?

Epidural analgesia has been safely used for perioperative and postoperative pain management but concerns for both hypotension and possible platelet dysfunction secondary to uremic platelets have decreased significantly the use of this type of pain management. The best approach is multimodal analgesia including non-opioids, opioids, NMDA receptor blockers, and local anesthetics at the incision site.

Perioperative opioids should be used with caution. Meperidine is not recommended due to accumulation of the active metabolite normeperidine, which decreases the seizure threshold and may cause convulsions. Morphine should be used with caution due to accumulation of morphine-6-glucuronide, an active metabolite that increases sedation and can cause respiratory depression. Morphine-3-glucuronide accumulation can cause neuroexcitation. Hydromorphone and fentanyl are the recommended opioids. Hydromorphone needs to be administered with caution as patients with ESRD can accumulate hydromorphone-3-glucuronide which may also cause neuroexcitation. Fentanyl is one of the opioids of choice for renal transplantation and is considered safe in ESRD with its lack of active metabolites. However, fentanyl clearance may be slightly decreased. Methadone is considered relatively safe, as it has no active metabolites and does not result in plasma accumulation.

Other analgesics have been used including: IV acetaminophen, NDMA receptor blockers, ketamine (0.5 mg/kg can be repeated every two hours or via infusion at 4–8 mcg/kg/min) in addition to other medications such as dexmedetomidine for their opioid sparing effects. Dexmedetomidine has the theoretical benefit of increasing urine output with the possible side effect of hypotension which is undesirable during renal transplantation.

How Would You Manage Intraoperative Fluids?

Intraoperative IV fluid management during pediatric renal transplant has been controversial. In the past, an isotonic solution without added potassium has been recommended to prevent hyperkalemia. Historically, normal saline 0.9% (NS 0.9%) has been used for this purpose. Potura et al., in a prospective randomized control trial in adults, demonstrated that use of NS

0.9% during deceased-donor renal transplant (DDRT) increased the incidence of hyperkalemia by 17% between groups compared to an acetate-buffered balanced crystalloid. This worsening hyperkalemia is likely secondary due to high chloride concentration, lack of base or buffer, low pH of 5.5, and high doses during transplant, producing a hyperchloremic metabolic acidosis.

We recommend the use of a buffered balanced solution, such as plasmalyte. IV fluids should be titrated to achieve euvolemia with a CVP of 8–10. Many transplant surgeons will request administration of supra-physiologic amounts of crystalloids and colloids in order to obtain a CVP 12–15 prior to unclamping vein and artery with the theoretical purpose of improving graft perfusion. However, Taylor et al. demonstrated that this practice may result in pulmonary edema.

After reanastomosis of the transplanted ureter, fluid management can be switched to two infusions, one at fixed rate for insensible losses (600 mL/m^2/day or about 2.5 mL/kg/h) and the other infusion to replace urine output at a rate of 1 ml of fluid per ml of urine output per hour. This fluid management will usually be adapted by the pediatric nephrologist in the pediatric intensive care unit to better maintain fluid homeostasis.

The Perioperative Immunosuppression Required for Renal Transplantation

Timing of the induction of immunosuppression is crucial in order to prevent acute graft rejection which is highest during the perioperative period. The choice of induction therapy remains controversial in children and is institution dependent. It generally includes intravenous/central anti T-cell antibodies combined with conventional immunosuppression agents. In some instances, it is initiated during the preoperative period by administering conventional oral immunosuppression agents like macrolides, such as tacrolimus or sirolimus along with antimetabolites like azathioprine or mycophenolate. Specific medications will be determined by institutional protocol. Again, good communication among the pediatric nephrologist, anesthesiologist, and transplant surgeon is key.

The pediatric anesthesiologist is involved by administering the perioperative antibody induction. These medications may include polyclonal antilymphocyte antibodies like rATG-thymoglobulin (Thymoglobulin, rabbit-derived) and antithymocyte globulin (ATGAM, horse-derived). The antiinterleukin-2 receptor monoclonal antibody (IL-2 RB) like basiliximab may also be used as an induction agent. Infusion of polyclonal antibodies may cause a massive cytokine release causing fever, rash, tachycardia, and chills. Pretreatment with acetaminophen, diphenhydramine and steroids usually prevents these side effects. IL-2 RB agents generally do not have this response.

The Specific Management Immediately Prior to Kidney Reperfusion

During the procedure, the surgeon may request heparin during recipient vessels cross-clamping. The patient will need to be well hydrated and obtain at least a normal CVP ~ 8–10 mmHg before reperfusion. Depending on center specific protocols, the surgeon may request supra-physiologic CVP ~12 along with mannitol and 1–2 mg/kg or furosemide and even a low dose dopamine infusion (1–5 mcg/kg/min) prior to unclamping of the vessels. However, none of these interventions have demonstrated improved outcomes on graft perfusion, prevention of delayed function, and graft survival.

Once the kidney is reperfused, urine output from the graft can be confirmed in the surgical field. The final stage is reanastomosing the graft ureter with the native ureter, which in some cases may be performed by a pediatric urologist. After an uncomplicated transplant course in the absence of severe pulmonary or cardiac disease, most patients may be extubated at the end of the case. If extubation criteria are not met or intraoperative complications like pulmonary edema or severe fluid shifts are present, extubation should be delayed and the patient transferred to the pediatric intensive care unit (PICU), intubated, and sedated. Most patients are usually managed in the PICU where adequate pain control and hemodynamic and fluid management are ensured.

How Would You Manage Hypotension During Ureteral Reimplantation?

Hypotension management during renal transplant is one of the most controversial subjects in the field. Patients with CKD 5 or ESRD are at high risk of hypotension during anesthesia due to calcification and decreased compliance in both arteries and veins.

Vasodilation due to inhaled anesthetics is more pronounced and response to vasoconstrictors such as direct peripheral Alpha-2 agonists like phenylephrine is decreased. These effects may be especially pronounced in patients taking antihypertensives such as ACEI or ARBII.

Historically, dopamine has been the medication of choice as the vasoconstriction effect is minimal at low doses and theoretically improves renal perfusion. This statement has been rejected by several publications although a recent review of the management in pediatric renal transplant patients demonstrated that intraoperative use of dopamine was an independent risk factor for delayed time to creatinine nadir in all grafts 9.5 days versus 6.5 days in patients without dopamine. In deceased donor grafts, the difference was even greater, 12.9 days versus 7.4 days.

The use of other vasoactive medications is not recommended due to possible renal artery constriction and decreased renal perfusion. Primary treatment of hypotension should initially be managed with intravenous crystalloid or colloid boluses to achieve normal CVP. Discussion with the surgeon should occur about starting vasopressor agents to treat hypotension after normal CVP is achieved with fluids. No specific agent has shown outcomes improvement versus the other, so the choice has to be made by the surgical and anesthesia team. Theoretical decreased graft perfusion due to vasoconstriction as a consequence of vasoactive medications has been described.

Suggested Reading

Kraut JA, Madias NE. Metabolic acidosis of CKD: an update. *Am J Kidney Dis.* 2016;67(2):307–17. PMID: 26477665.

McDonald SP, Craig JC; Australian and New Zealand Paediatric Nephrology Association. Long-term survival of children with end-stage renal disease. *N Engl J Med.* 2004;350 (26):2654–62. PMID: 15215481.

Warady BA, Chadha V. Chronic kidney disease in children: the global perspective. *Pediatr Nephrol.* 2007;22(12):1999–2009. PMID: 17310363.

Roshanov PS, Rochwerg B, Patel A, et al. Withholding versus continuing angiotensin-converting enzyme inhibitors or angiotensin II receptor blockers before noncardiac surgery: an analysis of the vascular events in noncardiac surgery patients cohort evaluation prospective cohort. *Anesthesiology.* 2017;126(1):16–27. PMID: 27775997.

Potura E, Lindner G, Biesenbach P, et al. An acetate-buffered balanced crystalloid versus 0.9% saline in patients with end-stage renal disease undergoing cadaveric renal transplantation: a prospective randomized controlled trial. *Anesth Analg.* 2015;120(1):123–9. PMID: 25185593.

Taylor K, Kim WT, Maharramova M, et al. Intraoperative management and early postoperative outcomes of pediatric renal transplants. *Paediatr Anaesth.* 2016;26(10):987–91. PMID: 27535492.

Myringotomy and Ear Tube Placement/Upper Respiratory Infection

Rebecca Evans and William D. Ryan

A two-year-old girl presents for myringotomy and ear tube placement. Over the past few days, she has had clear rhinorrhea and a nonproductive cough. On arrival her oral temperature is 38.0°C and the perioperative nurse discusses case cancellation with you. Lung auscultation is clear bilaterally.

What Are the Indications for Myringotomy and Ear Tubes?

Children with frequent ear infections (three ear infections in a six-month period or four ear infections within one year) should receive myringotomy and ear tubes to prevent chronic hearing loss and/or a cholesteatoma as a result of the accumulation of fluid in the middle ear with subsequent infection. The criteria can be shortened if the child has demonstrated diminished hearing.

What Will Your Anesthetic Plan Be for This Child?

Myringotomy and ear tube placement is a relatively minor and short procedure. Nearly all anesthetics consist of mask anesthesia with sevoflurane, without intravenous catheter placement, unless there are additional patient factors that warrant a more invasive strategy. Some children will awaken with severe ear pain that typically lasts an hour or two. Pain management varies between centers, and ranges from oral to intramuscular use of opioids and/or nonsteroidal antiinflammatory agents.

A study by Stricker et al. suggested that a combination of intramuscular fentanyl (1.5 mcg/kg) and ketorolac (1.0 mcg/kg) was associated with optimal outcomes with respect to analgesia and postoperative nausea and vomiting.

What Are the Implications of This Patient's Respiratory Symptoms?

Viral upper respiratory tract infections (URIs) are frequent in children, especially during the winter months. Typical symptoms include rhinorrhea, congestion, cough, fever, and malaise. Subclinical manifestations may include upper and lower airway edema, increased respiratory tract secretions, pneumonia, and bronchial irritability.

What Are the Increased Anesthetic Risks in Children with a URI?

Intraoperative airway complications during general anesthesia appear to be more common in children with a URI. These include coughing, laryngospasm, bronchospasm, and hypoxemia. Infants under 12 months of age tend to have more intraoperative complications than older children, and use of an endotracheal tube as compared with a facemask or laryngeal mask airway (LMA) increases the risk of these complications, but even LMA placement may be associated with complications in children with a URI. Passive exposure to cigarette smoke and a history of atopy are additional risk factors.

Transient postoperative hypoxemia, postintubation croup, and postoperative pneumonia are probably more likely to occur in children with a URI. Long-term complications and true outcomes are difficult to define and quantify and may not differ between normal children and those with a current or recent URI.

In infants and children with a URI, apneic oxygenation is less effective; thus oxyhemoglobin desaturation may occur when, during rapid sequence induction, the child is not receiving positive-pressure ventilation.

Should This Case Be Postponed Until a Later Date?

When a child presents with a URI, it is intuitive that an elective procedure requiring general anesthesia should be postponed until the child is well. But, because so many children have a concurrent URI at the time of their scheduled surgery, and long-term negative outcomes have not been demonstrated, this decision process is complex. How, then, should the anesthesiologist decide when to cancel an elective procedure in a child with a URI? First, one should assess the severity of the child's illness. The child with a runny nose without additional findings may be suffering from vasomotor or allergic rhinitis, which is usually not associated with perioperative airway complications. The following factors are associated with an increase in perioperative complications:

- Significant coexisting medical disease (especially cardiac, pulmonary, or severe neuromuscular disease);
- History of prematurity;
- Lower respiratory tract signs (e.g., wheezing, rales);
- High fever (>38.8°C);
- Productive cough;
- Major airway, abdominal, or thoracic surgery.

If any of these risk factors are present, it may be prudent to perform the procedure at a later date when the child is in better health.

On the other hand, there are a variety of additional factors that may influence your decision to proceed with surgery or cancel the case. The most common reason for proceeding with a case even though risk factors are present is the presence of a URI that will likely continue without surgical intervention. This occurs when children require adenoidectomy or myringotomy to relieve chronic middle ear fluid collections. Nonmedical factors that might sway you in favor of proceeding with the case are logistical family concerns, such as the parents taking a day off from work, difficulty obtaining day care, traveling a long distance at a great inconvenience to the family, etc. Since outcomes are not proven to be worse after surgery in children with a URI, these factors may play a role in the decision of whether or not to proceed. Most children who present with a URI have neither extremely mild symptoms nor severe symptoms. For these in-between children we must use our judgment to determine the proper course of action based on what we believe is best for the child.

How Would You Alter the Anesthetic Management of the Child with a URI Compared with a Healthy Child?

Anesthetic management of the child with an active or recent URI should be tailored to minimize airway irritability. Administration of a neuromuscular blocker to facilitate tracheal intubation will prevent laryngospasm. Humidification of airway gases may prevent the thickening of secretions that is commonly encountered in these children. Some pediatric anesthesiologists will administer an anticholinergic agent, such as atropine or glycopyrrolate, to attenuate vagally mediated airway complications; however, this remains untested. When feasible, facemask or LMA anesthesia is preferred over endotracheal intubation.

Some clues to the risks of URI can be gleaned by the results of a 2010 study in over 9,000 patients. A positive respiratory history (nocturnal dry cough, wheezing during exercise, wheezing more than three times in the past 12 months, or a history of present or past eczema) in a child with a URI was associated with an increased risk for intraoperative bronchospasm, laryngospasm, and perioperative cough, desaturation, or airway obstruction. In addition, a history of at least two family members having asthma, atopy, or smoking increased the risk for perioperative respiratory adverse events. In 2019, the REACT trial suggests a reduced incidence of peri-operative adverse events in children undergoing adenotonsillectomy following pre-treatment with albuterol. Those children having received pre-treatment with albuterol had reduced incidence of laryngospasm, coughing, and oxygen desaturation.

If You Decide to Postpone the Case, When Is It Safe to Proceed with This Procedure?

There is no consensus when to schedule elective surgery following an acute URI. In a 1979 publication that described the development of lower respiratory symptoms during general anesthesia in children with a URI, McGill and colleagues from DC Children's Hospital wrote: "the optimal period of recovery from the URI that should be allowed prior to considering the patient a candidate for an elective surgical procedure has not been defined." Nearly 40 years later, this is still true. Subclinical pathology, such as airway edema, atelectasis, and bronchial reactivity may remain for up to several weeks after the symptoms of the acute URI have resolved, depending on the specific type of viral agent. Three to four weeks seems to be a reasonable waiting time, but for many children this merely represents the period between successive illnesses.

Suggested Reading

Cohen MM, Cameron CB. Should you cancel the operation when a child has an upper respiratory tract infection? *Anesth Analg*. 1991;72 (3):282–8. PMID: 1994755.

Cote CJ. The upper respiratory tract infection (URI) dilemma: fear of a complication or litigation? *Anesthesiology*. 2001;95(2):283–5. PMID: 11506096.

Stricker PA, Muhly WT, Jantzen EC, et al. Intramuscular fentanyl and ketorolac associated with superior pain control after pediatric bilateral myringotomy and tube placement surgery: a retrospective cohort study. *Anesth Analg*. 2017;124 (1):245–53. PMID: 27861435.

Tait AR, Malviya S, Voepel-Lewis T, et al. Risk factors for perioperative adverse respiratory events in children with upper respiratory tract infections. *Anesthesiology*. 2001;95:299–306. PMID: 11506098.

von Ungern-Sternberg BS, Sommerfield D, Slevin L, et al. Effect of albuterol premedication vs placebo on the occurrence of respiratory adverse events in children undergoing tonsillectomies: The REACT randomized clinical trial. *JAMA Pediatr*. 2019 Apr 22. [Epub ahead of print] PMID: 31009034.

Chapter 31

Adenotonsillectomy

Rebecca Evans

A four-year-old child presents over winter break for a tonsillectomy, adenoidectomy, and bilateral ear tubes. When interviewing the patient, mom reports her child "snores all night long, sometimes stops breathing, and has fallen asleep in her preschool class." She has no neurologic or developmental delays.

She has had a series of ear infections, with the most recent infection last month. A hearing test was performed, showing diminished hearing which is causing her to fall behind her peers with regard to speech development.

In the preoperative area, she had clear rhinorrhea, non-productive cough. She complains of left ear pain. Her temperature is 38.0°C and the perioperative nurse discusses case cancellation with you. Lung auscultation is clear bilaterally.

How Common Is Pediatric Obstructive Sleep Apnea (OSA) Syndrome?

Currently 1–4% of children carry a diagnosis of OSA and with improved diagnostic techniques, the prevalence will continue to increase.

What Is the Difference Between Sleep Disordered Breathing and OSA?

Sleep disordered breathing is a generalized term that encompasses all abnormalities associated with breathing during sleep, ranging from snoring to obstructive sleep apnea.

Obstructive sleep apnea is a form of sleep disordered breathing with specific criteria including the symptoms of snoring, increased respiratory effort, periodic obstructive apnea, and oxygen desaturation.

What Is the Gold Standard for Diagnosing OSA?

The most reliable and validated way to diagnose OSA is by an overnight polysomnogram.

The diagnostic criteria for OSA in children include a child with an apnea duration of two breaths, hypopnea desaturation >3%, hypopnea duration of two breaths and hypopnea nasal pressure drop >50%.

How Do You Determine the Severity of OSA?

The severity of OSA is based on four criteria:

- Apnea-hypopnea index (AHI), number of hypopnea/apnea events secondary to obstructive events during sleep for 60 min as observed during polysomnography
- Nadir of oxygen saturation
- Percentage of sleep time with a P_{ETCO_2} > 50 mmHg
- Respiratory arousal index (RAI): the number of respiratory arousals per hour of sleep

Severe obstructive sleep apnea has an AHI >10, nadir SpO_2 <80%, P_{ETCO_2} >50 mm Hg >20% of the total sleep time, and RAI >8 per hour of total sleep time.

Commonly used severity classifications are the indices from the American Society of Anesthesiologists Task Force on Perioperative Management of Patients with Obstructive Sleep Apnea and the McGill Oximetry scoring system (Tables 31.1 and 31.2). In the absence of a sleep study, the clinical questionnaire OSA 18 can be used to determine the presence and severity of pediatric OSA.

What Are the Most Common Indications for Tonsillectomy in Children?

The most common indications for tonsillectomy include sleep-disordered breathing in younger age-group children and recurrent throat infections in older children. Both of these conditions can negatively impact the quality of a child's health. In the United States, tonsillectomy is one of the most common surgical procedures. There are more than 530,000 cases performed annually in children younger than 15 years. Most cases of tonsillectomy for sleep disordered breathing or OSA are performed in conjunction with an adenoidectomy.

When Are Tonsillectomy or Adenoidectomy Performed Alone?

Isolated tonsillectomy is indicated for recurrent pharyngo-tonsillitis, chronic tonsillitis, hemorrhagic tonsillitis, peritonsillar abscess, streptococcal carriage, dysphagia, abnormal dento-facial growth, halitosis, and suspicion of malignant disease. Isolated adenoidectomy is performed for recurrent or chronic rhinosinusitis or adenoiditis, and sometimes along with myringotomy tubes to treat recurrent otitis media.

INTRAOPERATIVE

Does the Presence of Sleep Disordered Breathing Affect Your Induction Plan?

Children with sleep-disordered breathing may have nasal airway obstruction as well. Ensuring that the mouth remains open and the use of an oral airway with a CPAP of 5–10 cm H_2O may aid in maintaining airway patency during inhalational induction.

Table 31.1 OSA severity scale by AHI between children and adults from the American Society of Anesthesiologists Task Force on Perioperative Management of Patients with Obstructive Sleep Apnea. AHI, apnea hypopnea index; OSA, obstructive sleep apnea

OSA severity	AHI in children	AHI in adults
None	0	0–5
Mild	1–5	6–20
Moderate	6–10	21–40
Severe	>10	>40

What Are Some Signs of Obstruction During Inhalation Induction?

Signs of respiratory obstruction include tachypnea; intercostal, sternal, and suprasternal retractions; grunting; nasal flaring; and oxygen desaturation.

How May You Adjust Your Pain Management Plan in a Patient Diagnosed with OSA?

The use of nonopioid adjunct pain medications will aid in ensuring a balance of pain control with appropriate respiratory ventilation in the postoperative period. Short-acting opioids such as fentanyl are easy to titrate to effect with less concern for respiratory depression in the post-anesthetic care unit (PACU). Patients with obstructive sleep apnea were found to require less pain medication than patients without obstructive sleep apnea who were undergoing a tonsillectomy and adenoidectomy. Some physicians prefer to administer approximately half of their normal opioid dosing regimen to patients with obstructive sleep apnea.

Other adjuncts such as acetaminophen, dexmedetomidine and high doses (1 mg/kg up to a total of 25 mg) of dexamethasone reduce postoperative pain without decreasing respiratory drive.

The use of NSAIDs, such as ketorolac, remains controversial. A meta-analysis revealed an increased number of patients returning to the operating room for postoperative bleeding in the setting of NSAID use. However, the study design was plagued by small sample sizes. Further meta-analyses revealed no

Table 31.2 The McGill Oximetry Scoring System. The severity of OSA is determined by the SpO_2 nadir and by the number of desaturation events during nocturnal oximetry. OSA, obstructive sleep apnea

Oximetry score	OSA classification	No. of desaturation events <90% SpO_2	No. of desaturation events <85% SpO_2	No. of desaturation events <80% SpO_2
1	Normal	<3	None	None
2	Mild	≥3	≤3	None
3	Moderate	≥3	>3	≤3
4	Severe	≥3	>3	>3

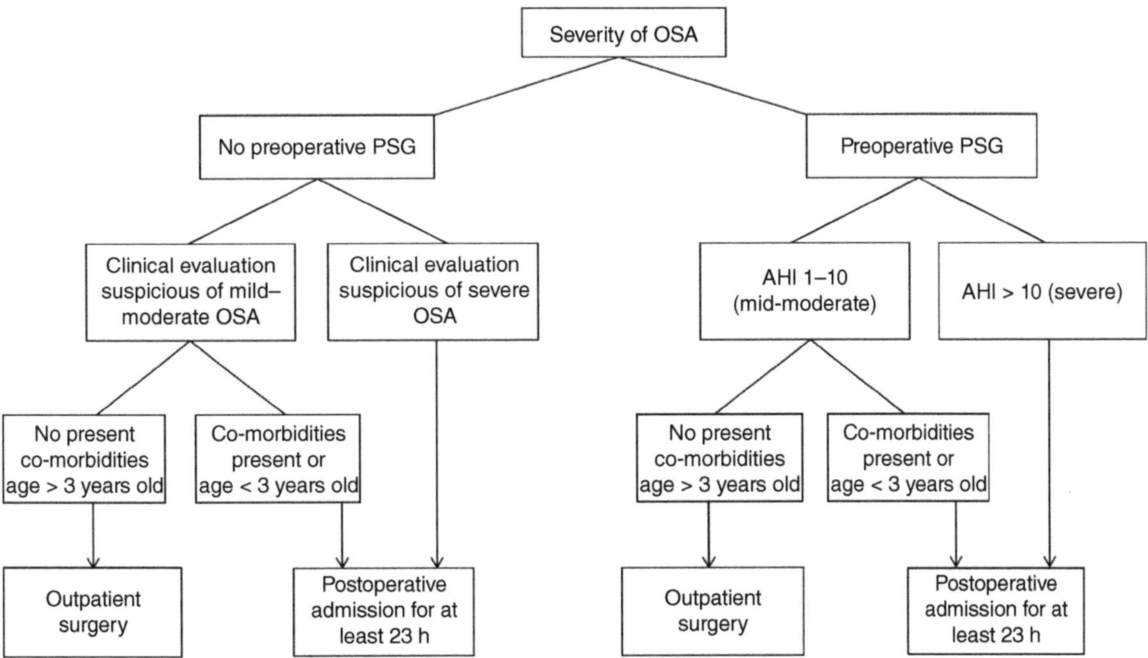

Figure 31.1 Postadenotonsillectomy disposition for children with OSA. PSG=polysomnography, AHI=apnea/hypopnea index. Reproduced with permission of Elsevier from: Patino M, et al. *Br J Anaesth* 2013;111 Suppl 1:i83–95. Copyright © 2012 M. Patino, S. Sadhasivam, M. Mahmoud.

increase in the risk of postoperative bleeding in the setting of NSAID use. Current practice varies among institutions.

POSTOPERATIVE

Which Patients Undergoing a Tonsillectomy and Adenoidectomy Should Remain in the Hospital Overnight for Observation?

The American Academy of Pediatrics (AAP) guidelines recommend postoperative admission for children with OSA who are under three years of age, are obese, or have serious comorbidities or severe OSA (AHI > 24/h, SpO_2 nadir $<80\%$, or peak $PCO_2 \geq$ 60 mm Hg).

Definitive studies have not yet determined set criteria for hospitalization and are generally based on expert consensus. However, most physicians use the following data as indication for hospitalization: children under three years old, diagnosis of severe OSA via polysomnogram, and/or presence of additional comorbidities such as hypotonia, obesity, failure to thrive, and/or severe structural airway abnormalities.

An excellent schematic for determining postoperative disposition may be found in Figure 31.1.

What Postoperative Complications Are Associated with Tonsillectomies and Adenoidectomies?

Complications can be divided into respiratory and non-respiratory:

Respiratory

- Hypoxemia and/or prolonged oxygen requirements
- Hypercapnia
- Postoperative pulmonary edema, which may require interventions such as intubation
- Anesthetic complications

Nonrespiratory Complications

- Pain
- Poor oral intake and dehydration
- Nausea and vomiting
- Airway hemorrhage

What Is the Incidence of Postoperative Tonsillar Bleeding? When Is It Most Likely to Occur?

Approximately 3–4% of tonsillectomies (16,000 cases) performed in the United States are associated with postoperative tonsillar bleeding.

A bimodal distribution of the onset of tonsillar bleeding is observed. The first 24 hours may be associated with a brisk, postoperative tonsillar bleed often associated with poor hemostasis or in a patient with an unknown bleeding disorder. The next most common time for a patient to present with a postoperative tonsillar bleed is 7–10 days postprocedure when the healing eschar falls off the tonsillar bed.

What Are the Anesthetic Considerations for a Postoperative Tonsillar Bleed?

Post-tonsillar bleeds can be separated into the acute and significant bleed and the slow oozing type bleed. A brisk and potentially arterial bleed can be a life threating emergency with numerous cases of patients exsanguinating from bleeding tonsillar pillars. Slow and progressive bleeds are often venous in nature and should be dealt with in a semi-emergent manner. In either case, patients should be considered to have a full stomach. IV induction is most appropriate with or without rapid sequence type intubation. The evidence on having a type and cross, especially for slow oozing bleeding, is lacking, as the incidence of transfusion in these patients is low. Certainly, for brisk and arterial bleed, a type and cross-match is advisable; however, an emergent case should not be delayed to wait for type specific blood.

When May the Parents Begin to Notice a Difference in Their Child's Breathing after a Tonsillectomy and Adenoidectomy Performed for Sleep Disordered Breathing or OSA?

Children often have increased airway obstruction in the immediate postoperative period. The reduction in obstruction during sleeping is often not appreciated for approximately two to four weeks postoperatively.

What Are Some Common Complications Associated with Children after General Anesthesia Who Have a Predisposition to Anxiety?

Children who were anxious in the preoperative period were found to have more postoperative pain, require more pain medications while hospitalized and during their first three days at home, and have a greater incidence of emergence delirium, postoperative anxiety, behavioral changes (apathy, withdrawal, enuresis, temper tantrums, eating disturbances), and sleep disturbances (see Chapter 6).

Suggested Reading

Cohen MM, Cameron CB. Should you cancel the operation when a child has an upper respiratory tract infection? *Anesth Analg.* 1991;72 (3):282–8. PMID: 1994755.

Cote CJ. The upper respiratory tract infection (URI) dilemma: fear of a complication or litigation? *Anesthesiology.* 2001;95:283–5. PMID: 11506096.

Marcus CL, Brooks LJ, Draper KA, et al. Diagnosis and management of childhood obstructive sleep apnea syndrome. *Pediatrics.* 2012;130 (3):576–84. PMID: 22926173.

Patino M, Sadhasivam S, Mahmoud M. Obstructive sleep apnoea in children: perioperative considerations. *Br J Anaesth.* 2013;111 Suppl 1:i83–95. PMID: 24335402.

Raghavendran S, Bagry H, Detheux G, et al. An anesthetic management protocol to decrease respiratory complications after adenotonsillectomy in children with severe sleep apnea. *Anesth Analg.* 2010;110(4):1093–101. PMID: 20142343.

Tait AR, Malviya S, Voepel-Lewis T, et al. Risk factors for perioperative adverse respiratory events in children with upper respiratory tract infections. *Anesthesiology.* 2001;95:299–306. PMID: 11506098.

Thongyam A, Marcus CL, Lockman JL, et al. Predictors of perioperative complications in higher risk children after adenotonsillectomy for obstructive sleep apnea: a prospective study. *Otolaryngol Head Neck Surg.* 2014;151(6):1046–54. PMID: 25301788.

Uliel S, Tauman R, Greenfeld M, et al. Normal polysomnographic respiratory values in children and adolescents. *Chest.* 2004;125 (3):872–8. PMID: 15006944.

Chapter 32

Tracheobronchial Foreign Body

Maura Berkelhamer and Kasia Rubin

An 18-month-old boy has sudden onset of tachypnea and coughing at home while playing with beads. Upon presentation to the emergency department, the child has right-sided wheezing and decreased air entry. The child is scheduled for bronchoscopy and removal of a presumed bronchially located bead.

What Is the Typical Presentation of Foreign Body (FB) Aspiration?

The majority of FB aspirations in small children are witnessed. Early symptoms include drooling, tachypnea, retractions, stridor, wheezing, and/or use of accessory muscles. Children with greater than 24 hours of symptoms may present with tachypnea, fever, and signs of respiratory distress.

What Is the Most Common Type of Aspirated FB?

Foods such as nuts and seeds, as well as other organic material in the bronchial tree, are the most commonly aspirated objects, but any small object, such as a bead, can be accidently inhaled when a toddler places it in his or her mouth. Because of their inability to coordinate swallowing and breathing movements, children under the age of four should not be fed any kind of small nut.

It is interesting to note the types of foreign bodies anesthesiologists *don't* see presenting for urgent bronchoscopic removal. Larger items such as hot dogs, balloons, and plastic wrappers can seal off the airway. They are not easily dislodged by either the Heimlich maneuver or coughing. Aspiration of these objects is associated with a high fatality rate.

How Does the Physical Exam Help to Locate the FB in the Airway?

The presence of stridor or wheezing may help you to determine the location of the FB. Stridor is produced by turbulent airflow through an obstructed airway. Inspiratory stridor usually indicates obstruction at or above the larynx. Expiratory or biphasic stridor generally points to obstruction below the larynx.

Decreased breath sounds are a very common finding and may help to determine the laterality of a bronchially placed FB. The incidence of right-sided foreign bodies is higher than foreign bodies in the left-sided bronchial tree. The absence of breath sounds over a portion of lung provides a clue to where you are likely to find the FB obstructing the airway: high in the hypopharynx obstructing the glottis opening, at the carina obstructing the mainstem bronchi or in the esophagus compressing the trachea.

Are Diagnostic Radiographs Necessary?

Not necessarily if the aspiration or sudden choking episode was witnessed. The vast majority of objects aspirated into the tracheobronchial tree are radiolucent, and chest radiographs are often not suggestive of pathologic changes in the first 24 hours after aspiration. A large review of airway FB cases found that only 11% of aspirated objects were radiopaque. Unilateral emphysema may be seen on chest X-ray due to the ball-valve effect of a distal obstruction. Radiographs are usually indicated when there is no history of a witnessed aspiration, and the child has an undiagnosed persistent cough or unilateral wheeze.

Radiographic signs of a lower bronchial obstruction may include:

- Air trapping on the side of occlusion by the FB exerting a ball-valve effect

- Flattened diaphragm
- Mediastinal shift to the unaffected side
- Bronchogram w/ cut-off
- Right middle lobe collapse
- Left upper lobe collapse

When Is Removal of a Bronchial FB a Surgical Emergency?

Conditions that warrant immediate bronchoscopy and removal of the FB include cyanosis/hypoxemia, or increased work of breathing. The suspicion of lipid pneumonitis due to an inhaled peanut, or tissue corrosion due to inhalation of a disc battery are also important reasons to attempt removal as soon as possible. When a peanut is aspirated, the patient's symptoms may worsen as the peanut oils initiate an inflammatory reaction. The peanut may swell and become more brittle, complicating removal.

What Is the Preferred Anesthetic Management Technique for FB Removal?

Most children presenting for removal of a bronchial FB will have an intravenous catheter *in situ* on arrival to the operating room. Midazolam can be titrated to achieve anxiolysis in the preoperative holding area under direct supervision of the anesthesiologist. An anticholinergic agent such as atropine or glycopyrrolate can also be administered to decrease secretions and block a vagal response. If a full stomach is suspected, rapid sequence induction and tracheal intubation may be performed prior to gastric evacuation; however, if there is suspicion that the FB could move distally with positive pressure ventilation, then spontaneous ventilation with an inhaled agent may be indicated.

There are advantages and disadvantages of both spontaneous and controlled ventilation methods during bronchoscopy. During spontaneous ventilation, interruptions in the anesthesia breathing circuit will not interfere with continuous oxygenation, and for some obstructive lesions with a ball-valve effect, negative pressure breathing may provide better oxygenation and ventilation. Disadvantages of spontaneous ventilation include the requirement to maintain a sufficient depth of anesthesia to obliterate airway reflexes and prevent patient movement during instrumentation yet maintain sufficient ventilatory function and hemodynamic stability. Thus, topical anesthesia to the airway is an important component of this technique.

A controlled ventilation technique, which may or may not consist of the administration of a neuromuscular blocker, relies on intermittent positive pressure breaths between apneic periods when the surgeon instruments the airway. Its advantages include the ability to provide optimal oxygenation and ventilation during the breathing phase, and assurance of lack of patient movement. Its obvious disadvantage is that during periods of apnea, even with preoxygenation, there is a limited time before oxyhemoglobin desaturation will occur, and the child will require additional positive pressure breaths. Another significant disadvantage is the lack of assurance that positive pressure ventilation will be successful with an obstructive lesion within the airway. In the case of a FB lodged within the bronchial tree, a theoretical disadvantage of positive pressure is the unintentional movement of the object distally. This can worsen airway exchange or create a ball-valve effect with hemodynamic consequences secondary to lung compression of vascular structures. This complication is rare.

What Complications Can Occur during Removal of the FB?

- Inadequate air exchange after the bronchoscope is inserted (spontaneous ventilation via the rigid bronchoscope increases dead space, work of breathing, and leakage of ventilating volumes resulting in reduced ventilation and oxygenation);
- Large objects may not fit through the rigid scope channel and may require excessive manipulation to remove
- Organic objects may crumble into pieces that need to be removed with multiple reinsertions of the bronchoscope and forceps
- Bronchospasm
- Pneumothorax or pneumomediastinum
- Tracheal or bronchial laceration
- Aspiration of gastric contents
- Hypoxemia and hypercarbia
- Arrhythmias or cardiac arrest

What Complications Can Occur after Removal of the Bronchial FB?

- Airway edema requiring continuous treatment with IV dexamethasone, inhaled racemic epinephrine, or humidified oxygen
- Pneumonitis from peanut oils if the diagnosis was delayed
- Post-obstructive pulmonary edema

Suggested Reading

Fidkowski CW, Zheng H, Firth PG. The anesthetic considerations of tracheobronchial foreign bodies in children: a literature review. *Anesth Anal.* 2010;111(4):1016–25. PMID: 20802055.

Zur KB, Litman RS. Pediatric airway foreign body retrieval: surgical and anesthetic perspectives. *Paediatr Anaesth.* 2009;19 Suppl 1:109–17. PMID: 19572850.

Chapter 33

Laryngotracheal Reconstruction Surgery

Lisa D. Heyden and Deepak K. Mehta

A six-year-old female, born at 26 weeks' gestation, presents for an aero-digestive evaluation (bronchoscopy, laryngoscopy, esophagoscopy) as part of her presurgical evaluation prior to laryngotracheal reconstruction (LTR).

At present, she is tracheostomy-dependent due to severe, grade 3 subglottic stenosis.

Medications include: albuterol by nebulizer and ranitidine.

She has a 4.0 uncuffed tracheostomy tube in place with a heat and moisture exchanger (HME).

What Are the Most Common Indications for Which Laryngotracheal Reconstruction (LTR) Is Performed?

An LTR is performed in cases of acquired or congenital subglottic stenosis.

What Is Subglottic Stenosis (SGS)?

Subglottic stenosis is narrowing of the airway between the lower border of the cricoid cartilage and extending up to below the vocal folds (Figure 33.1).

The most rigid and unyielding part of the airway is the cricoid cartilage.

What Are the Causes of Acquired SGS?

Trauma to the subglottis is the primary cause of acquired subglottic stenosis (SGS), most commonly resulting from prolonged or traumatic endotracheal intubation.

Prolonged intubation or intubation with an oversized tube or overinflated endotracheal cuff increases the risk of developing SGS, especially in the presence of underlying congenital anomalies.

Risk of developing SGS is increased in the presence of inflammatory conditions, such as persistent gastroesophageal reflux.

The incidence of SGS in intubated neonates is reported to be 0–2% although most neonates can tolerate long periods of intubation without injury to the subglottis (in stark contrast to adults).

What Are the Causes of Congenital SGS?

Congenital subglottic stenosis is a rare birth defect due to incomplete recanalization of the laryngotracheal tube during gestation and is frequently associated with other congenital head and neck lesions and syndromes including: 22q11 deletion, Down syndrome, and CHARGE syndrome.

What Are the Symptoms and Signs of SGS?

Signs of SGS include "noisy breathing" or stridor, respiratory distress, history of recurrent croup, and exercise intolerance. Stridor in SGS is biphasic because of fixed narrowing of the extra-thoracic airway. This is in contrast to inspiratory stridor, characteristic of supraglottic pathology, and expiratory stridor, characteristic of intrathoracic pathology.

What Is the Myer–Cotton Grading Scale for Determination of Severity of SGS?

The stenosis is based on age-appropriate airway size and degree of narrowing.

Mild stenoses (grades 1 and 2) are usually managed nonoperatively, whereas more severe stenoses (grades 3 and 4) often require surgical intervention (Figure 33.2).

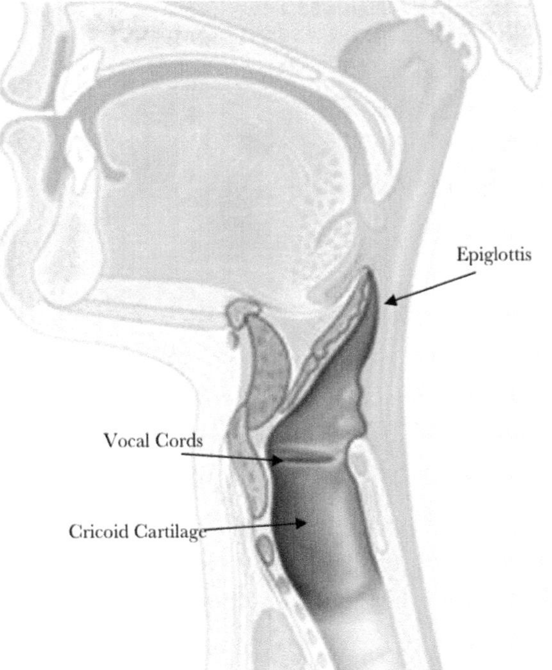

Figure 33.1 Schematic demonstrating the relationship between the vocal cords and cricoid cartilage

How Is the Airway Size Determined?

The airway is sized during suspension laryngoscopy. Under direct vision, the otolaryngologist places an uncuffed endotracheal tube through the vocal cords. A leak test is performed during which the insufflation is maintained at increasing pressures (e.g. 5, 10, 15 c H_2O) until a leak is visible under direct vision. The outer diameter of the uncuffed endotracheal tube determines the airway size. The largest tube that can be placed with an air leak less than 20 cm of water is recorded for staging.

What Is the Work-Up for SGS and Presurgical Planning?

A detailed history and physical exam is performed along with an assessment of voice quality.

A neck radiograph may demonstrate subglottic narrowing or masses (secondary stenosis which requires alternative treatment) and a CT scan may show complete tracheal rings (Figure 33.3).

Feeding abnormalities are evaluated and if there is suspicion of aspiration, a swallow evaluation is performed by a speech pathologist.

A comprehensive aero-digestive evaluation is performed during presurgical work up and planning.

The decision regarding whether or not to perform tracheal reconstruction is based on the degree of stenosis, the associated symptoms, and on the comorbidities. Children with a high risk for aspiration, severe tracheomalacia, or need for chronic ventilatory support are not good surgical candidates.

Preoperative diagnosis and treatment of conditions causing laryngeal inflammation, such as gastroesophageal reflux, eosinophilic esophagitis (EOE) or infection, is crucial as laryngeal inflammation affords a greater procedural failure rate.

During the evaluation, the otolaryngologist performs direct laryngoscopy and bronchoscopy to evaluate the degree of stenosis, as described above. A gastroenterologist performs an upper endoscopy with biopsy to screen for signs of inflammation suggestive of gastric reflux or EOE. Finally, a pulmonologist evaluates the lung status with flexible bronchoscopy and bronchial alveolar lavage.

The patient is considered suitable for airway surgery when the stenosis has matured (grade of stenosis is stable over time), there is no active inflammation, and ventilatory support is not needed.

What Is the Treatment for Mild SGS (Grade 1 and 2)?

Some cases of mild stenosis may be observed without intervention. Symptomatic but mild cases may need endoscopic treatment. A sickle knife can be used to divide thin tracheal webs. The stenosis is then dilated with a balloon. Lasers and micro-debriders are also sometimes used to remove scar tissue. Serial dilations, repeated at one- to three-week intervals, may be necessary. Children with thin, web-like, and soft stenosis consisting of immature scar tissue are likely to respond well to balloon dilation. Patients with mature, firm scars or cartilaginous narrowing are less likely to improve with conservative interventions.

What Is the Treatment for Severe Cases of SGS (Grade 3 and 4)?

Most patients with severe subglottic stenosis require a tracheostomy as the proximal airway is too narrow to accommodate the required flow. Speech therapy is often not tolerated as the airway doesn't provide sufficient flow to allow for the use of speaking valves or intermittent

Myer-Cotton Grading Scale for Subglottic Stenosis

Classification	From	To
Grade 1	No Obstruction	50% Obstruction
Grade 2	51% Obstruction	70% Obstruction
Grade 3	71% Obstruction	99% Obstruction
Grade 4	No Detectable Lumen	

Figure 33.2 Myer–Cotton grading system for degree of subglottic stenosis

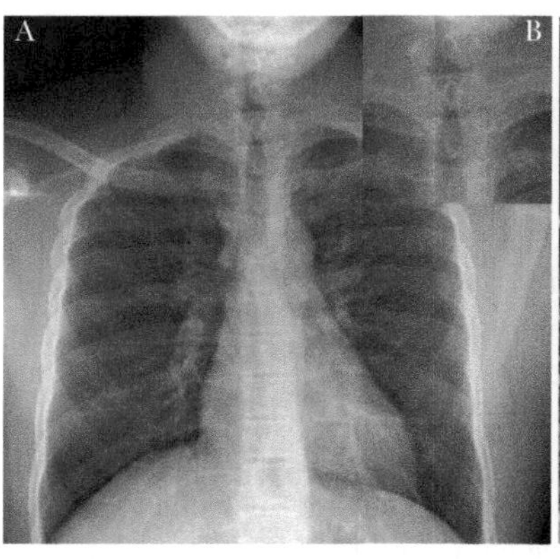

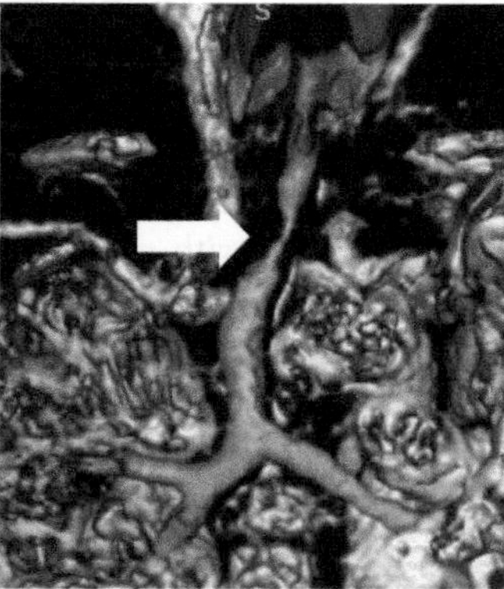

Figure 33.3 Radiographic appearance of severe tracheal narrowing by chest X-ray (A) with enlargement (B) (left) and CT 3D reconstruction of severe tracheal narrowing (white arrow) (right)

capping. Open surgical repair is often required to repair the stenosis and allow for tracheostomy decannulation. Decannulation rates after LTR are near 90%.

Laryngotracheal reconstruction can be performed as either a single or dual staged procedure. In both cases, a graft, usually costal cartilage, is inserted into the anterior and sometimes posterior tracheal wall to increase the diameter (Figure 33.4). In the single stage procedure, the tracheostomy tube is removed at the time of surgery. The patient remains intubated and sedated in the ICU for about seven days, then returns to the operating room for extubation. Another direct laryngoscopy and bronchoscopy are performed two weeks following the LTR procedure.

In the dual-staged procedure, the tracheostomy remains throughout the procedure and decannulation

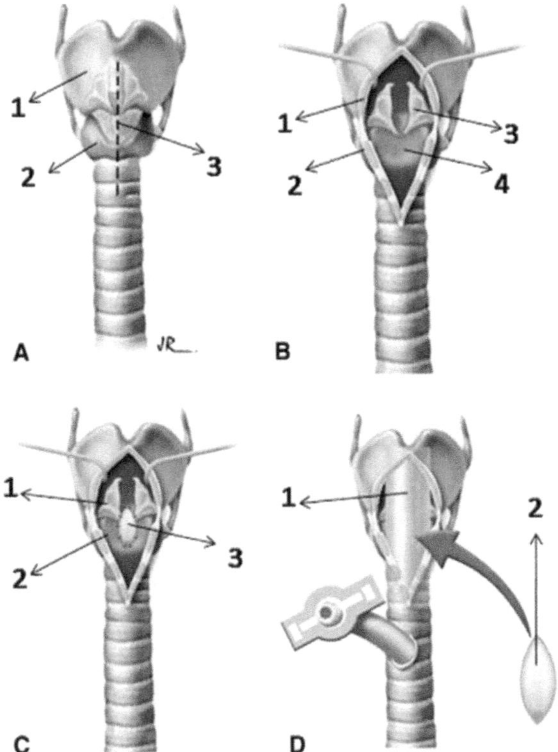

Figure 33.4 Schematic demonstrating the steps of standard laryngotracheal reconstruction. (A) Laryngotracheal anterior exposure: (1) thyroid cartilage; (2) cricoid cartilage; (3) incision site to perform anterior laryngeal split. (B) Airway exposure after anterior laryngeal split: (1) and (2) thyroid and cricoid cartilages split and retracted respectively; (3) arytenoids; (4) posterior cricoid plate, exposed and ready to be split. (C) Posterior larynx grafting and posterior cricoid split: (1) arytenoids; (2) posterior cricoid plate already opened; (3) rib cartilage graft filing posterior groove. (D) Laryngeal stent and anterior grafting: (1) solid stent inside the airway; (2) rib cartilage graft prepared to fill the anterior defect. Reproduced with permissions from Terra RM, et al., *J Thorac Cardiovasc Surg* 2009;137(4):818-23.

occurs at a later date after the airway size has been assessed for adequate patency. Double-stage repair may be advisable in cases of difficult intubation, poor pulmonary function, and those patients with prior failed reconstructions or sedation issues.

What Are Contraindications to LTR Surgery?

Contraindications to decannulation and surgery include: severe tracheomalacia, uncontrolled gastric reflux, asthma, active eosinophilic esophagitis, and tracheostomy tube dependence due to chronic pulmonary disease or neurologic impairment resulting in recurrent aspiration.

What Are the Major Anesthetic Considerations for Laryngotracheal Reconstruction?

Preoperative planning and close communication with the surgeon throughout the procedure are extremely important. To gain better surgical access to the neck, the tracheostomy tube is replaced by the surgeon with either a sterile wire-reinforced tube or an oral RAE tube that has been cut down by the surgeon to fit into the trachea. A Murphy eye may also need to be cut into the distal end of the altered RAE tube to limit the risk of tube obstruction. The stomal tube may need to be replaced by a nasal endotracheal tube after the airway is opened and the posterior graft is placed.

In single-stage procedures, without tracheostomy, an uncuffed nasal endotracheal tube is sutured in place by the surgeon. Sometimes balloon dilation of the airway is needed prior to intubation.

Total intravenous anesthesia is most commonly performed for maintenance with infusions being continued postoperatively to assure adequate sedations for airway protection.

Commonly used postoperative infusions at Texas Children's Hospital include: fentanyl (1–2 mcg/kg/hour), dexmedetomidine (0.3–1 mcg/kg/hour), and rocuronium (8–12 mcg/kg/minute).

Ketamine and/or midazolam infusions may be added in patients with a history of difficult sedation.

Complications from airway surgery can occur both intraoperatively or postoperatively. Intraoperative risks include tube dislodgement or obstruction, pneumothorax, and bleeding.

What Are the Postoperative Considerations with Regard to Ventilation and Sedation?

Postoperative sedation risks and benefits should be weighed. A limited period of sedation and immobilization may lower the risk of ventilator-acquired pneumonia, pressure ulcers, neuropathy and myopathy, as well as narcotic or benzodiazepine withdrawal. Sedation should eliminate anxiety and awareness in the initial postoperative period as well as decrease the risk of accidental extubation and manipulation of the surgical site. Often, the neck is kept in flexion to reduce tension on the airway anastomosis. The surgeon may elect to suture the endotracheal tube to the chest. Prolonged neck flexion results in significant neck spasms and may warrant scheduled diazepam during this period.

Paralysis with rocuronium, usually limited to the initial postoperative period (<24 hours), is administered to reduce the risk of airway granulation tissue formation resulting from mechanical sheer trauma (inadequately sedated patient resulting in friction from the tracheal tube with the surgical site). If neuromuscular blockade (NMB) is continued longer than 24 hours, NMB "holidays" should be incorporated in order to avoid patient muscle weakness.

Following a single-stage procedure with planned decannulation, the patient typically remains intubated in the PICU for one to three days after anterior grafting and five to seven days after anterior and/or posterior grafting.

Early postoperative complications also include wound infection, dehiscence, and graft dislodgement or displacement for both single- and double-stage reconstruction.

Extubation, along with direct laryngoscopy and bronchoscopy, is performed in the operating room. In the six- to twelve-hour period prior to going to the operating room, sedation protocols are converted to a propofol infusion at 50–100 mcg/kg/minute. Sedation boluses may be given, however, medications with long half-lives following continuous infusion should be stopped in the hours prior to the procedure. It is crucial that the patient not be overly sedated during extubation as this may contribute to failed extubation attempts. Steroids should be given prior to the operating room.

In the OR, the patient can be extubated to BiPAP or CPAP, although positive pressure may increase the risk of air leak and the development of subcutaneous air, pneumothorax, or pneumomediastinum.

Suggested Reading

Fauman KR, Durgham R, Duran CI, Vecchiotti MA, Scott AR. Sedation after airway reconstruction in children: a protocol to reduce withdrawal and length of stay. *Laryngoscope*. 2015;125:2216–19. PMID: 26152806.

Jefferson ND, Cohen AP, Rutter MJ. Subglottic stenosis. *Semi Pediatr Surg*. 2016;25:138–43. PMID: 27301599.

Maeda K. Pediatric airway surgery. *Pediatr Surg Int*. 2017;33:435–43. PMID: 28132084.

Terra RM, Minamoto H, Carneiro F, et al. Laryngeal split and rib cartilage interpositional grafting: treatment option for glottic/subglottic stenosis in adults. *J Thorac Cardiovasc Surg*. 2009;137 (4):818–23. PMID: 19327502.

Chapter 34

Thyroid Surgery

Adam C. Adler

> An 11-year-old female presents for subtotal thyroidectomy for Graves' disease. She has been treated with methimazole for the past three months and has a visibly enlarged anterior neck mass.

What Is Graves' Disease?

Graves' disease is the most common cause of hyperthyroidism in children. It is more common in females and often presents during the teenage years. It is an autoimmune disease in which thyroid-stimulating hormone (TSH)-receptor antibodies cause overproduction of TSH that activates the thyroid gland causing thyroid growth (goiter) and high levels of thyroid hormones. Common symptoms include tachycardia, tremors, weight loss, muscle weakness, heat intolerance, and insomnia. Some patients may demonstrate exophthalmos, an outward bulging of the eyes caused by periorbital inflammation, but this is less common in children. Medical management includes administration of antithyroid drugs, such as methimazole, radioactive iodine, or subtotal thyroidectomy when medical management fails or when the thyroid is large and unsightly. Surgical cure must be accompanied by lifetime administration of exogenous thyroid hormones. Beta blockers may be used to suppress palpitations, tachycardia, and tremors. In our patient, it is likely that her surgical intervention is mainly cosmetic and has been scheduled following a course of methimazole to ensure that her thyroid function is closer to normal at the time of surgery.

What Preoperative Laboratory Studies Are Indicated in This Patient?

Adequate thyroid suppression is evidenced by low or normal levels of circulating total T3 and free T4 as well as resolution of symptoms. A complete blood count should be obtained because of the rare occurrence of pancytopenia with antithyroid therapy.

Is a Cardiac Evaluation Warranted?

Depending on the duration of symptoms, Graves' disease patients are at risk for developing tachycardia-induced cardiomyopathy, but this is extremely rare in the pediatric population. Prolonged duration of untreated symptoms of tachycardia resulting from excessive circulating thyroid hormone can lead to dilated heart failure. Often, symptoms of heart failure can be identified by history. Chest radiograph can reveal an enlarged heart although in severe and prolonged cases, transthoracic echocardiography may be beneficial in identifying cardiac pathology prior to anesthesia.

How Is the Airway Evaluated in the Setting of a Large Thyroid Mass?

Patients should be questioned regarding their ability to lie supine and presence of dyspnea or dysphagia, which may reveal posterior compression of the airway and esophagus (Figure 34.1). A CT scan is helpful to assess upper airway compression. If significant airway compression exists, especially in the setting of dyspnea while supine, it may be prudent to perform tracheal intubation while the patient is breathing spontaneously (see Chapter 19). This is exceedingly rare in the pediatric population.

What Is a NIM Tube, and Why Is It Used for Thyroidectomy?

A neural integrity monitoring (NIM) tube is a specialized endotracheal tube for assessment of neural integrity during neck dissection. Electrodes on the endotracheal tube at the level of the vocal cords record stimulation of the laryngeal nerves. The proper

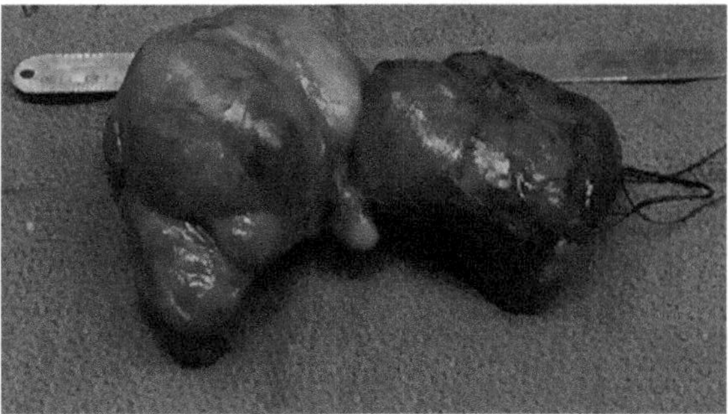

Figure 34.1 Gross thyroid specimen. The bulk of tissue seen here demonstrates the ability for the external mass to affect the airway. Additionally, this allows the provider to imagine the difficulty that would ensue during an attempted emergency tracheostomy trying to reach and identify the underlying trachea quickly and without causing significant bleeding. Courtesy of Adam C. Adler, MD

color-coded segment must be positioned between the vocal cords and is often done using a video laryngoscope to allow for visualization by surgical staff during placement.

What Is the Risk If a Recurrent Laryngeal Nerve Is Injured or Transected During the Surgical Procedure?

The recurrent laryngeal nerve is a branch of the vagus nerve and supplies all muscles of the larynx except the cricothyroid muscle. The cricothyroid muscle is a vocal cord tensor and is supplied by the superior laryngeal nerve. Recurrent laryngeal nerve damage results in unopposed action by the cricothyroid muscle causing closure of the vocal cords. Use of the NIM tube attempts to avoid accidental nerve damage by deliberate stimulation during dissection.

Identify the Timeframe and Causes of Postoperative Airway Obstruction

Immediate postoperative airway compromise following removal of the endotracheal tube is often the result of damage to the recurrent laryngeal nerves causing the vocal cords to obstruct the airway. As this complication is often unilateral, patients present with hoarseness or stridor.

Acute airway obstruction from a hematoma can occur immediately postoperatively and is the most frequent cause of airway obstruction in the first 24 hours. In the PACU, postoperative airway obstruction should raise immediate concern for a developing hematoma and may necessitate surgical reexploration.

Table 34.1 Symptoms and timeframe of airway obstruction following thyroid surgery

Postoperative timeframe	Cause	Symptoms
Acute onset	Recurrent laryngeal nerve injury	Unilateral: hoarseness Bilateral: aphona, airway obstruction
Acute to 24 hours	Hematoma formation	Acute to delayed hematoma formation resulting in external airway compression
24–48 hours	Hypocalcemia / trauma or complete parathyroidectomy	Signs of hypocalcemia

Twenty-four to forty-eight hours postoperatively, airway obstruction may be the result of accidental total parathyroidectomy or ischemia to the remaining parathyroid tissue. Hypoparathyroidism results in decreased production of parathyroid hormone resulting in decreased serum calcium. Hypocalcemia generally presents at 24–48 hours as laryngeal stridor and airway obstruction as calcium depletion does not occur immediately (Table 34.1).

What Are the Signs/Symptoms of Hypocalcemia?

Symptoms of hypocalcemia may include tingling of the lips and fingertips. Additional findings may develop, including carpopedal spasm, tetany, laryngospasm, seizures, QT prolongation, and cardiac arrest.

Examination: Chvostek's sign or elicited facial contraction following tapping the facial nerve in the per-auricular area and Trouseau's sign or carpal spasm on inflation of a blood pressure cuff.

Administration of one gram of calcium gluconate is generally sufficient in the immediate setting.

What Is Thyroid Storm?

Thyroid storm is a hypermetabolic state characterized by excessive thyroid hormone levels. This leads to excessive oxygen consumption and systemic sympathetic activation causing multiorgan failure. Thyroid storm is life threatening and requires immediate recognition and treatment. Recognition of thyroid storm in patients under general anesthesia can be challenging and requires a high level of suspicion.

Symptoms encompass nearly every organ system and can include: high fever, agitation, tachycardia, sweating, severe dehydration, peripheral edema, abdominal pain, nausea, vomiting, cardiac arrhythmia, cardiac failure, and pulmonary edema.

What Are the Causes of Thyroid Storm?

Most commonly, thyroid storm can result from: medication non-compliance, infection, trauma, surgery, myocardial infarction, diabetic ketoacidosis, and pregnancy.

What Is Treatment for Thyroid Storm?

Treatment is generally supportive: initiation of cooling, aggressive IV fluid administration, and electrolyte repletion. Cardioversion may be necessary if arrhythmia is present. Invasive or noninvasive ventilation should be considered as suggested by arterial blood gas results.

An endocrinology specialist should be consulted to guide thyroid suppression treatment. For achieving thyroid suppression, one should consider the five 'Bs': Block synthesis (i.e., antithyroid drugs); Block release (i.e., iodine); Block T4 into T3 conversion (i.e., high-dose propylthiouracil, propranolol, corticosteroid; Beta-blocker); and Block enterohepatic circulation (i.e., cholestyramine).

Suggested Reading

Bajwa SJ, Sehgal V. Anesthesia and thyroid surgery: the never ending challenges. *Indian J Endocrinol Metab.* 2013;17(2):228–34. PMID: 23776893.

Carroll R, Matfin G. Endocrine and metabolic emergencies: thyroid storm. *Ther Adv Endocrinol Metab.* 2010;1:139–45. PMID: 23148158.

Malhotra S, Sodhi V. Anaesthesia for thyroid and parathyroid surgery. *Cont Educ Anaesth Crit Car Pain.* 2007;7(2):55–8. https://doi.org/10.1093/bjaceaccp/mkm006.

Sinclair CF, Téllez MJ, Tapia OR, et al. A novel methodology for assessing laryngeal and vagus nerve integrity in patients under general anesthesia. *Clin Neurophysiol.* 2017;128(7):1399–405. PMID: 28395952.

Chapter 35

Myelomeningocele and Hydrocephalus

Adam C. Adler

> A four-year-old child presents for replacement of her ventriculo-peritoneal (VP) shunt. She has spina bifida diagnosed postnatally and has mild developmental delays. Over the last day, she was lethargic at home and "not acting herself" prompting a trip to the emergency department by her parents.
>
> In the preoperative area, she is responsive but very sleepy. Vitals include: Temp 37.6°C, BP 107/62, HR 67 bpm, SpO_2 100%. She is your next case to follow.
>
> Two hours later, the nurse in the preoperative holding area calls you concerned that she seems "sleepier" and not very arousable. She is also concerned that the patient's heart rate is only 49.

What Are the Types of Spina Bifida?

Spina bifida is a broad term encompassing defects of the skin (spina bifida occulta), vertebrae, meninges (meningocele), and spinal cord (myelomeningocele [MMC]).

What Are the Predisposing Risk Factors Related to Spina Bifida?

Maternal folate deficiency has been associated with a two- to eight-fold increased risk for developing spina bifida. Other maternal factors include vitamin B12 deficiency, pregestational diabetes, obesity, and antiepileptic use (carbamazepine and valproic acid). History of previous pregnancy (with the same partner) complicated by spina bifida affords significant increased risk.

What Prenatal Studies Are Performed to Assess for Spina Bifida and the Degree of Neurologic Involvement?

Elevated levels of maternal serum alpha-fetoprotein are suggestive of spina bifida or anencephaly. Amniocentesis allows for measurement of alpha-fetoprotein in the amniotic fluid and fetal karyotyping for associated chromosomal abnormalities. When the diagnosis is suspected, ultrasound or fetal MRI can assess for neurologic defects and presence of a Chiari malformation. Ultrasound of the lower extremities is used to assess fetal leg and foot movement and associated limb deformities.

What Is the Incidence of Myelomeningocele (MMC)?

The incidence of MMC is around 0.5–1:1,000 live births.

What Are the Etiologies of MMC?

The exact etiology of MMC remains unknown. Failure of closure of the neural tube or mesenchymal closure of the caudal neuropore during development has been suggested. Exposure of unprotected neural tissue may result in traumatization of the spinal cord. In addition, it is thought that prolonged exposure of the spinal cord tissue to amniotic fluid throughout gestation leads to damage.

What Is the Defect That Occurs with a MMC?

A defect in the vertebral arches leads to protrusion of the meninges and spinal cord (neural tissue).

What Are the Most Common Locations of MMC Defects?

Most commonly, the defect occurs in the lumbar region, although it can occur at any location along the spinal cord. Anencephaly occurs when the cerebral portion of the primary neural tube fails to close.

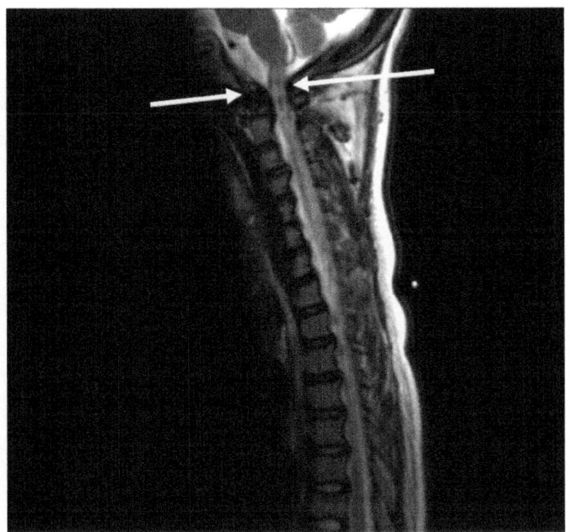

Figure 35.1 MRI of brain with herniation of cerebellar tonsil tissue at the level of the foramen magnum (arrows)

What Are the Potential Causes of Neurologic Morbidity in Patients with MMC?

Long-term sequelae relate to immobility leading to pressure-related ulcerations, venous thrombosis leading to deep venous thrombosis/pulmonary embolism, urinary tract infection from frequent bladder catheterizations, and issues relating to hydrocephalus and shunt function.

Hydrocephalus is common in children with MMC especially in the presence of Chiari malformations and may be related to obstruction of CSF flow by the herniated cerebellum (Figure 35.1).

What Are the Associated Neurologic Disabilities Attributed to a MMC?

Neurologic manifestations include: varying degrees of mental retardation, bowel and bladder dysfunction, and orthopedic-related disability. The degree of bowel and bladder dysfunction and extremity paralysis correlates with the level of herniated spinal cord tissue.

What Is the Rationale for Midgestation Fetal Repair of MMC?

Prolonged fetal exposure of the developing spinal cord to amniotic fluid is thought to contribute to significant neurologic morbidity. Fetal correction via a midgestational procedure has been shown to significantly improve neurologic function and reduce the morbidity from hydrocephalus and the Arnold–Chiari malformation. Fetal repair lends a significant reduction in the need for VP shunt, a major cause of morbidity for these patients. The considerations for fetal intervention are discussed in Chapter 46.

What Other Conditions Are Associated with a MMC?

Patients with spina bifida have a high incidence of Arnold–Chiari II malformation. The Chiari II malformation is herniation of the hindbrain (cerebellum and brainstem) through the foramen magnum. Fetal correction of MMC is associated with a reduced incidence of Chiari II malformations. Chiari II malformations are corrected by surgical decompression to remove the bone surrounding the hindbrain. The repair is performed in the prone position, is generally extradural and with the assistance of neurologic evoked potential monitoring.

What Is the Classic Allergy Triad in MMC Patients?

Patients with MMC are typically assigned an empiric latex allergy. Historically, latex-based products were used during the patient's surgical procedures in addition to the latex-based urinary catheters which led to sensitization and subsequent allergy. Latex is a rubber derivative. Additionally, a syndrome known as latex-fruit syndrome exists in which certain fruits (banana, kiwi, mango, pineapple, chestnuts, strawberry, and soy) produce a substance similar to that of latex which can also lead to allergic reaction. Approximately 30–50% of patients with latex allergy have cross allergic reactions to these fruits.

What Are the Signs and Symptoms of Patients with Chiari II Malformations?

Neonates with Chiari II malformations may present with swallowing difficulties, stridor, apneic spells, weak cry, or arm weakness. Older children and adults may present with bilateral limb weakness, muscle wasting, and sensory disturbances. Less commonly, dysphagia and ataxia can also be present.

What Are the Anesthetic Issues Associated with MMC Repairs?

Children with large MMCs generally undergo surgical repair in the first days of life as the exposed neural tissue is at risk for infection. Large open MMC should be kept covered and moist to prevent significant evaporative losses. When intubating these children, care must be taken to avoid pressure on neural tissue in the supine position. Foam or gel donuts are used under the patient to avoid pressure on the exposed spinal cord.

What Are Evoked Potentials?

Evoked potentials provide testing of the continuity of major neurologic tracts in the brain and spinal cord. The tracts are evaluated by application of an external stimulus and measurement of the signals propagated by the neurologic pathway. Testing of evoked potentials is generally reserved for surgical procedures during which a high risk of neurologic pathway disruption exists.

There are four main types of evoked potentials monitored in the operating room setting: visual, auditory, somatosensory, and motor potentials.

- Somatosensory evoked potentials (SSEP) involve a stimulus applied to the extremities with signal propagation sampled at the cortex.
- Motor evoked potentials (MEP) involve stimulation of the motor cortex with measurement of signal propagation at the extremities.

SSEP and MEP monitoring allow for monitoring of the posterior spinal cord and dorsal columns (SSEP) and the anterior spinal cord and corticospinal tract (MEP) respectively.

Evoked potentials measure a baseline amplitude (signal strength) and latency (time between signal transmissions). Continuous monitoring throughout the case is performed with changes from baseline signifying a potential disruption of neural tissue. Decreases in amplitude of >50% or increases in latency of >10% are usually considered significant. Corticospinal tract assessments (MEP) are assessed intermittently to assure tract integrity especially after hardware placement.

Table 35.1 Changes to measured amplitude and latency expected with commonly used anesthetic agents

	Amplitude	Latency
Volatile agents	↓	↑
Nitrous oxide	↓	–
Propofol	↓	↑
Benzodiazepines	–	–
Ketamine	↑	–
Etomidate	↑	↑
Opioids	–	–
Barbiturates	↓	↑

How Do Anesthetics Affect Evoked Potentials?

Commonly used anesthetic drugs have varying effects on the monitoring of evoked potentials (Table 35.1).

Neuromuscular blocking drugs preclude the monitoring of motor evoked potentials. Volatile agents generally affect evoked potential monitoring on a dose dependent basis. Maintenance of a continuous plane of anesthesia is paramount. Major changes to infusion levels or bolus doses can cause large changes in evoked potentials.

During the Surgical Procedure, the Neuromonitoring Technician Reports Loss of Signals. What Are the Next Steps in Management?

- The first step is to be certain that all team members, especially the surgeon, are aware of the signal change.
- Change to total intravenous anaesthesia (TIVA) technique if not already in progress.
- Consider reversing the last step of the procedure when appropriate (removal of pedicle screw, distraction of spine, etc.).
- Increase perfusion pressure using vasopressors to elevate the mean arterial pressure (and hence the spinal cord perfusion pressure).
- Consider placing arterial line/central line if pressor infusion to be continued postoperatively.
- Transfuse packed red blood cells (PRBC) if anemic.
- Maintain normocarbia.

- Reduce PEEP to optimize spinal cord perfusion.
- Maintain normothermia.
- Consider a wake-up test to assess neurologic function.
- Consider high dose corticosteroids.

What Are the Signs and Symptoms of Raised Intracranial Pressure?

Signs and symptoms of raised intracranial pressure (ICP) in children may include large head size, cognitive delays or regression, headache, incontinence, irritability, memory loss, decreased appetite, poor coordination, regression of milestones, seizures, visual disturbances.

What Are the Causes of Hydrocephalus in Children?

Hydrocephalus, or enlargement of the intracranial ventricles, is attributed to excess CSF production, disturbance of flow, or impaired reabsorption. Most commonly, the etiology of hydrocephalus involves impaired flow of CSF (obstructive hydrocephalus) and may be isolated or associated with other congenital or acquired malformations or tumors.

Prior to closure of the fontanelle, the infant skull can accommodate to ventricular enlargement. Once the fontanelle has closed, ventricular enlargement can lead to rapid and life threatening elevations in intracranial pressure if left untreated.

What Is Hydrocephalus Ex-Vacuo?

Hydrocephalus ex-vacuo refers to dilation of the ventricles due to surrounding brain atrophy and not the result of CSF flow obstruction.

Identify the Pathway from CSF Production to Reabsorption

CSF is produced by ependymal cells in the choroid plexus of the lateral ventricles. From there, CSF flows through the interventricular foramen into the third ventricle, through the cerebral aqueduct and into the fourth ventricle. The fourth ventricle, in communication with the spinal cord, allows CSF to flow in the subarachnoid space.

CSF is reabsorbed by the vascular system through dural venous sinuses in the spinal cord via arachnoid granulations.

What Is a Shunt?

A shunt is a valved conduit placed in the ventricle to allow drainage of CSF.

What Are the Indications for Shunt Placement?

Shunt requirement is based on symptomatology and/or the inability for CSF to flow properly.

What Are the Possible Locations for CSF Shunt Placement?

Shunts have their proximal end within the lateral ventricle (Figure 35.2). The distal end most commonly is placed in the peritoneal cavity. Other places for distal shunt placement are intra-pleural and intra-atrial. Intra-abdominal infection is the most common reason to avoid peritoneal shunt placement.

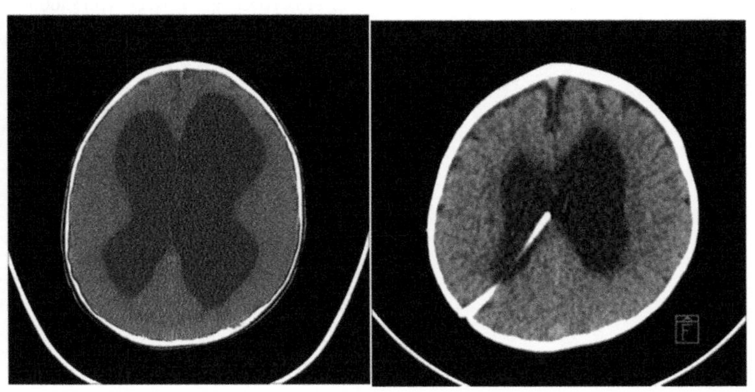

Figure 35.2 CT scan demonstrating hydrocephalus of the lateral ventricle pre (left) and post (right) decompression with a midline crossing VP shunt

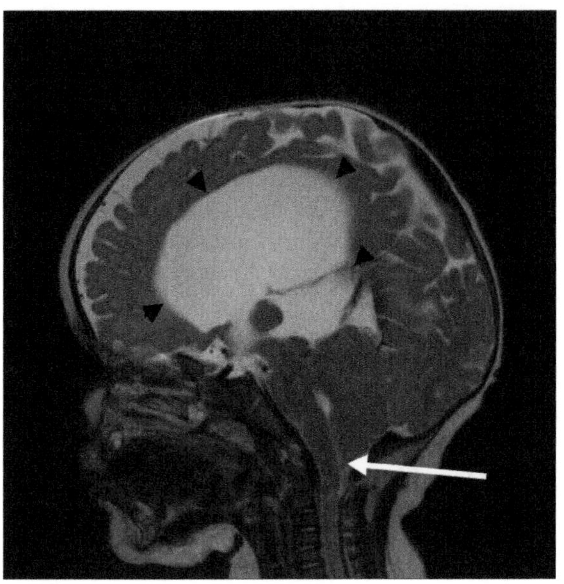

Figure 35.3 Brain MRI demonstrating enlargement of the lateral ventricle (arrow heads) and herniation of cerebellar tonsil (white arrow)

Describe the Symptoms and Signs Associated with Shunt Malfunction

Shunt malfunction in children with open fontanelle can be masked by enlargement of the head to accommodate the excess CSF (Figure 35.3).

In children with closed fontanelle, or those who have exhausted their compensatory mechanism, behavioral changes, somnolence, setting sun eyes, vomiting, and when severe, Cushing's reflex, may be present.

What Is the Cushing Reflex/Triad?

The Cushing reflex, described by famed neurosurgeon Dr. Harvey Cushing, is a physiologic response to elevated intracranial pressure. The reflex consists of hypertension, bradycardia, and an abnormal respiratory pattern. Hypertension may be a compensatory mechanism for preservation of cerebral perfusion in the setting of elevated ICP.

A Pre Op Nurse Calls You, Concerned for Bradycardia in a Patient Coming for VP Shunt Malfunction. What Is the Appropriate Plan of Action?

Bradycardia in this child may be the result of significant elevations in ICP. The neurosurgical team should be notified immediately, and the patient taken to the operating room emergently for decompression. CSF can be removed if an external ventricular drain is present. Drainage of CSF may be possible via needle insertion into a shunt with a reservoir by the neurosurgeon.

Suggested Reading

Adzick NS. Fetal myelomeningocele: natural history, pathophysiology, and in-utero intervention. *Semin Fetal Neonatal Med.* 2010;15 (1):9–14. PMID: 19540177.

Fetal surgery for spina bifida: past, present, future. *Semin Pediatr Surg.* 2013;22(1):10–17. PMID: 23395140.

Hadley DM. The Chiari malformations. *J Neurol Neurosurg Psychiatry.* 2002;72 Suppl 2: ii38–ii40. PMID: 12122202.

Kumar A, Bhattacharya A, Makhija N. Evoked potential monitoring in anaesthesia and analgesia. *Anaesthesia.* 2000;55(3):225–41. PMID: 10671840.

Mitchell LE, Adzick NS, Melchionne J, et al. Spina bifida. *Lancet.* 2004;364 (9448):1885–95. PMID: 15555669.

Chapter 36

Pediatric Neurological Tumors

Arvind Chandrakantan

A seven-year-old girl presents to the emergency department with recent onset of severe headaches, nausea and vomiting. Her vital signs include: BP 98/68, HR 122, RR 26/minute. An urgent CT scan demonstrates a large infra-tentorial mass. An MRI of the head with and without contrast is booked.

What Are the Different Types of Pediatric Intracranial Tumors? What Are Their Presenting Symptoms?

There are numerous types of intracranial tumors, but they can be divided into basic regions of supra-tentorial, infra-tentorial, posterior fossa tumors, and brain stem tumors. Subdivisions and common presenting symptoms are noted in the graphic, often with overlap. The most common pathologies based on intracranial location are noted in Figure 36.1 and Table 36.1.

What Are the Signs of Increased Intracranial Pressure in Children?

Increased intracranial pressure is often insidious and the signs are often subtle. These include irritability, crying, headaches, diplopia, nausea, stiff neck, vomiting, and motor weakness. The classic Cushing's triad is a more advanced stage of untreated increased ICP consisting of hypertension, bradycardia, and irregular breathing/bradypnea. Cushing's triad is potentially deleterious and requires immediate assessment and decompression to prevent morbidity/mortality.

What Is the Monro–Kellie Hypothesis?

This hypothesis states that the cranium has a fixed volume of brain tissue, blood, and CSF. Therefore, any increase in one compartment, such as tumor, is offset by decreases in one or more of the other compartments. Any increase in intracranial pressure due to tumor for example, has to be offset by either decreasing cerebral blood volume or CSF.

Since dural punctures can lead to herniation in this scenario, manipulation of the blood flow compartment through $PaCO_2$ management has been a mainstay of anesthetic management. The conundrum in these cases is that reducing the coronary blood flow (CBF) also reduces cerebral perfusion pressure (CPP). This is explained in the following equation:

$$\begin{aligned}&\text{CPP} = \text{Mean Arterial Pressure (MAP)}\\&(\text{MAP} - \text{Intracranial Pressure (ICP)}\\&\text{or Central Venous Pressure (CVP)}\\&(\text{whichever is greater})).\end{aligned}$$

By transposition:

$$\text{ICP} = \text{MAP} - \text{CPP}$$

Therefore, any increase in the MAP will directly translate to an increase in ICP. This balance however, is critical. In adult studies, reducing the MAP to decrease ICP causes secondary neuronal death due to ischemic/ischemic-reperfusion injuries.

Decreasing the CO_2 through hyperventilation compounds the problem by reducing blood return to the right side of the heart (and hence cardiac output and MAP), as well as reducing cerebral blood flow.

What Is the Optimal $PaCO_2$ for Neurosurgical Procedures?

The $EtCO_2$ is used as a surrogate for $PaCO_2$ provided that there isn't a significant Alveolar-arterial

Table 36.1 Common neurological tumor pathologies and presenting symptoms in children by anatomic region (numbers correlate with Figure 36.1)

	Anatomic region	Common tumor subtypes	Common symptoms
1	Suprasellar/ chiasmatic	Optic glioma, cranopharyngioma, germinoma, prolactinoma, pituitary adenoma, pliomyxoid astrocytoma	Headache, nausea, vomiting, visual field deficits, precocious or delayed puberty, anorexia, diabetes insipidus
2	Pons	Pontine glioma	Diplopia, cranial nerve palsy, incoordination, headache
3	Pineal/ midbrain	Glioma, pineoblastoma, pineocytoma, germinoma, primitive neuroectodermal tumor (pNET)	Upwards gaze paralysis, vomiting, nystagmus, diplopia, tremors
4	Cerebellum	Medulloblastoma, ependymoma, pilocytic astrocytoma, atypical teratoid rhabdoid tumor (ATRT), glioma	Headache, vomiting, ataxia, tremors, nystagmus
5	Basal ganglia/ thalamus	Gliomas, germinoma, oligodendroglioma	Movement disorder, weakness, hemisensory deficit, visual field deficit
6	Cerebral cortex	Gliomas, dysembroplastic neuroectodermal tumor (dNET), pNET, ependymoma, oligodendroglioma, ganglioglioma	Elevation of intracranial pressure (ICP), seizures, weakness, language disorder, encephalopathy, visual field deficit, headache
7	Ventricular system	Choroid plexus papilloma/carcinoma, ependymoma, ATRT, astrocytoma, desmoplastic infantile ganglioglioma	Nausea, vomiting, elevated ICP
8	Meninges	Meningioma	Seizures, headache

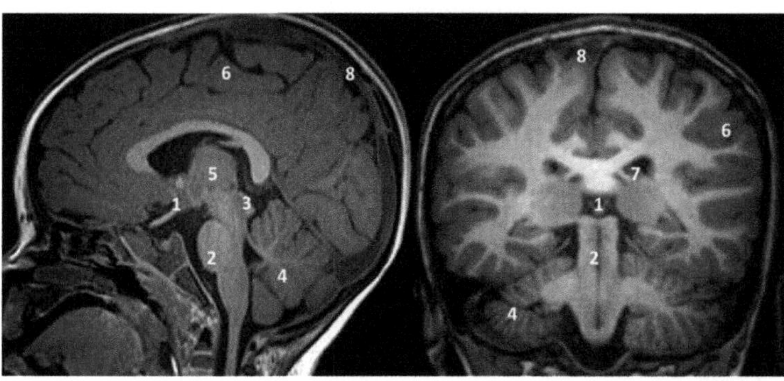

Figure 36.1 Sagittal and coronal CT images demonstrating the most common pediatric brain tumor pathologies by anatomic region (see Table 36.1 for region-specific descriptions)

(A-a) gradient. This is clinically checked with an ABG at the beginning of the procedure prior to incision and compared against the $EtCO_2$. In general, while reducing the $PaCO_2$ reduces cerebral blood flow due to cerebral vasoconstriction, this has to be balanced against maintaining CBF to critical areas. While most maintain the $PaCO_2$ around 30 mmHg, decreasing the $PaCO_2$ below 25 mmHg is not advisable.

The MRI Demonstrates a Posterior Fossa Tumor Which Is Poorly Circumscribed, Suggestive of Medulloblastoma. The Neurosurgeon Books a Tumor Resection. What Are Your Intraoperative Concerns?

It is important to look at the patient's electrolyte and volume status based on how long the child has been vomiting and has had poor oral intake. In cases of severe disturbances, temporization with a ventricular drain may allow for better medical optimization prior to a lengthy resection.

Monitoring should include addition of arterial lines with consideration for central venous access. Urinary output monitoring is critical for maintenance in cases where diuretics are used (mannitol/furosemide) or for the development of diabetes insipidus (DI) or syndrome of inappropriate antidiuretic hormone (SIADH).

Surgical pinning using the Mayfield pins causes an intense but very short-lasting stimulation. Specific considerations for the prone position include pressure on the eyes/nose, endotracheal tube dislodgement, and especially venous air embolism. Blood products should be readily available, especially in small children.

The Surgeon States that the Dura Is "Tight." What Is the Appropriate Management?

Bulging dura is a sign of elevated ICP. Intraoperative management includes: elevation of the head of bed, hyperventilation, avoidance of inhaled anesthetics, administration of diuretics (furosemide and/or mannitol), use of hypertonic 3% saline.

What Are the Positioning Concerns with Pediatric Neurosurgical Patients?

Based on the location of the tumor, there are multiple possible positions for pediatric patients. This includes but is not limited to prone, lateral, and head up positioning. Patients in the prone position are more prone towards facial/lingual swelling, especially in longer cases. Patients in the lateral position are prone towards brachial plexus stretching, and arm/neck positioning demands careful attention. Patients in the head up position, specifically with the head above the heart, are more prone towards venous air embolisms.

Why Is the Incidence of Venous Air Embolism (VAE) Greater in Posterior Fossa Surgery?

VAE is associated with sitting craniotomies. The incidence in pediatric neurosurgeries is less than in adult neurosurgeries. The highly vascular nature of the posterior fossa due to the presence of numerous low pressure dural sinuses predisposes this area to air entrainment. Entrained air can reduce or block blood flow in the right ventricle. If VAE is suspected, the area should be flooded with saline to prevent further air entrapment, and attempts should be made to limit travel of the embolism with jugular compression. Supportive hemodynamic management is also necessary, as hemodynamic consequences often ensue especially with large embolisms. These can lodge themselves in the right ventricular outflow tract, in the pulmonary circulation, or travel through a patent foramen ovale into the brain.

Copious urine output in this patient could be due to a number of factors, including excess hydration, use of diuretics, nephrogenic DI, and centrally mediated disorders including central DI and cerebral salt wasting (Table 36.2).

> The patient is extubated without incident and is transported to the pediatric intensive care unit. The patient begins to have copious urine output. What is the differential diagnosis? What is the difference between cerebral salt wasting, DI, and SIADH?

A fractional excretion of sodium (FeNa) is useful in this circumstance. The fractional excretion of Na is calculated by obtaining both the serum and urine Na simultaneously and using the serum Na as the numerator. If it is very low, then that is suggestive of SIADH or cerebral salt wasting (CSW). DI manifests with a high FeNa. Assessment of the patient's volume status is also critical; hypovolemic patients require fluid resuscitation (rather than restriction).

The treatment regimens similarly vary between the diagnoses. SIADH is primarily treated through fluid restriction to reduce water balance, as it is viewed as an excess of free water due to excessive water retention. Cerebral salt wasting, on the other hand, is characterized by excessive urinary Na wasting, and following the principles of osmolarity, free water loss as well. Therefore, the patients are intravascularly volume depleted with severe electrolyte disturbances. DI can be classified into either nephrogenic or central DI. For the purposes of this discussion, we are considering central DI which is

Table 36.2 Characteristics associated with syndrome of inappropriate antidiuretic hormone, diabetes insipidus, and cerebral salt wasting syndrome

	Syndrome of inappropriate antidiuretic hormone	Cerebral salt wasting syndrome	Diabetes insipidus
Intravascular volume	Hypervolemia	Hypovolemia	Hypovolemia
Serum sodium	Low	Low	High
Urine sodium	High	High	Normal
Urine output	Low	High	High
Primary treatment	Fluid restriction	Sodium and fluid resuscitation	Fluid resuscitation

characterized by free water wasting due to concentrating defects in the renal tubules. Fluid resuscitation is the first line of therapy, and failing this, desmopressin should be considered.

Suggested Reading

Crawford J. Childhood brain tumors. *Pediatr Rev.* 2013;34(2):63–78. PMID: 23378614.

Sathyanarayanan J, Krovvidi H. Anaesthetic considerations for posterior fossa surgery. *Cont Educ Anaesth Crit Car Pain.* 2013;14 (5):202–6. doi:10.1093/bjaceaccp/mkt056.

Chapter 37

Epilepsy Surgery

Matthew D. James and Adam C. Adler

> A nine-month-old boy born at 39 weeks of gestation was noted to have "seizure like" activity at three weeks of age and was found to have a hypothalamic hamartoma.
>
> His current vital signs are: blood pressure 90/52 mmHg; heart rate 116/min; respiratory rate 24; SpO_2 100% on room air. Weight is 8.6 kg. The patient is taking levetiracetam.

What Is the Incidence of Seizures in the Pediatric Population?

In 2015, 1.2% of the total US population had active epilepsy; this includes about 470,000 children. About 0.6% of children aged 0–17 years have active epilepsy, such that an elementary school with 500 students would have 3 children with epilepsy.

What Are the Treatment Options for Subcortical Epilepsy?

Treatment includes medical therapy and is usually the first option including: antiepilepsy drugs (AEDs), and maintenance of a ketogenic diet. Surgical options vary greatly from implantation of a vagal nerve stimulator to gamma knife radiosurgery, stereotactic thermoablation (radiofrequency or laser, with or without MR thermography), transcallosal interforniceal resection, transventricular endoscopic resection, or pterional (orbitozygomatic) resection.

What Is the Incidence of Hypothalamic Hamartoma?

Hypothalamic hamartomas (HH) are relatively rare. HH with epilepsy occurs in 1 of 200,000 children. A small number of patients with HH only have precocious puberty and are much less likely to have cognitive disabilities. Males appear to have a slightly higher risk than females (approximately 1.3:1) for HH with epilepsy. There are no identified maternal risk factors for developing HH, and there are no known geographical or ethnic concentrations.

How Is a Ketogenic Diet Employed in Epilepsy Patients?

Originally developed in the 1920s for control of seizures prior to development of AEDs, the ketogenic diet has made a resurgence when seizures are refractory to medical treatment. It consists of a high fat and low protein and carbohydrate diet to produce ketosis. The mechanism of action in treating seizures is highly multifactorial but centers around reduced neuronal firing and activation and can have a profound effect on seizure frequency.

What Is a Vagal Nerve Stimulator?

Vagal nerve stimulators (VNS) have been used as an adjunct to treat intractable epilepsy in children. The exact mechanism of action remains unknown but may be related to changes in regional blood flow during stimulation. Most vagal nerve stimulators are MRI compatible and each institution should have protocols involving the pre- and postinterrogation of these devices in relation to the MRI. At Texas Children's Hospital, the VNS is turned off immediately prior to the MRI and restarted on completion of the scan.

Who Is a Candidate for Laser Ablation?

Any patient with medically refractory epilepsy and MRI discrete lesions like an HH is a candidate for laser ablation therapy.

What Are the Major Anesthetic Considerations for Laser Ablation Procedures?

Most of the anesthetic considerations for seizure ablation surgery have to do with the intraoperative imaging. If intraoperative MRI is not available then there are major considerations with respect to both transporting the patient, and the time spent in the remote location. Depending on your facility, transportation may be required from the OR to CT and MRI. The MRI metal screening sheet should be completed by the parents prior to the procedure. Neuromuscular blockade is requested throughout because of the stereotactic nature of the procedure. Intravenous steroids are requested to treat expected swelling of the treated and surrounding tissues; usually a single dose of dexamethasone is given at the initiation of ablation.

Do Laser Ablation Cases Require Intraoperative Neuromonitoring?

Because of technologic limitations, as of 2018, a total intravenous anesthetic (TIVA) is not required. But in the near future there may be MR-compatible tools for intraoperative neuromonitoring.

What Are the Considerations Involved with Transporting a Patient Between Surgery and MRI?

Patients often lose heat and may become hypothermic during transport outside of the OR and while in the MRI machine. Warm blankets and disposable gel heating pads should be applied just before leaving each location. If possible, an MRI-compatible stretcher should be brought to the OR to avoid additional patient transfers which may increase the likelihood for laser lead malposition.

Supplies, medications, and airway equipment should accompany these patients during transport.

TIVA should be started to assure continued anesthesia and amnesia during transport.

What Are the Possible Complications Involved with an Extended Anesthetic Taking Place in the MRI?

Temperature maintenance remains an important focus in this phase of the case. After the patient is positioned in the MRI the surgical team will discourage touching of the patient – including reapplying new blankets or wrapping of the extremities. The ablation may be affected if the patient's temperature changes significantly over the course of the time in MRI if the degree of ablation is based on thermography. Inability to adjust the patient's position during the lengthy ablation may increase the risk of pressure ulcers and deep venous thrombosis. Careful padding when the patient is first placed into the scanner is important because repositioning may not be allowed for several hours.

What Are the Postoperative Considerations Following Ablation Surgery?

One of the major advantages of laser ablation over open surgery is a faster recovery. If the operation was uncomplicated then usually the patient can go to a regular inpatient floor. Occasionally, these patients may be discharged on postoperative day one. A postablation MRI scan is generally done to confirm absence of intracranial bleeding. If your MRI is at a site remote from the operating room, then there is always the question of whether or not to transport the patient back to the OR to manage the airway versus extubating in the MRI suite. The risks versus benefits of remote airway management must be considered.

What Is Electrocorticography (ECOG)?

Electrocorticography (ECOG) is a technique in which a grid is placed on the brain surface to allow for epileptic foci to be mapped for surgical excision.

What Are the Important Anesthetic Implications for ECOG?

Unless the grids are in place and the seizure foci have been well localized, all benzodiazepines should be avoided. If possible, propofol should be avoided in cases where seizures need to be stimulated. In cases where "light anesthesia" is required to stimulate seizure activity, patients should be well secured to avoid injury or dislodgement of tubes and lines.

Volatiles should be discontinued prior to electrocorticography.

Commonly, infusions of opioids and dexmedetomidine are used after pinning and exposure, during times of seizure stimulation. Ketamine may be added when required to enhance sedation and should be discussed with the surgeon and neuromonitoring staff when used.

When motor evoked potentials are not employed, muscle relaxation may be used. However, soft bite blocks such as rolled gauze should be carefully placed prior to any motor evoked potential to assure protection to the tongue and oral structures.

During surgical resection of the seizure focus, a volatile agent may be used; however, occasionally, the surgeon will perform a post resection ECOG, in which case TIVA should be resumed.

Suggested Reading

Chui J, Manninen P, Valiante T, et al. The anesthetic considerations of intraoperative electrocorticography during epilepsy surgery. *Anesth Analg*. 2013;117(2):479–86. PMID: 23780418.

Curry DJ, Gowda A, McNichols RJ, et al. MR-guided stereotactic laser ablation of epileptogenic foci in children. *Epilepsy Behav*. 2012;24 (4):408–14. PMID: 22687387.

Russ SA, Larson K, Halfon N. A national profile of childhood epilepsy and seizure disorder. *Pediatrics*. 2012;129:256–64. PMID: 22271699.

Zack MM, Kobau R. National and state estimates of the numbers of adults and children with active epilepsy United States, 2015. *MMWR Morb Mortal Wkly Rep*. 2017;66 (31):821–5. PMID: 28796763.

Moyamoya Disease

Elyse C. Parchmont and Adam C. Adler

A three-year-old boy presents for preoperative evaluation prior to pial synangiosis. A recent angiogram under general anesthesia to evaluate his cerebral circulation following recurrent transient ischemic attacks confirmed the diagnosis of Moyamoya disease. Current medications include aspirin. The nurse practitioner calls to determine what work-up and patient recommendations are appropriate prior to surgery.

What Are the Anatomic Changes and Pathophysiology Associated with Moyamoya Disease (MMD)?

Moyamoya is a Japanese word meaning "puff of smoke," which describes the web-like vascularity depicted when viewing the reticular anastomosis and collateral formations between the internal and external carotid arteries on cerebral angiography (Figure 38.1).

The disease involves a progressive stenosis of the internal carotid artery and its branches with gradual development of collaterals from the base of the brain and through the skull from the external carotid artery. Intimal thickening and hyperplasia result in vascular occlusion and consequent proliferation of collateral vessels at variant planes such as leptomeningeal, basal ganglia, and/or transdural. The result of this collateral vessel formation can be critically diminished blood flow in the cerebral vasculature which can lead to eventual ischemic crisis.

What Is the Epidemiology of MMD?

Moyamoya disease was originally reported by Takeuchi and Shimizui in 1957. In the United States, the ethnically specific breakdown of incidence ratio per 100,000 includes 4.6 in the Asian population, 2.2 for African Americans, and 0.5 for the Hispanic population. MMD is likely genetically inherited as there is a 9–12% incidence in those with a family history of the disease. There is a female predominance, with the female to male ratio being 1.8:1. Though the syndrome is thought to be genetically influenced, radiation and various infectious processes have been suggested as possible causes of pathogenicity.

What Disorders Are Associated with MMD?

Table 38.1 Disorders most commonly associated with Moyamoya development.

Congenital syndromes	Apert syndrome Hirschsprung disease Marfan syndrome Neurofibromatosis – type 1 Trisomy 21
Immunological disorders	Graves' disease
Hematological disorders	Aplastic anemia Fanconi anemia Sickle cell anemia Thalassemia
Neoplasia	Wilms tumor Craniopharyngiomas
Infectious	Tuberculous meningitis Leptospirosis
Vascular disorders	Atherosclerotic disease Cardiomyopathy Coarctation of the aorta Hypertension
Others	Radiation Pulmonary sarcoidosis Nephrotic syndrome

What Is the Most Likely Age for Presentation?

Disease may be acquired as an autosomal dominant process and can even present in early infancy, while a chronic and progressive disease presentation occurs with the highest incidence within the first decade of life.

What Are the Signs and Symptoms of MMD?

In early childhood, MMD usually presents with ischemic symptoms, whereas adults may present with intracranial hemorrhage. In children, MMD often manifests with transient ischemic attacks or ischemic strokes. Symptoms may include headache, dizziness, and seizures, although some patients are asymptomatic. Decline in neurological function and/or cognition, choreiform movements, growth hormone deficiency, and visual impairment may occur as the disease progresses.

What Are the Disease Stages of MMD?

The dynamic and continual disease process is a slow progression ultimately leading to complete occlusion of the internal carotid artery. Early on, suprasellar carotid stenosis occurs followed by formation of basal collaterals. As stenosis worsens to include occlusion at the Circle of Willis vessels, extracranial collaterals form. With progressing stenosis, these extracranial collaterals enlarge and eventually provide nearly all flow.

What Factors Affect Prognosis?

A worse prognosis is associated with younger age at presentation (under six years), severe neurological deficits at presentation, and advanced angiographic changes.

How Is MMD Diagnosed?

If intracranial hemorrhage is suspected, then computed tomography (CT) of the head is indicated. Acute and chronic infarcts and areas of cortical ischemia will be revealed by magnetic resonance imaging (MRI) and magnetic resonance angiography (MRA) with roughly 90% sensitivity. Angiography is the gold standard for diagnosis, allowing for assessment of the internal and external carotid systems independently.

What Are the Angiographic Stages of MMD?

Table 38.2 Angiographic staging of Moyamoya disease.

Grade I	Carotid stenosis without collateral vessels
Grade II	Basal collateral vessels seen
Grade III	Prominent basal collateral vessels
Grade IV	Stenotic or occluded Circle of Willis and posterior cerebral arteries
Grade V	Extra cranial collateral network
Grade VI	Total carotid occlusion

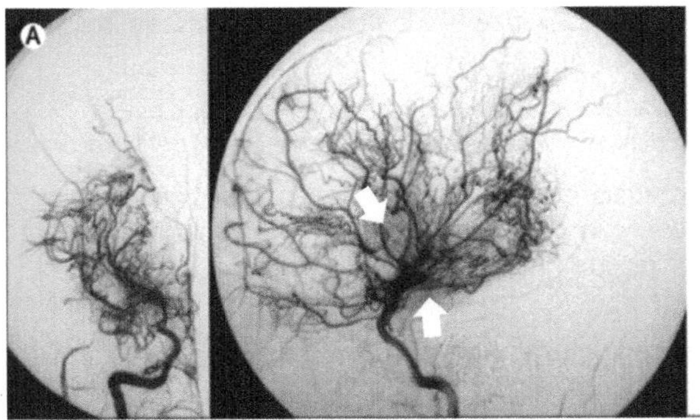

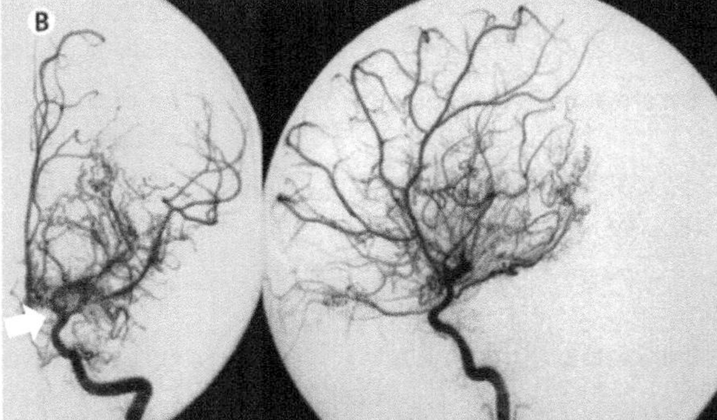

Figure 38.1 Cerebral angiogram of the right internal carotid artery (A) and left internal carotid artery (B) showing the classic Moyamoya vessels "puffs of smoke" (arrows). Reproduced from: *Lancet Neurol.* 2008 Nov;7(11):1056–66 with permission of Elsevier.

What Are the Available Medical Therapies for MMD?

Most patients with MMD benefit from medical therapy for symptom relief. However, nearly all patients have disease progression and ultimately require surgical intervention. Medical management includes: calcium channel blockers (nimodipine or nicardipine), antiplatelet agents (aspirin or ticlopidine), and coagulation modifiers such as pentoxifylline. Patients experiencing seizures can be placed on anticonvulsant therapy.

What Are the Available Surgical Therapies for MMD?

There are many variations of surgical interventions aimed to revascularize areas of decreased cerebral perfusion that have shown subsequent ischemia and recurrent cerebral ischemic events. These procedures are generally focused on increasing collateral blood flow, or directly or indirectly bypassing the occluded areas. Up to 87% of surgical patients can obtain systemic benefits and relief from surgical intervention.

Access to the surgical field is obtained through the removal of dural flaps, craniotomy, or via burr holes. Variables in surgical procedure choice can be patient age, comorbidities, signs and symptoms, and surgeon preference and experience.

What Are the Major Anesthetic Considerations for Patients with MMD?

Preoperatively, detailed examination should be performed with attention to neurological deficits including frequency of ischemic attacks that may alert the provider to the extent of compromise of the cerebral vasculature. A reliable baseline blood pressure reading should be assessed. Routine laboratory examinations including CBC, electrolytes, coagulation studies, and type-and-screen should follow the same protocol as for craniotomies. Calcium-channel blockers or antiseizure medications should be continued until the day of surgery. Low dose aspirin may be continued perioperatively or stopped according to hospital or surgical guidelines, whereby then some facilities replace aspirin therapy with low molecular weight heparin.

Table 38.3 Common surgical procedures for Moyamoya disease

Direct bypass techniques	Most commonly done with a superficial temporal artery (STA) to middle cerebral artery (MCA) bypass. This procedure provides immediate increase in blood flow to ischemic brain, usually done in adults, and is technically difficult to conduct in children.
Encephaloduroarteriosynangiosis (EDAS)	Preferred indirect revascularization procedure in which the STA is mobilized and anastomosed to the edges of the opened dura. This is usually done in children but in adults is combined with STA-MCA bypass technique
Pial synangiosis	A modification of EDAS in which the surface of the dura is exposed and the pial surface is increased by opening it into multiple flaps to increase collateral vessel development from the dural vessels. A branch of the STA is sutured directly into the pial surface. Results from studies indicate majority of pediatric patients have significant halting of disease progression
Encephalomyosynangiosis (EMS)	An indirect revascularization procedure in which temporalis muscle is attached to the surface of the brain to promote collateral vessel formation
Encephaloduroarteriomyosynangiosis (EDAMS)	Combination of EDAS and EMS. Dural flaps created are folded into the dural/ epi-arachnoid space with middle meningeal artery promoting angiogenesis. Neovascularization reported in 50–90% cases in different studies. Incidence of postoperative strokes is reduced when combined with STA–MCA bypass
Combination procedures	Encephalomyoarteriosynangiosis (EMAS), a combination of EDAS and EMS; encephaloduromyoarteriopericranial synangiosis
Other surgical procedures	Craniotomy with dural inversion, cervical sympathectomy, and omental transposition

Preoperative intravenous access should be obtained when possible, avoiding pain and anxiety with the use of topical local anesthetic spray or creams, along with adequate oral premed to reduce anxiety. Prehydration with at least 20 cc/kg of crystalloid should be administered.

Premedication for sedation to decrease stress or crying is a consideration, as both can cause hyperventilation, decreasing cerebral blood flow due to hypocapnia, and can subsequently increase ischemic risk. The premedication should be adequate, but not excessive, as hypoventilation and hypercarbia will increase ischemic risk.

Anesthetic management must focus on maintaining cerebral perfusion and oxygen delivery throughout the perioperative period. The anesthesia goals for patients with MMD include:

- Maintaining a balance between cerebral oxygen supply and demand
- Maintaining normotension/avoiding hypotension (MAP at or above patient's baseline)
- Maintaining normocarbia or mild hypocarbia
- Maintaining normovolemia
- Avoiding hyperviscosity
- Avoiding anemia (Hct below 30%)
- Maintaining normothermia or mild hypothermia
- Avoidance of preoperative anxiety/stress
- Avoidance of postoperative pain (without causing hypoventilation)

What Are the Effects of Commonly Used Anesthetics on Cerebral Blood Flow (CBF) and Metabolic Rate ($CMRO_2$)?

While most agents have been used successfully in patients with MMD, it is most critical to avoid uncontrolled swings of blood pressure while being mindful of the various effects of agents on CBF and $CMRO_2$ as stated in Table 38.4.

Monitoring includes standard ASA monitors in addition to arterial blood pressure, urinary catheter and central body temperature. Transcranial EEG, near-infrared spectroscopy (NIRS), somatosensory evoked potentials (SEP), and transcranial Doppler (TCD) are useful for monitoring cerebral ischemia and are institution specific.

Mild hypothermia can offer some degree of neuroprotection by reducing the cerebral metabolic rate; however, there is not sufficient evidence to secure this as an evidence-based practice. Conversely, hyperthermia increases oxygen consumption and demand and can increase risk for ischemia. Normothermia is most often the goal for body temperature to avoid any cerebral vascular spasm that could occur from a hypothermic state, which could decrease flow in the brain. Heating blankets, underbody fluid mat systems, and fluid warmers can be used perioperatively to raise or lower body temperature.

Table 38.4 Effects of anesthetics on cerebral blood flow and metabolic rate; NC=no change

Anesthetic agent	Cerebral blood flow (CBF)	Cerebral metabolic rate ($CMRO_2$)
Volatile agents	⇧	⇩
Nitrous oxide	⇧	⇧/NC
IV anesthetics (propofol)	⇩	⇩
Ketamine	⇧	⇧
Dexmedetomidine	⇩	⇩
Opioids	NC	NC

Blood pressure should be maintained at or slightly above the baseline preoperative blood pressure perioperatively to avoid decrease in cerebral blood flow and cerebral perfusion pressure. Regional anesthesia in the form of a skull block may be considered with the theoretical risk of causing cerebral steal from regional vasodilation.

What Is the Risk of Cerebral Steal in MMD Surgery?

Collateral vessels in patients with MMD lack typical responses to CO_2. Thus, normal vessels with intact CO_2 activity will dilate with hypercarbia and potentially "steal" or shunt blood flow from collateral vessels. On the contrary, collateral vessels lack the ability to dilate with hypercarbia and are unable to increase blood flow to areas supplied by these vessels by altering CO_2. The baseline $PaCO_2/EtCO_2$ should be maintained to minimize steal or diversion away from the collaterals.

Complications during surgical interventions may include: blood pressure lability, seizures, and symptomatic postoperative hyper-perfusion injury (re-perfusion injury). Perioperative risks can involve varied ischemic neurological events, transient ischemic attacks (TIAs) or strokes, intracranial hemorrhage, or infection.

What Are the Important Postoperative Considerations in Patients with MMD?

Sedation and adequate pain control should be used to avoid crying, hyperventilation, and stress responses. In children, parental presence can be beneficial.

Pain control is crucial as pain is associated with an increase in cerebral metabolism as inadequate analgesia increases $CMRO_2$ and CBF. Patients are at high risk for postoperative cerebral infarction necessitating close monitoring, usually best accomplished by ICU admission. Postoperative opioid administration such as morphine can be titrated with keen observation to avoid hypoventilation. Neurological status must be assessed and intervened upon if abrupt changes occur. Appropriate nonopioid pain adjuncts should be considered.

After revascularization procedures, months are required to develop the necessary "bypass" collaterals and medical management should continue during this time to avoid complications, especially aspirin therapy.

Suggested Reading

Baaj AA, Agazzi S, Sayed ZA, et al. Surgical management of moyamoya disease: a review. *Neurosurg Focus.* 2009 Apr;26(4):E7. PMID: 19335133.

Baykan N, Zgen SO, Ustalar S, et al. Moyamoya disease and anesthesia. *Pediatr Anesth.* 2005;15: 1111–15. PMID: 16324034.

Kuroda S, Houkin K. Moyamoya disease: current concepts and future perspectives. *Lancet Neurol.* 2008 Nov;7(11):1056–66.

Parray T, Martin TW, Siddiqui S. Moyamoya disease: A review of the disease and anesthetic management. *J Neurosurg Anesthesiol.* 2011 Apr;23(2):100–9. PMID: 20924291.

Tho-Calvi SC, Thompson D, Saunders D, et al. Clinical features, course, and outcomes of a UK cohort of pediatric moyamoya. *Neurology.* 2018;90(9):e763–70. PMID: 29483323.

Chapter 39

Cleft Lip and Palate

Julia H. Chen and Sudha Bidani

A 12-month-old male presents for a primary cleft palate repair. The patient was recently adopted, and no significant medical history has been documented.

In the preoperative holding area, the patient is being held and appears calm. The patient's preoperative vital signs are: weight 10 kg, T 36.7°C, pulse 110 bpm, BP 90/54, RR 28, SpO_2 99% on room air. On physical exam, the patient is noted to have a right-sided cleft palate. The patient appears to have slight micrognathia. The remainder of the physical exam is within normal limits.

When Does Development of the Face and Lip Occur? When Does Development of the Palate Occur?

The development of the lip occurs during weeks four to eight of gestation. The primary palate (palate that is anterior to the incisive foramen) forms during week six of gestation with the secondary palate formed during weeks six to twelve. Cleft lip and alveolus results from failure of fusion of the nasal and maxillary prominences, whereas cleft palate (secondary palate) results from failure of fusion of the palatal shelves.

What Are the Predisposing Risk Factors Related to Cleft Lip and Palate?

Causes of cleft lip and palate are multifactorial and reported etiologies include genetics, maternal exposures and risk factors (smoking, alcohol, gestational diabetes, folate deficiency), as well as teratogens (retinoic acid, valproic acid, phenytoin).

What Is the Incidence of Cleft Lip and Palate?

The incidence of orofacial clefts is 1 in 700 live births. Cleft lip with or without cleft palate is more common in males (2:1) and certain ethnic populations (Asian, Native American). Nonsyndromic forms of cleft lip with or without cleft palate account for 70% of all cases.

How Are Different Types of Cleft Lip and Palate Classified?

The classification of craniofacial clefts was described by Dr. Tessier in 1976. Orofacial clefts are the most common craniofacial cleft deformity, and multiple classification systems for orofacial clefts exist. Cleft lip and palate can occur in combination or in isolation. Cleft lip is commonly described as unilateral or bilateral, and complete or incomplete. The clinical severity of cleft palate ranges from a submucosal, often undetectable, cleft to a complete bilateral cleft of the primary and secondary palate.

What Physiological Problems Are Common for Patients with Cleft Palate?

In cleft palate patients, improper closure between the palate and nasopharynx can lead to physiological problems of feeding (unable to generate negative pressure for swallowing and sucking) and difficulties with speech and language development. Eustachian tube dysfunction and middle ear disease related to abnormal insertion of the tensor veli palatini can result in conductive hearing loss. Inability to oppose maxillary and mandibular teeth leads to the inability to properly chew food.

When Is a Cleft Lip and/or Palate Typically Repaired?

Primary cleft lip repair is typically performed at around age 10–12 weeks. Historically, the "rule of 10s" described the preoperative parameters of weight over 10 lbs, hemoglobin over 10 g/dL, and age over 10 weeks. Primary cleft palate repair is typically performed around age 9–12 months in order to optimize speech and language development.

What Other Procedures Are Common for These Patients?

Eustachian tube dysfunction, middle ear disease, and conductive hearing loss may be associated with cleft palate; these patients often require placement of myringotomy tubes. In the long term, these patients may require multiple procedures including lip and nasal revisions, additional palate surgery for velopharyngeal insufficiency, alveolar bone grafting, dental procedures, maxillary advancement, and cosmetic septorhinoplasty. Orthodontic intervention is usually required following palate repair to improve maxillary hypoplasia and crowding of the teeth.

What Is Velopharyngeal Insufficiency, and How Is It Treated?

Velopharyngeal insufficiency (VPI) is the insufficient separation of the nasopharynx from the oropharynx due to a shortened palate. During speech, escape of air through the nose can lead to several speech disorders including hypernasal speech and inability to produce specific speech sounds. Surgical treatment for VPI involves lengthening of the palate by palatal revision, pharyngeal flap, or pharyngoplasty (bringing the posterior pharyngeal wall forward with an artificial implant or fat injection).

What Are the Important Preoperative Considerations for Cleft Lip or Palate Repair?

Preoperative evaluation of all pediatric patients includes a detailed history of birth and family history, review of systems, and recent illnesses. Cleft patients may have chronic congestion that should be differentiated from an acute illness. A thorough physical examination should be performed, with a focus on the head and neck examination, as well as possible associated malformations. Attention should be placed on facial asymmetry, external ear anomalies, and crowding of maxillary teeth in teenage patients. If a particular syndrome or genetic diagnosis is suspected, further preoperative workup may be warranted. Laboratory studies are typically not warranted unless clinically indicated.

What Are the Important Components of a Pediatric Airway Exam?

Physical exam findings that might indicate a possible difficult airway include micrognathia, limited mouth opening, limited neck extension, and facial asymmetry. Micrognathia is associated with posterior regression of the tongue and a small hyomental space, making laryngoscopy difficult. Certain ophthalmic, auricular, and facial anomalies can occur in specific syndromes associated with difficulty with ventilation or tracheal intubation. Cleft alveolus, protruding premaxilla, and high-vaulted arch deformities contribute to difficult intubation in pediatric patients. Intubation may be challenging in patients with combined bilateral cleft lip and alveolus.

What Syndromes Are Commonly Associated with Cleft Lip/Palate?

Many syndromes are known to be associated with orofacial clefts. They include Trisomy 21 (Down syndrome), Nager syndrome, Treacher Collins syndrome, Stickler syndrome, hemifacial microsomia, 22q deletion syndromes, Goldenhar syndrome, and Pierre Robin sequence.

Clinical features of Pierre Robin sequence include micrognathia, glossoptosis, downward displacement of the base of tongue, and airway obstruction. Clinical features of Treacher Collins syndrome include mandibular hypoplasia, microtia, and eye colobomas.

Does This Child Need Premedication?

Stranger anxiety typically occurs around six to eight months of age. Premedication may be of benefit in older children, as these patients often require multiple surgical procedures throughout their lifetime and may have anxiety related to perioperative experiences. Although there are several choices of anxiolytic pre-medications, midazolam is most often chosen because of its relative safety, rapid onset with oral or nasal administration (5–10 minutes), and rapid offset (within 30 minutes). Premedication should be used with caution in patients at risk for airway obstruction as well as those with anticipated difficult airway.

How Would You Induce General Anesthesia?

Although most children's hospitals would use inhalational induction with sevoflurane in oxygen, with or without nitrous oxide, IV induction is an acceptable alternative and is used in some centers. Administration of a neuromuscular blocker to facilitate tracheal intubation is optional, though only after the proven ability to provide positive pressure ventilation. Many centers use an oral Ring-Adair-Elwyn (RAE) preformed tracheal tube that sits along the midline of the chin. It avoids distortion of the upper lip and angles of the mouth, and can accommodate the Dingman mouth gag used by the surgeon to facilitate access to the palate during surgery. Bilateral breath sounds should be confirmed in both flexion and extension positions to ensure adequate depth of the endotracheal tube (ETT) below the vocal cords with changes in positioning.

What Are the Most Important Intraoperative Considerations?

Intraoperative airway complications during cleft lip and palate repair include accidental extubation, and tracheal tube obstruction from kinking or from compression by the Dingman mouth gag. An abrupt change in the end tidal carbon dioxide tracing should prompt assessment of the tracheal tube and adequacy of ventilation. Communication with the surgical team is important as the surgical field and the airway occupy the same surgical space and are often accessed with difficulty during the procedure.

What Is Your Plan for Intraoperative Analgesia? What Nerve Blocks Are Available for This Procedure?

Because of the young age of these patients and their propensity toward upper airway obstruction, intraoperative and postoperative opioids should be used with caution. These patients are at increased risk of unplanned emergency tracheal intubation in the postoperative period as a result of respiratory depression from the use of opioids. Therefore, many centers will use an infraorbital nerve block with local anesthesia. This nerve is easily accessible as it exits the infraorbital foramen.

How Would You Prepare This Patient for Extubation? Awake or Deep Extubation? How Do You Protect the Airway Postoperatively?

Since these patients are at risk for postoperative airway complications, an awake extubation is preferred. Airway obstruction can occur secondary to tissue edema, or tongue swelling from the Dingman mouth gag. Increased oral secretions and airway manipulation can increase the risk of laryngospasm following extubation. Oropharyngeal airways should be avoided in these patients as placement could disrupt surgical suture lines and irritate mucosal flaps. Aggressive suctioning of the mouth and nose should be avoided for similar reasons and preferably done under direct visualization by the surgeon at the end of the procedure. If used, removal of mouth gag should be confirmed. In patients with a history of difficult mask ventilation or intubation, or concern for postoperative airway obstruction, the surgeon can place a traction suture through the tongue that when pulled can decrease airway obstruction and improve ventilation. In addition, the surgeon can place and secure a nasopharyngeal airway at the end of surgery under direct visualization.

What Postoperative Preparations Should Be Made? Can This Patient Be Discharged after PACU Discharge Criteria Are Met?

Postoperatively, younger patients can be placed in elbow immobilizers to avoid disruption of surgical sutures. The patient can be placed in prone or lateral positioning (recovery position) to improve ventilation and enable blood and secretions to pool into the cheek or out of the mouth. If there are concerns for postoperative airway edema or obstruction (pharyngeal flap, pharyngoplasty), admission to an intensive care unit and continued pulse oximetry is warranted.

Acknowledgments

We wish to acknowledge the image contributions to this chapter of Laura Monson, MD, and John Wirthlin, DDS, MSD.

Suggested Reading

Arosarena OA. Cleft lip and palate. *Otolaryngol Clin North Am.* 2007;40(1):27–60. PMID: 17346560.

Nargozian C, Ririe DG, Bennun RD, et al. Hemifacial microsomia: anatomical prediction of difficult intubation. *Paediatr Anaesth.* 1999;9(5):393–8. PMID: 10447900.

Sheeran PW, Walsh BK, Finley AM, et al. Management of difficult airway patients and the use of a difficult airway registry at a tertiary care pediatric hospital. *Paediatr Anaesth.* 2014;24(8):819–24. PMID: 24471869.

Shkoukani MA, Chen M, Vong A. Cleft lip: a comprehensive review. *Front Pediatr.* 2013;1:53. PMID: 24400297.

Xue FS, Zhang GH, Li P, et al. The clinical observation of difficult laryngoscopy and difficult intubation in infants with cleft lip and palate. *Paediatr Anaesth.* 2006;16 (3):283–9. PMID: 16490092.

Craniosynostosis

Rebecca Evans and Grace Hsu

A 12-month-old, 9.2 kg healthy child presents for an open cranial vault repair for sagittal synostosis. All preoperative laboratory studies (CBC, electrolyte panel, coagulation studies) are normal, with the exception of an elevated PTT (46.0, normal 22.0–36.0).

Physical examination, family history, and review of systems are unremarkable. There was no history of prior general anesthesia, and his surgical history was notable for an uneventful circumcision at birth. A repeat PTT was drawn the morning of surgery and remained elevated (41.0).

DIAGNOSIS

What Is Craniosynostosis?

Craniosynostosis is a premature closure of one or more of the cranial sutures.

What Is the Incidence of Craniosynostosis in Children?

The incidence is 1:2000 births, males more commonly affected than females.

What Is the Natural Progression of Cranial Suture Closure?

The anterolateral fontanelle closes by approximately three months of age, the posterior fontanelle by three to six months, the anterior fontanelle by 9–18 months, posterolateral fontanelle by two years.

What Are the Four Cranial Sutures Involved in Craniosynostosis?

The four cranial sutures are sagittal, coronal, lamboid, and metopic. The premature closure of the sagittal suture is the most common simple craniosynostosis (50%) followed by coronal (20%) and metopic (10%) (Figure 40.1).

The growth of the skull is in the direction perpendicular to the fused suture, resulting in characteristic skull appearances.

Simple versus Complex Craniosynostosis

Simple Synostosis. Nonsyndromic or one suture prematurely closed, 80% of diagnoses.
Complex Synostosis. Syndromic or involving the premature closure of two or more sutures, 20% of diagnoses.

Which Syndromes Are Most Commonly Associated with Craniosynostosis?

Craniosynostosis can be a component of many named syndromes; however, the most common syndromes encountered are: Crouzon, Apert, Pfeiffer, Saethre-Chotzen, and Carpenter.

What Are the Common Clinical Characteristics of Apert Syndrome?

Apert syndrome is a spontaneously occurring autosomal dominant syndrome occurring in approximately 1:100,000–1:160,000 patients. A multitude of systems can be affected including:

- Cranio-facial with coronal synostosis, proptosis, hypertelorism, midfacial hypoplasia, cleft palate, choanal or tracheal stenosis (Figure 40.2).
- Respiratory with a 40–50% incidence of obstructive sleep apnea.
- Cardiac with a 10% incidence of congenital heart disease, especially ventricular septal defect (VSD) and pulmonary stenosis.
- Genitourinary with cryptorchidism and hydronephrosis.
- Musculoskeletal with syndactyly.
- Neurologic with developmental delay, and elevated intracranial pressures.

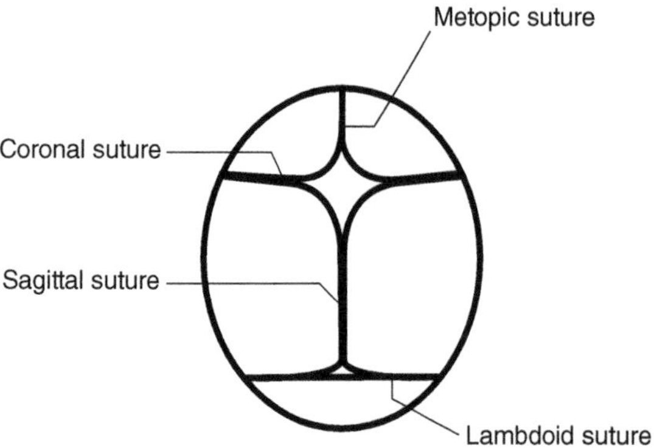

Figure 40.1 Pictorial representation of cranial sutures. Image by Estrellita and Rob Swenker, reproduced here under CC BY 3.0 license https://creativecommons.org/licenses/by/3.0/

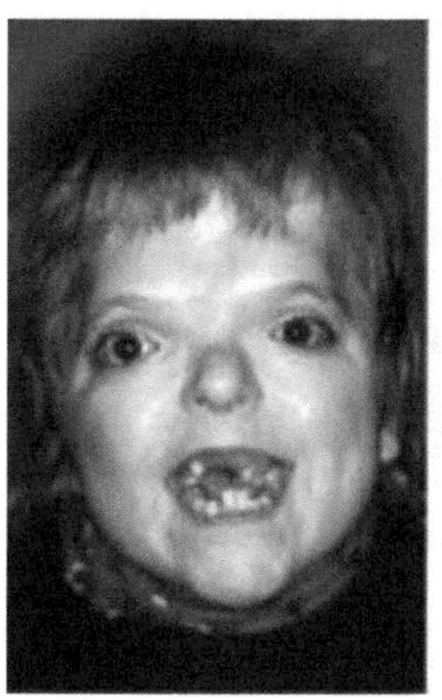
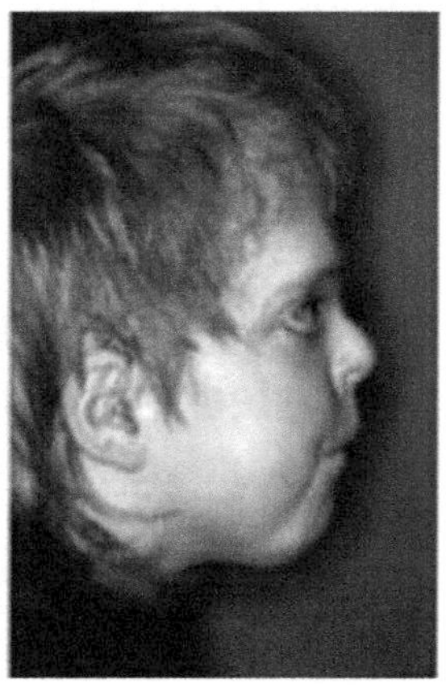

Figure 40.2 Child with Apert syndrome, hypertelorism, and midfacial hypoplasia. Reproduced from: Hohoff A., et al . The spectrum of Apert syndrome: phenotype, particularities in orthodontic treatment, and characteristics of orthognathic surgery. *Head & Face Medicine* (2007) 3:10 reproduced here under CC BY 2.0 license https://creativecommons.org/licenses/by/2.0/

What Are the Common Clinical Characteristics of Crouzon Syndrome?

Crouzon syndrome can be sporadically occurring or inherited. A multitude of systems can be affected including:

- Craniofacial including cranial synostosis (most commonly coronal and lamboid), fontal bossing, midface hypoplasia, and airway obstruction leading to obstructive sleep apnea (Figure 40.3).
- Optic atrophy occurs in roughly 20% of patients.
- Neurologic: these patients can have mild developmental delay and increased intracranial pressure.

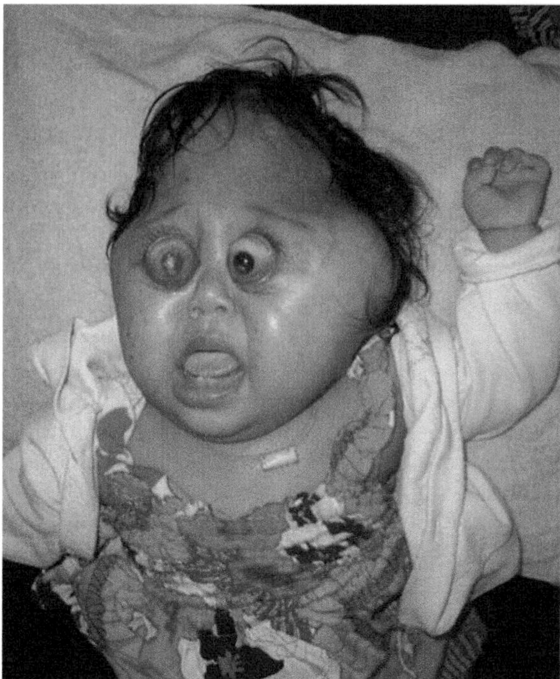

Figure 40.3 Child with a severe case of Crouzon syndrome. Reproduced under CC0 license

These patients can be difficult to mask ventilate due to their facial features.

What Are the Common Clinical Characteristics of Saethre–Chotzen Syndrome?

Saethre–Chotzen syndrome is a rare syndrome causing craniosynostosis (most commonly coronal), brachycephaly, maxillary hypoplasia, renal anomalies, cryptorchidism, and mild developmental delays. These patients can be difficult to intubate especially due to the maxillary hypoplasia.

Which Structure Is Most Commonly Associated with Syndromic Craniosynostosis?

The coronal suture is most commonly associated with syndromic craniosynstosis.

What Are Some Indications for Cranial Vault Reconstruction?

Indications for cranial vault reconstruction include poor or slowed brain growth, increased intracranial pressure (ICP), severe exophthalmos, obstructive sleep apnea, craniofacial deformity, and psychosocial and cosmetic reasons.

Why Do Surgeons Recommend Surgical Repair in Children by One Year of Age?

Patients without correction of craniosynostosis are at an increased risk for visual loss and developmental delay. Children repaired after the age of one year were found to have a lower IQ than those repaired prior to one year of age. In addition, better cosmetic results can be achieved if corrected during the first year of life when rapid brain and skull growth occurs.

PREOPERATIVE TESTING

What Preoperative Laboratory Tests Are Required for a Craniosynostosis Repair?

Most centers require a baseline hematocrit and blood type and cross-match as the minimum laboratory studies. Some centers perform other testing including a CBC, electrolyte panel, and coagulation studies.

What Would You Expect the Hemoglobin of a Term Neonate to Be? Two-Month-Old? Six-Month-Old? What Causes This Difference?

Neonates are born with a hemoglobin of approximately 17 g/dL composed solely of fetal hemoglobin. The increased density of hemoglobin in the newborn is a residual from the child's need to extract oxygen from its mother's blood across the placenta while in utero.

Between the two- to three-month-old period, the fetal hemoglobin present at birth has reached the end of its lifespan (approximately 90 days) and the adult hemoglobin has not reached its full production capability. Therefore, it is normal for children aged two to three months to have a hemoglobin of 10 g/dL. Adult levels of hemoglobin are reached by four to six months of age.

INTRAOPERATIVE MANAGEMENT

What Procedures Are Performed to Repair Craniosynostosis? What Are the Benefits/Risks Associated with Each?

- Endoscopic strip craniectomy: performed on children within the first four months of life, least invasive repair, requires a protective helmet to be worn after surgery, many discharged postoperative day one, may avoid intensive care unit admission (institution dependent).
- Spring-assisted cranioplasty: for sagittal suture craniosynostosis only, reduced intraoperative blood loss, short hospital stay.
- Total cranial vault reconstruction: endoscopic or open, associated with 50–100% blood volume loss, 90–100% of infants require transfusion, PICU care postoperatively, no protective helmet required (Figure 40.4).

A Z-shaped opening allows for tension-free approximation and later coverage by hair growth which improves cosmetic outcomes (Figure 40.4).

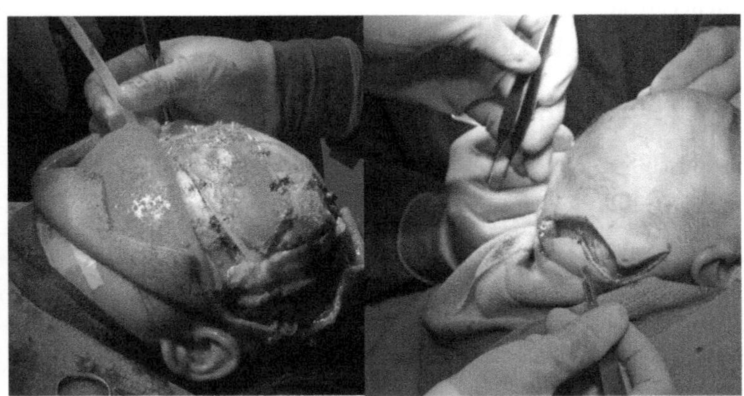

Figure 40.4 (Left) Anterior cranial vault remodeling showing the retraction of the skin and muscle and removal of bone and replacement of the remodeled skull bones with absorbable plastic spacers to allow for bony growth. (Right) Z-shaped opening allows for tension free approximation and later coverage by hair growth. Courtesy of Adam C. Adler, MD

What Are the Anesthetic Concerns Related to Craniosynostosis Repair?

- Potential for difficult airway, especially if the child is syndromic, diagnosed with obstructive sleep apnea, has abnormal neck mobility, or midface hypoplasia.
- Blood loss: open cranial vault reconstruction is associated with a 50–100% blood volume loss. Less blood loss is associated with other repairs; however, laceration of the sagittal sinus during any type of repair can be catastrophic.
- Cardiac arrest: increased incidence, particularly in total cranial vault reconstructions, secondary to sudden massive blood loss or venous air embolism.
- Hypothermia: secondary to exposure of the head during surgery, resuscitation with large quantities of fluids/blood.
- Other organ involvement in syndromic patients (example: congenital heart disease occurs in 10% of patients with Apert syndrome)
- Increased ICP: more common in syndromic craniosynostosis, associated with greater hemodynamic instability than patients without elevated ICP, may require elevated mean arterial pressure (MAP) to maintain adequate cerebral perfusion.

What Are the Risk Factors and Treatment for Venous Air Embolism (VAE)?

Craniofacial procedures are high risk for development of VAE. VAE occurs when air is entrained into the venous system which can collect in the right ventricular outflow and impede cardiac output. Patients are at increased risk with head-up position, exposed dural venous sinuses, and relative hypovolemia.

The most sensitive method for detection of VAE is transesophageal echocardiograph. Precordial Doppler can be applied to the chest for continuous auscultation and the mill wheel murmur sound can be heard when air is being entrained.

Treatment includes stopping surgery by flooding the surgical field with saline, returning the table to a flat or head down (Trendelenburg) position. Treatment is supportive with volume resuscitation, 100% oxygen, addition of inotropic support as needed, institution of positive end-expiratory pressure (PEEP) to raise intrathoracic pressure, and advanced cardiac life support/pediatric advanced life support as needed for cardiac arrest.

How Does Positioning Influence Anesthetic Management?

- Reverse Trendelenburg: reduces blood loss, increased risk for venous air embolism.
- Trendelenburg: increased blood loss, reduced risk of venous air embolism.
- Prone: skin break down, pressure on the eyes/face/nose.
- Superman: extubation with extension of the head/neck.

What Are Some Risk Factors for Increased Intraoperative Bleeding?

Risk factors are weight less than 5 kg, age <18 months, earlier surgery date, syndromic craniosynostosis, surgical time >5 h.

What Is the Incidence of Blood Transfusion in Craniosynostosis Repairs?

Incidence is variable depending upon the surgical procedure, simple vs. complex craniosynostosis, and the surgeon's expertise. Performing a cranial vault reconstruction without resuscitation with blood products is rare; 90–100% of infants in a literature review required transfusion for this procedure. A minimum of 2 units of cross-matched packed red blood cells (PRBCs) is recommended prior to initiation of the case.

BLOOD TRANSFUSIONS

What Are the Current Recommended Ratios of PRBC:FFP:Platelets for Transfusion of a Child?

FFP and platelets are recommended if the blood loss is greater than 1 blood volume. A variety of resuscitation practices have been described for craniosynostosis repair including the use of whole blood, reconstituted PRBC and fresh frozen plasma (FFP), PRBC, crystalloids and colloids. Individual institutions maintain their own protocols for these procedures.

What Are the Risks of Resuscitating with Only PRBC or Crystalloid?

Dilution coagulopathy is a risk if the blood loss is greater than one blood volume.

What Surgical and Pharmacological Adjuncts Help Reduce the Rate of Transfusion?

- Preoperative management strategies: Preoperative recombinant human erythropoietin in combination with the use of cell saver results in decreased allogeneic blood transfusions. Directed blood donation from older children or from a family member may also help reduce the number of blood unit exposures.
- Intraoperative management strategies: Techniques such as acute normovolemic hemodilution, antifibrinolytics, induced hypotension, and cell salvage are used to help reduce intraoperative blood loss.
- Surgeon specific: Placement of blocking stitches or surgical clips on the skin flaps helps minimize blood loss during open cranial vault reconstruction. Additional techniques such as infiltrating the subcutaneous tissue with epinephrine, needle tip cautery, and bone wax have also aided in reducing blood loss.

POSTOPERATIVE MANAGEMENT

What Are Common Postoperative Complications Related to Craniosynostosis Repair?

Ongoing blood loss possibly requiring transfusion, cerebral edema, visual changes, cerebrospinal leak, infection, and transfusion reactions have all been reported in the postoperative period.

What Electrolyte Abnormalities May Be Present Postoperatively?

1. Hyponatremia secondary to cerebral salt wasting syndrome.
2. Hyperchloremic metabolic acidosis in large volumes of normal saline were used for resuscitation.

Suggested Reading

Buchanan EP, Xue AS, Hollier LH Jr. Craniofacial syndromes. *Plast Reconstr Surg.* 2014;134(1):128e–53e. PMID: 25028828.

Goobie SM, Haas T. Bleeding management for pediatric craniotomies and craniofacial surgery. *Paediatr Anaesth.* 2014;24 (7):678–89. PMID: 24815192.

Murad GJ, Clayman M, Seagle MB, White S, Perkins LA, Pincus DW. Endoscopic-assisted repair of craniosynostosis. *Neurosurg Focus.* 2005;19(6):E6. PMID: 16398483.

Stricker PA, Fiadjoe JE. Anesthesia for craniofacial surgery in infancy. *Anesthesiol Clin.* 2014;32(1):215–35. PMID: 24491658.

Anesthesia for Dental Procedures

Esther Y. Yang and Arvind Chandrakantan

A three-year-old child presents for dental extractions and rehabilitation. Previous attempts to treat for a malodor and broken tooth in the dentist's office were unsuccessful.

What Criteria Does a Dentist Use to Decide Whether to Treat a Child in the Office or Under General Anesthesia?

Many factors enter into this decision and include the age of patient, treatment requirements (extraction, crowns, rehabilitation), behavior, and additional medical history.

Younger patients tend to have less cognitive and emotional ability to cooperate for an exam, radiographs, local anesthetic administration, and dental procedures in the office. Their attention span and ability to open their mouths for a prolonged amount of time are still being developed. Such children have often failed attempts at "conscious" sedation in the dentist's office.

Depending on the amount and extent of treatment necessary, the patient's ability to tolerate the treatment will vary. The average pediatric patient will have 20 primary teeth and, depending on the location of their cavities, may require multiple areas of local anesthetic. Therefore, a child who has a cavity on the lower right and also lower left quadrants of the mouth may need two separate injections. A patient who has anywhere from 8 to 12 cavities may require multiple dental procedures. Cooperation from a child often decreases with increased number of procedures. This can be consolidated into a single operating room visit under general anesthesia.

The presence of oral or perioral pathology, anatomical anomalies, or trauma that requires surgical intervention and requires stabilization and splinting will be facilitated by the use of general anesthesia.

Infections or abscesses that cause swelling or dysphagia will predispose to airway obstruction during sedation, and should instead be referred for general anesthesia.

Patients with comorbidities that require medical management, or unique management of sedation, should be referred for pediatric anesthesia consultation. These include congenital heart disease, bleeding disorders, craniofacial abnormalities with a compromised airway, severely developmentally delayed and combative patients, to name a few.

What Type of Tracheal Intubation Is Indicated for Dental Procedures?

A nasal intubation with a cuffed Ring-Adair-Elwyn (RAE) tube is preferred because it allows the dentist a clear view of the oral cavity and maximal working space in a limited area. Nasotracheal intubation is safe in children of all ages. The size of the nasal tube should be a half size smaller than the appropriate oral route size. The most common complication from nasotracheal intubation is bleeding that results from the tube shearing off friable nasal or adenoidal tissue. This can be decreased by softening the tube by presoaking it in hot water and using the red rubber catheter technique. This consists of preinsertion of a lubricated, appropriately sized red rubber catheter through the nasal passage and into the oropharynx. (It is initially used as a "sound" in each nasal passage to determine if one side is more patent than the other.) The nonleading flanged end of the rubber tube is attached to the beveled end of the nasotracheal tube to provide a nontraumatic leading edge through the nasopharynx, and then detached when the tracheal tube passes into the oropharynx. Prior to insertion of the nasotracheal tube, 0.05% oxymetazoline should be administered into each nasal passage to further attenuate bleeding. Nasotracheal tube insertion in children is not technically different than that for adults, except that the unique angling of the child's oropharynx usually necessitates the assistance of a Magill forceps to feed the tracheal tube in an anterior direction toward the glottic inlet.

When Should Antibiotics for Endocarditis Prophylaxis Be Administered?

Since nasotracheal intubation may result in a transient bacteremia, antibiotics for endocarditis prophylaxis should be administered to certain high-risk susceptible children. These include patients with:

- Prosthetic heart valves, including mechanical, bioprosthetic, and homograft valves (transcatheter-implanted as well as surgically implanted valves are included), and patients with prosthetic material used for cardiac valve repair, such as annuloplasty rings and chords;
- Prior history of endocarditis;
- Unrepaired cyanotic congenital heart disease;
- Repaired congenital heart disease with residual shunts or valvular regurgitation at the site or adjacent to the site of the prosthetic patch or prosthetic device;
- Repaired congenital heart defects with catheter-based intervention involving an occlusion device or stent during the first six months after the procedure; and
- Valve regurgitation due to a structurally abnormal valve in a transplanted heart

What Are the Contraindications to Nasal Intubation?

Certain medical circumstances may necessitate avoidance of a nasal intubation. These include bleeding disorders such as hemophilia, use of anticoagulants, and a previous cleft palate repair with a pharyngeal flap between the palate and the nasopharynx. An oral tracheal tube is then used, and the dentist, in collaboration with the anesthesia practitioner, moves it from side to side during the procedure to optimize surgical exposure.

Suggested Reading

Watt S, Pickhardt D, Lerman J, Armstrong J, Creighton PR, Feldman L. Telescoping tracheal tubes into catheters minimizes epistaxis during nasotracheal intubation in children. *Anesthesiology*. 2007;106:238–42. PMID: 17264716.

Wilson W, Taubert KA, Gewitz M, et al. Prevention of infective endocarditis: guidelines from the American Heart Association: a guideline from the American Heart Association Rheumatic Fever, Endocarditis, and Kawasaki Disease Committee, Council on Cardiovascular Disease in the Young, and the Council on Clinical Cardiology, Council on Cardiovascular Surgery and Anesthesia, and the Quality of Care and Outcomes Research Interdisciplinary Working Group. *Circulation*. 2007;116:1736. PMID: 17446442.

Strabismus Surgery

Chris D. Glover and Christian Balabanoff-Acosta

> A three-year-old child with Trisomy 21 presents for right strabismus repair. Past medical history is significant for a ventricular septal defect (VSD) and a persistent inward deviation of the right eye that the parents report is constant over the last year. She is not currently on any medications and the parents report no allergies.

What Is Strabismus? What Is Amblyopia?

Strabismus is the misalignment or deviation of the eyes. The prevalence in children ranges from 2% to 7%. This misalignment can be associated with diplopia, decreased vision, and headaches. Neonatal strabismus usually resolves by three months of age. Strabismus found in school age children is considered aberrant and usually warrants an evaluation. A general understanding of the more common diagnosis will facilitate this discussion. *Esotropia* is the inward deviation of the nonfixed eye. *Exotropia* is the outward deviation of the non-fixed eye. *Hypertropia* is an upward vertical deviation of the non-fixed eye while *hypotropia* is defined as the downward vertical deviation of the non-fixed eye.

Amblyopia or lazy eye is defined by decreased vision in an eye when it fails to work properly with the brain. It is commonly caused by strabismus and usually treated with patching or through the use of atropine eye drops, which blur vision in the stronger eye forcing a child to predominantly use the weaker eye.

Given the FDA's Concerns with Neurodevelopment, Is It Imperative to Correct Strabismus at This Time or Could This Case Be Considered Elective and Be Performed When the Child Is Older?

While the FDA's concerns on anesthetic neurotoxicity continue to be debated, it is imperative that this child receives treatment in the form of corrective lenses, pharmacologic aids, or surgical correction. Visual maturity usually occurs through age five and this must be weighed when deciding on corrective action. The primary reason for surgically correcting strabismus at an early age is to restore binocular vision to maintain visual acuity, to improve depth perception, and to eliminate double vision. Earlier correction may prevent amblyopia and visual loss given the higher risk children with strabismus pose. This is further supported by evidence that the duration of the misalignment is a major predictor of the outcome.

What Are Considerations Associated with the Preoperative Assessment in Children Presenting for Strabismus Repair?

Strabismus surgery remains quite common in pediatric ophthalmology practice. While most children with strabismus are healthy, the preoperative assessment should attempt to elucidate coexisting syndromes. This can include cerebral palsy, craniofacial syndromes, neurofibromatosis, and hydrocephalus. Outside of that, the risk of postoperative nausea and vomiting should also be discussed.

Syndromes Associated with Strabismus

- Craniosynostosis syndromes: Apert and Crouzon syndromes
- Goldenhar syndrome
- Marfan syndrome/Homocystinuria
- Myotonic dystrophy
- Down syndrome
- Hydrocephalus
- Neurofibromatosis
- Cerebral palsy
- Prematurity

How Will You Secure the Airway in This Patient?

Several options are available for airway management during strabismus repair, including a supraglottic airway (SGA) or tracheal intubation. When using an SGA, it is most convenient for the surgeon if a flexible shaft is used, that can be secured to the chin. If tracheal intubation is chosen, an oral RAE tube should be used, when available, for the same reasons to facilitate the surgical approach.

How Will You Maintain General Anesthesia?

Inhaled anesthesia with volatile anesthetics, total intravenous anaesthesia (TIVA) with propofol, or a combination of both can be used for strabismus surgery. The use of propofol may decrease the risk of postoperative nausea and vomiting (PONV). Since these surgeries are at a relatively higher risk of OR fires because of the proximity to the airway, a low FIO_2 (<30%) should be maintained. PONV is discussed in detail in Chapter 5.

After Induction, the Surgeon Informs You that She Would Like to Perform a Forced Duction Test and Would Like Paralysis. What Is a Forced Duction Test and What Is Its Purpose? Is Succinylcholine an Appropriate Choice for This Patient?

The forced duction test (FDT) tests ocular muscle range of motion to differentiate between a mechanical or paralytic etiology for the strabismus. Surgeons may request nondepolarizing muscle relaxants to have the muscles completely relaxed, but this seems rare in practice. Use of succinylcholine should be avoided as it may result in erroneous information obtained during the FDT potentialy altering surgical management.

Is There a Malignant Hyperthermia (MH) Risk Associated with Strabismus Repair? What about Masseter Muscle Spasm?

By most accounts, the answer is that no correlation exists between malignant hyperthermia (MH) and patients undergoing strabismus repair. A review of MH susceptibility in over 2,500 patients revealed no association between MH and strabismus. When looking at masseter spasm, children with strabismus have traditionally had a fourfold higher incidence when compared to children without strabismus following a single exposure to succinylcholine. However, given the difficulty in diagnosing masseter muscle spasm and the lack of objective findings associated with this disorder, an association between strabismus and masseter spasm remains difficult.

What Is the Oculocardiac Reflex (OCR)? What Are the Risk Factors Associated with OCR? Please Delineate an Algorithm for Treating OCR? Are There Ways to Prevent OCR from Occurring?

First described in 1908 by Bernard Ashner and Guiseppe Dagnini, the oculocardiac reflex can occur from extraocular and intraocular causes. Traction of the ocular muscles and pressure on or around the globe are readily apparent extraocular causes. Intraocular causes can include ocular trauma, increases in ocular pressure from injections, or an evolving hematoma. The OCR is a trigeminal-vagal nerve reflex arc that results in a significant decrease in the heart rate. The afferent limb travels via the long and short ciliary nerves to the ciliary ganglion and then continues to the gasserian ganglion along the ophthalmological division of the trigeminal nerve. The efferent impulse travels by way of the nucleus of the vagus nerve to the cardiac depressor nerve, which produces the negative inotropic and conduction effects seen with this reflex.

Left untreated, this reflex can manifest in a number of dysrhythmias including junctional bradycardia, atrioventricular block, premature ventricular contractions or asystole. Of note, the OCR is more severe and sustained if the stimulus is abrupt or sustained. The occurrence of the oculocardiac reflex has been quoted to be as high as 90% depending on the anesthetic and the use of anticholinergics.

The OCR usually resolves with removal of the surgical stimulus and this should be the first step in treating OCR-induced bradycardia. Ventilatory status should be assessed as apnea can accompany OCR. Depth of anesthesia should also be assessed. If there is hemodynamic instability or the presence of aberrant underlying cardiac rhythms, atropine should be the first line agent administered.

There are some principles that can mitigate the prevalence of OCR. They include:

- Surgeon/anesthesia communication: to coordinate when the surgical stimulus occurs as well as ensuring adequate depth of anesthesia.
- Avoidance of hypercarbia and hypoxia.
- Administration of anticholinergics: this has been shown to statistically decrease the incidence of OCR.

Another possibility is the oculocardiac reflex that presents itself in this surgery is secondary to the pressure on the eyes. The net effect is a vagal response with bradycardia and hypotension. This vagal response occurs by stimulation of the afferent nerves from the V1 portion of the trigeminal nerve which extend to the midbrain with efferent response from the vagal nerve. If it presents the surgeon should be told to halt surgery and pressure on the eyes. Having a syringe of atropine (0.02 mg/kg) and glycopyrrolate on hand will be helpful to treat the vagal response.

What Is Your Plan for Emergence and Extubation?

Most surgeons prefer deep extubation. To perform deep extubation, you will have to have the patient breathing at a steady rate and deep enough either with TIVA or sevoflurane to blunt the response to oral suctioning.

As this surgery has a high risk for nausea, dexamethasone 0.15 mg/kg should be administered after induction. Ondansetron 0.1 mg/kg 30 minutes before the end of the case should always be given.

As mentioned earlier a sub-hypnotic infusion with IV propofol 15–20 mcg/kg/min during the procedure will prove helpful in patients with known PONV.

Other antiemetics that can be used are metoclopramide 0.1 mg/kg (maximum dose of 10 mg) and/or promethazine in patients over 24 months 0.25–1 mg (max dose 25 mg). Suppression of PONV is critical as retching and vomiting result in significant increases in intra-ocular pressure.

The Child Wakes Up in the Recovery Room a Little Agitated and Vomits Later in Recovery. What Are the Risk Factors in Children for the Development of Postoperative Nausea and Vomiting (PONV)? What Are Risk Factors Specific to Strabismus Surgery that Increase the Risk of Developing PONV?

Vomiting following strabismus surgery remains problematic and usually occurs in two-thirds of patients undergoing strabismus repair, if untreated. Untreated PONV can result in dehydration, delayed discharge, and decreased patient and parental satisfaction. Surgical specific complications including: subconjunctival hemorrhage and surgical wound dehiscence are possible.

Risk factors in the development of pediatric PONV have been identified in Table 42.1. Risk factors specific to strabismus surgery include initiation of an emetic reflex associated with ocular muscle manipulation, the occurrence of OCR during strabismus repair, altered postoperative vision, and the number of repaired muscles.

Describe an Optimum Intraoperative Strategy to Mitigate the Development of PONV? Can the Anesthetic Technique Be Optimized to Limit the Incidence of PONV?

Postoperative nausea is remarkably difficult to diagnose in the pediatric population so this will specifically describe a prophylactic strategy using anti-emetics. Metoclopramide at doses between 0.15 mg/kg and 0.25 mg/kg has been shown to be more effective than placebo in preventing early vomiting up to six hours following strabismus repair. The same study found that droperidol at 0.075 mg/kg was most effective in preventing postoperative vomiting (POV). Given the black box warning issued on the use of droperidol in 2001 secondary to prolonged QT issues, its use as an antiemetic has all but ceased. Ondansetron and droperidol are more effective than metoclopramide in reducing PONV.

The two most common agents used currently in strabismus surgery are dexamethasone and

Table 42.1 Pediatric PONV risk factors

High-risk surgery • Strabismus • Tonsillectomy • Mastoidectomy
Age ≥ 3 years old
Personal or family history of motion sickness or PONV
Surgery ≥ 45 minutes in duration
Repeated doses of opioid

ondansetron. Dexamethasone has effectiveness starting at a dose of 0.05–0.5 mg/kg. Ondansetron has been shown to be effective from 0.05 to 0.2 mg/kg. Ondansetron has been found to be consistent in reducing the incidence of PONV regardless of when administered in regards to surgical stimulus. High-risk patients such as those undergoing strabismus repair should receive multimodal antiemetic therapy. Dexamethasone and ondansetron in combination are more effective than either drug administered alone in reducing postoperative vomiting (9% vs. 28%).

The use of different anesthetic techniques has been found to impact the potential development of PONV in patients undergoing strabismus repair. While anticholinergic administration decreases the incidence of the OCR, it does little in the face of preventing PONV. Benzodiazepine as a premedication has been shown to reduce PONV. Nitrous oxide use in pediatric strabismus surgery has not been shown to increase PONV risk, although studies in adults have shown benefit with its exclusion. Propofol used as maintenance after induction does reduce postoperative vomiting, but this must be weighed with the finding of increasing the potential of developing OCR in strabismus patients. Aggressive intraoperative fluid therapy at 30 mL/kg has shown decreases in the incidence of PONV.

An optimal analgesic strategy should be pursued as it may further contribute to PONV, emotional distress, and delayed discharge. Opioids should be minimized if possible given their direct contribution to increased PONV. This is difficult, as ophthalmic blocks are not commonly performed in children. Nonsteroidal anti-inflammatories should be part of an analgesic regimen for pediatric patients undergoing strabismus surgery.

What Can You Do for Emergence Delirium in These Patients?

In pediatric anesthesia, emergence delirium is a common event and more likely to occur in children if with pain and those waking up with either one eye shut or both. Alpha adrenergic medications such as clonidine 1–2 mcg/kg or dexmedetomidine 0.25–1 mcg/kg can be used. As pain is one of the likely culprits, a subtenon block performed by the surgeon during the procedure can alleviate much of the pain that the patients can have. An adequate intraoperative dose of opioids will reduce the risk of delirium. Once the patient is awake, propofol or other fast-acting opiates like fentanyl can be used if signs of delirium show up. Emergence delirium is discussed in Chapter 6.

Suggested Reading

Chisakuta AM, Mirakhur RK. Anticholinergic prophylaxis does not prevent emesis following strabismus surgery in children. *Paediatr Anaesth.* 1995;5:97–100. PMID: 7489431.

Donahue SP. Clinical practice. Pediatric strabismus. *N Engl J Med.* 2007;356:1040–7. PMID: 17347457.

Gayer S, Tutiven J. Anesthesia for pediatric ocular surgery. *Ophthalmol Clin North Am.* 2006; 19:269–78. PMID: 16701164.

Hopkins PM. Malignant hyperthermia: advances in clinical management and diagnosis. *Br J Anaesth.* 2000;85:118–28. PMID: 10928000.

Kuhn I, Scheifler G, Wissing H. Incidence of nausea and vomiting in children after strabismus surgery following desflurane anaesthesia. *Paediatr Anaesth.* 1999;9(6):521–6. PMID: 10597556.

Robaei D, Rose KA, Kifley A, et al. Factors associated with childhood strabismus: findings from a population-based study. *Ophthalmology.* 2006;113:1146–53. PMID: 16675019.

Anesthesia for Penile Procedures

Kathleen Chen, Ann Ng, Kayla McGrath, and Donald A. Schwartz

An 18-month-old boy with phimosis presents for circumcision. He is otherwise healthy. In your preoperative discussion with the parents, you describe performing general anesthesia with a caudal block. The parents seem concerned about "sticking a needle near the spine" as the patient's mother reports a bad experience with her labor epidural. They ask you to explain the benefits and risks of a caudal block and how it is placed.

What Are the Indications for a Circumcision?

Circumcision is the most common surgical procedure performed in males. This can be performed for medical reasons (e.g., phimosis, balanitis, chronic urinary tract infection), religious practice, societal norms, and/or aesthetic reasons. Commonly, circumcision is performed in the neonatal period; however, it can be delayed for a variety of reasons including prematurity, genitourinary anomalies (e.g., hypospadias) or religious practice.

Medical indications for circumcision include phimosis due to balanitis xerotica obliterans (with a reported incidence of 1.5%) and recurrent balanoposthitis, which is inflammation of the glans and foreskin (1.0% incidence). Other relative indications for circumcision are based on retrospective data that suggests the prevention of sexually transmitted diseases, and a reduced incidence of penile cancer and urinary tract infections, especially in patients with urologic abnormalities who are prone to infections.

Risks of circumcision are rare and include inadequate foreskin removal, inadequate cosmetic appearance, retained plastic ring when using the Plastibell device, infection, and glans or urethral injury.

What Is the Sensory Innervation of the Penis?

The sensory innervation of the penis is supplied by the dorsal nerve of the penis, a branch of the pudendal nerve. The pudendal nerve supplies the entire perineum and originates from the ventral rami of the sacral nerve roots S2, S3, and S4. The pudendal nerve appears in the pudendal canal where it travels anteriorly into the deep perineal pouch. It continues along the dorsum of the penis terminating in two dorsal nerves, located at 10- and 2-o'clock, which are targeted during a dorsal penile nerve block.

Describe the Anatomy of the Caudal Epidural Space and the Sacral Hiatus

The caudal epidural space is the most distal portion of the epidural space at the level of the sacrum. The sacrum is made up of five fused vertebrae (S1–S5) that join the lumbar vertebrae with the coccyx. All of the sacral laminae are fused in the midline with the exception of the S5 lamina, which form the sacral cornua. This defines the sacral hiatus, which is a midline opening in the sacral vertebrae S4 and S5. The sacral hiatus is covered by a membranous layer that extends downward to the coccyx (the sacrococcygeal ligament). It is through this ligament that the caudal space can be entered during a caudal block.

Is a Caudal Block a Good Adjunct to General Anesthesia for Postcircumcision Pain?

Circumcision can cause significant postoperative pain and discomfort. Therefore, it is important to provide postoperative analgesia, the most efficacious of which is a nerve block to provide total anesthesia. Caudal blocks are the most common regional anesthetic performed in infants and children. They consistently demonstrate effectiveness as an adjunct to general anesthesia for surgeries below the umbilicus in children, including circumcision, by lowering the perioperative narcotic requirement.

How Is a Caudal Block Performed?

A caudal block is placed during general anesthesia while the child is in a flexed lateral decubitus position. The sacral cornu can be palpated at the midline just above the gluteal cleft. Once the sacral hiatus is found, a needle (butterfly, straight, or angiocatheter) can be inserted into the hiatus. The needle will pierce skin, a subcutaneous fatty layer, and the sacrococcygeal ligament/membrane. Many experienced practitioners will describe feeling a loss of resistance into the epidural space and the needle should then be advanced several millimeters further into the space. Aspiration of the catheter should occur to decrease the risk of intravascular injection.

What Is a Test Dose in Relation to a Caudal Block?

A test dose is performed to assess if a block is intravascular prior to injection of the local anesthetic. Epinephrine (0.5 mcg/kg) may be used to identify intravascular injection. Most providers use lidocaine 1.5% with 1:200,000 epinephrine for this purpose.

A positive test dose is evidenced as shown in Table 43.1.

Table 43.1 Signs and sensitivity for positive test dose using epinephrine for caudal block

Sign	Sensitivity for intravascular injection (%)
T-wave amplitude increase >25% from baseline	100
Systolic blood pressure increase > 15 mmHg	95
Heart rate increase > 10 beats per minute	71

What Are Indications for a Caudal Block?

- Lower abdominal surgery – e.g., inguinal hernia repair
- Testicular procedures – e.g., hydrocele
- Penile surgery – e.g., hypospadias/circumcisions
- Hip – e.g., manipulations/pinning
- Lower limb – various orthopedic procedures

What Are Contraindications to a Caudal Block?

Contraindications to caudal anesthesia are similar to that of epidurals and/or spinals and include:

- Patient or legal guardian refusal
- Sepsis or infection at the site of injection (diaper rash)
- Coagulopathy
- Congenital anomaly of the lower spine

What Is the Significance of a Sacral Dimple and How Does It Affect Your Decision to Place a Caudal Block?

Sacral dimples and other skin abnormalities of the lower back are seen in 2–3% of newborns. Most dimples are harmless, but some may indicate underlying spinal or bony pathology. Dimples that are associated with skin tags, hair tufts, discolored skin patches or that are located distant from the gluteal fold are more likely to indicate pathology, and imaging with ultrasound and MRI is usually done during infancy. A sacral dimple may indicate the presence of spina bifida occulta – a relatively common condition in which there may be downward displacement of the spinal cord or dural sac, tethering of the cord structures, or the presence of a mass (Figure 43.1). While most cases are asymptomatic, neurologic problems involving the lower extremities and bladder may be present and progress with age. In

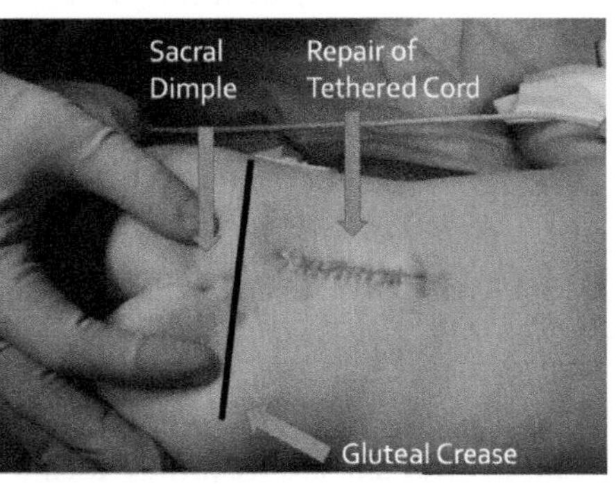

Figure 43.1 Anatomic view of sacral dimple in the presence of a repaired tethered cord. Courtesy of Adam C. Adler, MD

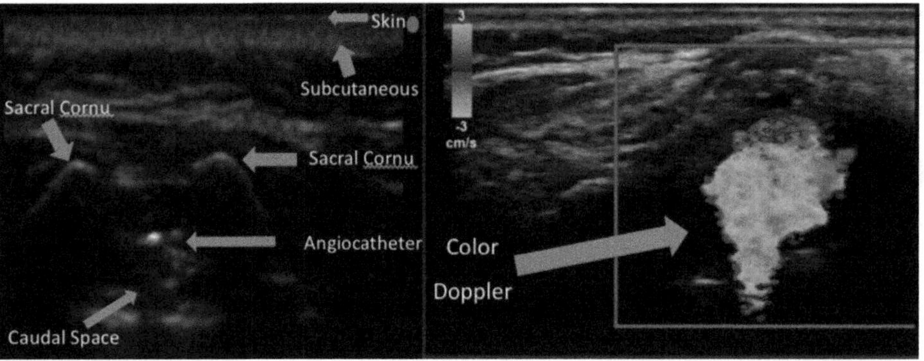

Figure 43.2 Left: Ultrasound guidance for visualization of caudal block placement. Right: Use of Doppler ultrasound to identify location of injection. Courtesy of Adam C. Adler, MD

the absence of an MRI or ultrasound that demonstrates normal underlying anatomy, it is prudent to avoid placing a caudal block.

What Confirmatory Tests Are Available for Caudal Blocks?

Methods to confirm correct placement of the caudal epidural injection include a "whoosh" test, which involves auscultation over the sacrum during injection of air, or nerve stimulation tests. Several groups have described using real-time ultrasound to confirm dural displacement, placing the probe either in the sagittal or transverse axis. Subcutaneous infiltration or ECG changes during the test dose suggest improper needle placement.

What Role Can Ultrasound Play in Performing a Caudal Block?

The availability of portable ultrasonography is proving to be useful for the placement of caudal blocks, including real time assessment of injection in addition to identification of the sacral hiatus when palpation is difficult (Figure 43.2).

How Would You Dose the Local Anesthetic in a Caudal Block and How Does the Dose Affect the Level of Analgesia?

Ropivacaine and bupivacaine are frequently used as the local anesthetics for caudal blocks in the pediatric population. Ropivacaine 0.2% provides similar analgesia to bupivacaine with less motor blockade. Bupivacaine 0.125% does not cause a significant motor blockade. Suggested doses are provided in Table 43.2.

Table 43.2 Dose of local anesthetic for caudal block based on surgical procedure

Surgery	Dose (ropivacaine 0.2% or bupivacaine 0.25%)
Lower extremity	1 mL/kg
Penile/anal surgery	0.7–1 mL/kg
Abdominal incision	1–1.25 mL/kg

- A 0.5 mL/kg dose of 0.25% bupivacaine typically produces analgesia at the lumbo-sacral level;
- A 1.0 mL/kg dose of 0.25% bupivacaine typically produces analgesia to the thoraco-lumbar level;
- A 1.25 mL/kg dose of 0.25% bupivacaine typically produces analgesia to the midthoracic level.

What Adjunct Medication Can You Use to Prolong a Caudal Block?

Clonidine (1 mcg/kg) can prolong caudal blocks with minimal side effects. Higher doses may result in sedation, hypotension, and bradycardia. Clonidine has been avoided in neonates and premature infants due to concerns of postoperative apnea and given careful consideration for those with congenital heart disease.

Opioids can be used to prolong a caudal block, but their use is limited by opioid-related side effects, including sedation, urinary retention, itching, and nausea. Morphine (preservative-free) provides long-lasting analgesia, but the risk of respiratory depression necessitates prolonged monitoring in an inpatient setting. Fentanyl and other lipophilic opioids have not been shown to prolong a caudal block in a clinically significant way.

Ketamine can triple the duration of a caudal block at doses of 0.5 mg/kg without concerns for motor blockade or sedation. However, animal studies have shown that ketamine can cause apoptotic degeneration in the developing brain, thus concerns for neurotoxicity have limited its use.

Intravenous dexamethasone 0.5 mg/kg when given with a caudal block results in longer block duration and reduced requirement for additional analgesics.

What Is the Safety Record for Caudal Blocks?

As a single shot block, a caudal block is a highly reliable and safer alternative compared with other neuraxial techniques in children with no reports of epidural hematoma, abscess, or paraplegia. The reported issues based on the pediatric regional anesthesia network database include:

- Block failure or patchy block (most common at 1%)
- Blood aspiration (0.6%) or positive test dose (0.1%)
- Accidental dural puncture or "wet tap": 0.1%
- Severe local anesthetic toxicity (seizures or cardiac arrest): 0.008%

Caudal blocks can produce a dense motor block which depending on the surgical setting (outpatient/ambulatory) may be highly undesirable. Use of ropivacaine 0.2% or dilute bupivacaine 0.125% helps to minimize motor block occurrence.

What Are the Options for Postoperative Analgesia Using a Peripheral Penile Nerve Block?

The dorsal penile nerves can be anesthetized by injecting 1–2 mL of local anesthetic solution below the deep fascia at the base of the penis at the 2- and 10-o'clock positions. This is commonly referred to as a dorsal penile nerve block (DPNB). Complications of DPNB include subcutaneous hematoma at the site of injection (fairly common), and rarely, arterial injection.

Alternatively, a penile block can be accomplished with one injection into the subpubic space, which contains the pudendal nerve as it exits from beneath the pubic bone. The base of the penis is gently stretched downward with one hand while the block needle is advanced along the caudal edge of the pubic bone in the midline. Initially, a "give" is felt as the needle pierces the superficial fascial layer. The needle is further advanced until another more marked give is felt as the needle pierces Scarpa's fascia to enter the subpubic space. After gentle aspiration to rule out an intravascular injection, 3–5 mL of 0.25–0.5% plain bupivacaine is injected. Occasionally a small subcutaneous hematoma will develop, but no other complications from this block have been reported. As this is an end-arterial system, epinephrine is never used in the local anesthetic solution.

Risks of the dorsal penile block include local hematoma formation, local anesthetic toxicity, and potentially ischemia of the penis if epinephrine is used. Ischemia has also been reported at the glans penis when a hematoma at the injection site caused decreased perfusion.

Local infiltration of the penis is distinguished from a specific nerve block and is traditionally referred to as a ring block. Between 2 and 3 mL of local anesthetic solution are injected below the deep fascial level at the base of the penis in a circumferential fashion. Practitioners who prefer the ring block to the DPNB cite the inconsistent anatomical location of the dorsal penile nerves.

Is There a Difference between Penile and Caudal Blocks with Respect to Efficacy?

Multiple studies comparing caudal blocks and penile nerve blocks have found that they have similar efficacy with regard to perioperative analgesia. One study reported that caudal blocks are "more successful" for postoperative analgesia, increasing the duration of time to supplemental "rescue" analgesic agents. Another study demonstrated that caudal blocks are superior in children under six years old (or <25 kg) for hypospadias repair when compared to a penile block. The most recent meta-analysis comparing caudal blocks and penile nerve blocks suggests that both offer similar analgesic success rates for pediatric patients undergoing circumcision with caudal blocks providing a longer duration of analgesia.

Aside from Caudal or Penile Blocks, What Other Means of Analgesia Is Available?

Topical anesthesia with local anesthetic creams is another option for pain management and has been described more commonly in the neonatal population for circumcisions. One common product used is eutectic mixture of local anesthetics (EMLA) cream, a water-based mixture containing 2.5% lidocaine and 2.5% prilocaine. For adequate absorption and efficacy, sixty minutes is required. In studies that looked at EMLA cream application compared to placebo, infants had lower heart rates and less crying. Risks of using EMLA cream include local skin reactions and methemoglobinemia due to the metabolism of prilocaine. Methemoglobinemia has been found to be low risk in infants. A randomized, blinded trial compared EMLA cream applied one hour prior to surgery to penile blocks placed intraoperatively on children 2–12 years of age. This study showed no difference in pain scale between the two groups although no studies have compared the use of EMLA cream to caudal blocks.

Suggested Reading

Adler AC, Belon CA, Guffey DM, et al. Real-time ultrasound improves accuracy of caudal block in children. *Anesth Analg.* 2019;Feb 27. [Epub ahead of print]. PMID: 30829666.

Cyna AM, Middleton P. Caudal epidural block versus other methods of postoperative pain relief for circumcision in boys. *Cochrane Database Syst Rev.* 2008;8(4):1–38. PMID: 18843636.

Hong J-Y, Han SW, Kim WO, Kim EJ, Kil HK. Effect of dexamethasone in combination with caudal analgesia on postoperative pain control in day-care paediatric orchiopexy. *Br J Anaesth.* 2010 July;105(4):506–10. PMID: 20659915.

Johr M, Berger TM. Caudal blocks. *Pediatr Anesth.* 2012;22:44–50. PMID: 21824215.

Schwartz D, Raghunathan K, Dunn S, Connelly NR. Ultrasonography and pediatric caudals. *Anesth Analg.* 2008;106:97–9. PMID: 18165561.

Tsui BC, Berde CB. Caudal analgesia and anesthesia techniques in children. *Curr Opin Anesthesiol.* 2005;18:283–8. PMID: 16534352.

Walker BJ, Long JB, Sathyamoorthy M, et al. Complications in pediatric regional anesthesia: an analysis of more than 100,000 blocks from the Pediatric Regional Anesthesia Network. *Anesthesiology.* 2018 Jul 30. doi: 10.1097/ALN.0000000000002372. [Epub ahead of print]. PMID: 30074928.

Bladder Exstrophy

Kim-Phuong Nguyen

A two-month-old, 5.5 kg infant presents for complete primary repair of classic bladder exstrophy. The infant was born to a 35-year-old G2P1 at 40 5/7 weeks of gestation with good prenatal care. Prenatal bladder exstrophy was diagnosed during an anatomical ultrasound at 22 weeks gestational age.

What Is Bladder Exstrophy?

The bladder exstrophy-epispadias complex consists of rare congenital defects involving the genitourinary and gastrointestinal systems, abdominal wall muscles, pelvic structures, and sometimes the spine and anus. The combined incidence of exstrophy-epispadias complex is approximately 2.15 per 100,000 live births with twice (and up to six times) as many males being affected. Reduction in the expression of p63, a member of the p53 tumor suppressor family, may be a risk factor for development of exstrophy-epispadias complex. During the first weeks of fetal life, exstrophy-epispadias complex results from a derangement in mesodermal layer fusion. The defect in the abdominal wall is widely believed to be the result of overdevelopment of the cloacal membrane which prevents medial migration of the mesenchymal tissue towards midline. The rupture of the cloacal membrane results in herniation of the lower abdominal components to the surface of the abdominal wall.

The severity of the exstrophy-epispadias depends on whether the rupture occurs before or after the separation of the genitourinary and gastrointestinal tracts. The exstrophy-epispadias complex covers a range of severity from epispadias (least severe) to classic bladder exstrophy to cloacal exstrophy (most severe). Classic bladder exstrophy has an incidence of 1 per 10,000 to 50,000 live births and is characterized by an open bladder, exposed dorsal urethra, diastasis of the pubic symphysis, anteriorly displaced anus, inguinal hernia, and genitalia defects. Classic male and female exstrophy is demonstrated by Figure 44.1.

Only 25% of exstrophy-epispadias complex cases are diagnosed prenatally with fetal ultrasound between 15 and 32 weeks of pregnancy, and the remainder are diagnosed during the postnatal examination. Prenatal diagnosis warrants referral to a specialized center with expertise in managing this complex anomaly. Likewise, any infants diagnosed at birth should be sent expeditiously to these centers for experienced evaluation and treatment. Nelson et al. described improved clinical outcomes, lower hospitalization costs, and lower morbidity and mortality rates when patients were treated at specialized hospitals.

What Other Anomalies May Be Associated with Bladder Exstrophy?

While epispadias occurs in isolation, cloacal exstrophy usually occurs with other anomalies. These include malformations of the gastrointestinal, musculoskeletal, and central nervous systems, known as the OEIS complex (omphalocele, exstrophy, imperforate anus, spinal abnormalities). Additionally, patients with classic exstrophy may have skeletal and limb deformities such as clubfoot, congenital hip dislocations, and tibial malformations. Horseshoe kidney and other renal anomalies are more common in children with classic bladder exstrophy (CBE). CBE are rarely associated with omphalocele, imperforate anus, and rectal stenosis. Approximately 7% of CBE patients may have spinal abnormalities such as spina bifida, scoliosis, and hemi-vertebrae.

What Are the Current Treatment Options for Classic Bladder Exstrophy?

Historically, bladder exstrophy patients underwent a cystectomy with high morbidity in the first year of life due to complications from renal failure. Advanced

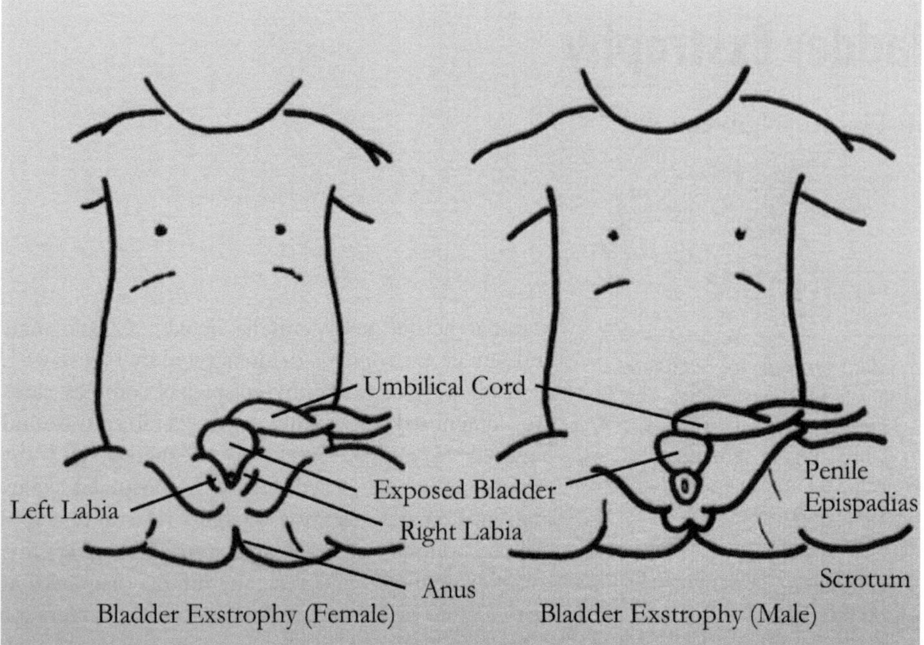

Figure 44.1 Classic features of bladder exstrophy by gender. Illustration by Sandra Perez

surgical techniques have greatly improved survival rates to nearly 100%. The primary reconstructive goal is closure of the bony pelvis, bladder, and abdominal wall defects, followed by epispadias repair; however, long-term goals include preserving renal function, obtaining urinary continence, achieving sexual function, and cosmesis.

The immediate management of bladder exstrophy consists of covering the extruding viscera with sterile silicon gauzes and occlusive dressing to prevent dehydration of the exstrophic plaque and keeping the areas clean with saline washes to reduce risk of infection. There are two main surgical approaches to bladder exstrophy repair: complete primary repair of exstrophy (CPRE) versus modern staged repair of exstrophy (MSRE). As the name implies, the staged repair involves several stages of repair. The first stage is closure of the abdomen and bladder during the newborn period. The second stage is closure of the urethral epispadias. The third stage is a continence procedure and delayed until between ages five to nine, so that the patient achieves an adequate bladder capacity. The complete primary repair combines the first two stages of MSRE. Proponents of CPRE suggest that combining the first two stages stimulates bladder growth and reduces cost by decreasing the number of operations.

PREOPERATIVE EVALUATION

What Preoperative Workup Should Be Considered?

Assessment of all organ systems to ensure absence of associated anomalies is a crucial part of preoperative preparation. Patients with cloacal exstrophy should have cardiac, spinal, and renal ultrasounds to evaluate for associated anomalies. For patients with classic bladder exstrophy, the minimum workup should include a basic metabolic panel to assess baseline renal function before any urinary tract reconstruction. Complete blood count is usually obtained and type/cross-match is recommended if pelvic osteotomies are necessary. For surgical planning, a renal ultrasound screen for other congenital anomalies of the kidney and urinary tract and an abdominal plain X-ray measures the degree of pubic diastasis.

What Preoperative Metabolic Derangements Would Be Expected?

Generally, patients with classic bladder exstrophy have normal kidneys and renal function. For cloacal exstrophy, an inherent short gut syndrome can result in significant fluid and electrolyte losses (sodium, chloride, calcium, and magnesium) from the terminal ileum. Patients with short gut syndrome may have significant fat, fat-soluble vitamins, and bile acid malabsorption.

INTRAOPERATIVE MANAGEMENT

What Monitors and Access Would You Require for This Case?

This infant is presenting for complete closure of abdominal and bladder defects, repair of epispadias, and pelvic osteotomies. The complexity and prolonged duration of the procedure with potential for large blood and insensible losses would require large bore peripheral intravenous catheter, arterial catheter, and central venous catheter along with the routine American Society of Anesthesiology (ASA) monitors. Arterial catheterization allows for sampling of electrolytes, blood glucose, arterial blood gases, and hematocrit levels. Due to the open bladder, urine output is not easily measured. Current noninvasive hemodynamic monitoring systems have not been validated for infants. Central venous pressure monitoring allows for continuous assessment of fluid status and postoperatively, the catheter is used for infusion of parenteral nutrition. Arterial and central line placement can be particularly challenging in small infants. Ultrasound guidance is recommended for insertion of arterial and central venous catheters. Special consideration should be given to pressure point padding given the long procedure, especially the sacrum.

What Intraoperative Fluids Would You Deliver? The Infant Was Breastfed Four Hours Prior to Surgery

Determination of intraoperative fluids requires calculation of the maintenance, replacement of ongoing losses, and correction of any specific electrolyte abnormalities. Maintenance is calculated using the "4-2-1 rule" which was first developed by Holliday and Segar in 1957. The formula is derived by calculating water maintenance based on energy expenditure. For decades, their recommendations for the maintenance fluid of choice has been the use of dextrose 5% with 0.2% normal saline. For this patient under 10 kg, the calculated hourly rate equals 22 mL/h (4 mL/kg × 5.5 kg). Large abdominal surgery with exposed bladder or peritoneum requires 10–50 mL/kg/h of nonglucose-containing isotonic crystalloid to compensate for the insensible losses. Either normal saline or lactated Ringer's solution is routinely used for replacement of volume deficits or blood losses.

What Is Your Plan for Perioperative Pain Management?

Regional anesthesia techniques, especially epidural catheter placement, combined with narcotic and non-narcotic analgesics and sedatives are often utilized. Oftentimes, these infants are managed in the pediatric intensive care unit for the first few postoperative days due to respiratory depressive effects of analgesics and sedatives. Children with continuous epidural analgesia required six- to ten-fold lower doses of intravenous morphine intra- and postoperatively than those without an epidural. Non-narcotic analgesics such as acetaminophen and ketorolac may be helpful alternatives to avoid respiratory depression. Additionally, opioids can reduce GI motility and delay oral feeding. Although ketorolac has been used safely in infants of this age, renal function and postoperative bleeding should be monitored. Despite a well-positioned epidural catheter, additional analgesia or sedation with opioids, diphenhydramine, and benzodiazepines may be required for optimal pain management.

POSTOPERATIVE MANAGEMENT

What Are Some Unique Considerations for Postoperative Pain Management?

The use of pelvic osteotomies during primary closure improves the success of the closure by reducing the tension on the approximation of the pelvis symphysis and abdominal wall and results in deeper placement of the bladder into the pelvis. Fixator pins and external fixation devices are left postoperatively for four to six weeks and the patient is kept immobilized during that time period using modified Buck's traction. Plain film X-rays are obtained to check the degree of pubic diastasis seven to ten days after surgery. If pubic diastasis is significant, the external pins are adjusted gradually to reapproximate the pubic symphysis. A spica cast has been used for pelvic and lower extremity immobilization, but it is associated with lower primary closure success rates and higher skin breakdown. The mean length of stay among bladder exstrophy patients is approximately 30 days.

Effective analgesia is critical to the success of this procedure; however young infants are more vulnerable to the respiratory and hemodynamic effects of opioids and sedative drugs. Epidural anesthesia has multiple benefits as alluded to earlier. Risks of epidural analgesia in very young infants include local anesthetic toxicity, and bacterial colonization of the catheters. Short-term non-tunneled catheters have been demonstrated to be colonized with *Staphylococcus epidermidis* at a rate of 9–11% in the lumbar region versus 29% in the caudal region. The duration of the indwelling epidural catheter can be extended by tunneling the catheter subcutaneously, thereby reducing the risks of bacterial colonization and accidental dislodgement. Kost-Byerly and colleagues reported a case series where tunneled epidural catheters were maintained for up to 30 days in infants undergoing bladder exstrophy repair without increased risk. The lumbar or caudal epidural catheter can be easily tunneled using an 18-gauge angiocatheter or Tuohy needle to the flank of the infant. The entry point of the catheter is covered with steri-strips or topical skin adhesive device. It is recommended to examine the site twice a day to ensure no localized infection or fecal contamination.

What Local Anesthetic Dose and Rate Would You Use for the Epidural?

Bupivacaine and ropivacaine 0.1% to 0.2% are the most commonly used local anesthetics for epidural analgesia in pediatrics. The steady state volume of distribution for amides is greater in children, which prolongs the elimination half-life, and thus, the risk of drug accumulation with repeated doses and/or continuous infusion is increased in infants and children. Bupivacaine must be used with caution as rising serum levels between 1 and 24 hours have been demonstrated with infusions of 0.2 mg/kg/h in neonates when infusing up to 48 hours. In pharmacokinetic studies of ropivacaine in infants under 1 year of age, Bosenberg et al. demonstrated ropivacaine plasma concentrations reached steady state within 24 hours for infusion rates of 0.2 mg/kg/h for up to 72 hours with no adverse side effects.

There is scant data on the safety of epidural beyond 72 hours in infants. A safe level of ropivacaine is considered a maximum serum of 4 mcg/mL or an infusion rate less than 0.4 mg/kg/h. Titration by the measurement of ropivacaine blood levels is not possible as these samples require a lengthy analysis. One recent case report has described the postoperative management of an infant with bladder exstrophy using a tunneled lumbar epidural infusing ropivacaine 0.1% at 3 mL/h (0.4 mg/kg/h) for 26 days. The ropivacaine levels for all samples remained below 4 mcg/mL. For this patient, 0.1% ropivacaine at 2.2 mL/h (0.4 mg/kg/h x 5.5 kg) would be an appropriate rate.

Serum lidocaine levels can be easily measured in most hospital's laboratories and used to guide therapy, alerting clinicians of potential toxic levels. Epidural lidocaine infused at a rate 0.8 mg/kg/h through a tunneled caudal epidural was used safely in neonates with bladder exstrophy. The rate for this patient is calculated at 4.4 mL/h (0.8 mg/kg/h x 5.5 kg) of 0.1% lidocaine.

Suggested Reading

Kost-Byerly S, Jackson EV, Yaster M, et al. Perioperative anesthetic and analgesic management of newborn bladder exstrophy repair. *J Pediatr Urol.* 2008;4(4):280–5. PMID: 18644530.

Meldrum KK, Baird AD, Gearheart JP. Pelvic and extremity immobilization after bladder exstrophy: complications and impact on success. *Urology.* 2003;62 (6):1109–13. PMID: 14665365.

Nelson CP, Dunn RL, Wei JT. Contemporary epidemiology of bladder exstrophy in the United States. *J Urol.* 2005;173(5):1728–31. PMID: 15821570.

Nelson CP, Dunn RL, Wei JT, Gearheart JP. Surgical repair of bladder exstrophy in the modern era: contemporary practice patterns and the role of hospital case volume. *J Urol.* 2005;174:1099–122. PMID: 16094068.

Wilkins S, Zhang KW, Mahfuz I, et al. Insertion/deletion polymorphisms in the Delta Np63 protmor are a risk factor for bladder exstrophy epispadias complex. *PLoS Genet.* 2012;8(12):e1003070. PMID: 23284286.

Chapter 45

Anesthesia for Ex Utero Intrapartum Therapy (EXIT)

Vibha Mahendra and Caitlin D. Sutton

A healthy 26-year-old gravida 2 para 1 female was referred for evaluation by her primary obstetrician after an 18-week ultrasound revealed fetal hydrops associated with enlarged lungs and dilated distal trachea. Magnetic resonance imaging (MRI) of the fetus confirmed a diagnosis of laryngeal atresia with no other apparent anomalies, and a diagnosis of congenital high airway obstruction syndrome (CHAOS) was made. A multidisciplinary team consisting of a pediatric surgeon, otolaryngologist, maternal fetal medicine (MFM) specialist, obstetric anesthesiologist, pediatric anesthesiologist, and neonatologist was assembled to review the case. All team members agreed that known laryngeal atresia made successful endotracheal intubation unlikely, and an ex utero intrapartum therapy (EXIT) procedure was deemed the most appropriate approach to delivery.

What Is an EXIT Procedure?

An EXIT procedure is a coordinated surgical procedure performed via cesarean delivery during which fetal oxygenation is maintained by the utero-placental circulation. These procedures are most commonly performed in fetuses with known congenital anomalies that are unlikely to have a successful transition from fetal to neonatal life without medical intervention. Common indications include airway, pulmonary, and cardiac abnormalities. An EXIT-to-airway procedure allows for placental oxygenation to continue while intubation and/or tracheostomy are attempted. An EXIT-to-resection procedure may be performed for pulmonary abnormalities while taking advantage of the ability to operate while on placental support, such as for resection of a congenital pulmonary mass. EXIT-to-ECMO (extracorporeal membrane oxygenation) allows for continued cardiopulmonary support after placental support is discontinued, such as for severe cardiac anomalies. Common indications for each procedure are listed in Table 45.1. Advances in diagnostic and surgical techniques are rapidly expanding the list of indications for EXIT procedures, but the anesthetic principles and considerations remain largely the same.

How Are Patients Selected for an EXIT Procedure?

A mother and fetus are considered appropriate candidates for an EXIT procedure when the risk of extrauterine death or disability to the fetus outweighs the risk of no prenatal intervention, and the risk to the mother is low. These patients should be evaluated by a multidisciplinary team, including pediatric surgeons, MFM specialists, obstetric and pediatric anesthesiologists, and neonatologists. Ideal patients are a mother with an otherwise uncomplicated pregnancy, and a fetus whose indication for surgery is an isolated defect. Relative contraindications include serious maternal comorbidities or the presence of multiple fetal congenital anomalies or a lethal genetic mutation.

What Should the Anesthesiologist's Preoperative Evaluation Include?

Maternal Preoperative Concerns

A thorough history and physical exam should be performed on the mother with special attention to medical comorbidities, pregnancy-related conditions, past abdominal or gynecologic surgeries, complications with general or neuraxial anesthesia, and information about previous deliveries. The anesthesiologist should be aware of any procedures performed during the pregnancy (e.g., cerclage, amnioreductions), as well as any current medications (e.g., tocolytics, antihypertensives, anticoagulation). Physical examination should focus on the cardiopulmonary system and an

Table 45.1 Common indications for EXIT procedure

Airway/Head and Neck anomalies **(EXIT-to-airway)**	Large cervical masses (cervical teratomas, cervical lymphangioma, large goiters) Retro-micrognathia/agnathia Congenital high airway obstruction syndrome (CHAOS)
Lung or mediastinal masses **(EXIT-to-resection)**	Congenital cystic adenomatoid malformation (CCAM) Bronchopulmonary sequestration Compressing mediastinal masses
Cardiopulmonary conditions **EXIT to extracorporeal membrane oxygenation (ECMO)**	Severe congenital diaphragmatic hernia Certain types of congenital heart disease

assessment of the back in preparation for placement of neuraxial anesthesia.

What Are the Fetal Preoperative Concerns?

For EXIT procedures, the fetus should be as close to term as possible, but some cases such as severe fetal hydrops may require an earlier procedure and delivery. Fetal genetic testing and imaging should be reviewed to ensure there are no contraindications to performing the procedure. The fetal anesthesiologist should be aware of fetal anomalies such as isolated limb abnormalities, as this may affect ease of obtaining IV access. Additionally, discussion with the MFM specialist should include assessment of placental location, fetal presentation, and estimated fetal weight, as these factors can alter the plan for surgical access as well as medication dosing.

The pediatric anesthesiologist's role perioperatively includes preparation of fetal resuscitation drugs, ensuring adequate fetal monitoring with pulse oximetry, administration of medications (intramuscular or intravenous), evaluating and/or managing the neonate's airway, as well as overseeing neonatal resuscitation intraoperatively. In cases where surgical intervention is planned immediately after delivery (such as for resection of pulmonary masses), the pediatric anesthesiologist typically transports the neonate to an adjacent operating room to care for the baby during the procedure.

Describe the Logistical Concerns with an EXIT Procedure

EXIT procedures may occur in adult or pediatric hospitals, primarily based on local institution practices. Given the fact that the anesthesiologists are caring for both an adult and a fetus/neonate, it is not unusual that at least one of the anesthesiologists will find themselves in an unfamiliar environment with different institutional protocols regarding medication availability, transfusion medicine, and overall interdisciplinary teamwork and practices. As such, logistical planning should focus on familiarizing all involved anesthesiologists with the operating room setting, blood bank and pharmacy practices, and equipment and medications in order to minimize complications and delays with intraoperative resuscitation. For example, uterotonics may not be routinely available in a pediatric OR setting. All surgical steps and equipment as well as medications should be explicitly planned and evaluated prior to the procedure in order to identify potential logistic complexities before the day of surgery.

What Are the Maternal Anesthetic Goals?

While cesarean deliveries are typically performed under neuraxial anesthesia alone, EXIT procedures are most often performed using general anesthesia, typically with volatile anesthetics due to their ability to reliably decrease uterine tone.

Maternal goals include preservation of adequate utero-placental perfusion and maintenance of adequate uterine relaxation, typically achieved at volatile anesthetic concentrations of up to 2–3 times minimum alveolar concentration (MAC) of a pregnant woman. Concerns regarding fetal cardiac depression at these high levels of volatile anesthetic have led to increasing interest in the use of other techniques such as supplemental IV anesthesia (SIVA) or neuraxial anesthesia in combination with intravenous medication for uterine relaxation such as nitroglycerin. The patient should be positioned with left uterine displacement (15–30 degree tilt) to prevent aortocaval compression. Blood pressure should be monitored with an arterial line, with the goal of maintaining maternal blood pressure at baseline, and end-tidal carbon dioxide should be maintained at physiological levels for pregnancy, approximately 30 mmHg. Large bore IV catheters may be advantageous for rapid fluid or blood administration.

The volatile anesthetic concentrations required to preserve uterine relaxation for the duration of the EXIT procedure may have the unintended consequence of also decreasing maternal mean arterial pressure (MAP) secondary to decreasing systemic vascular resistance. Uterine flow is not autoregulated, and as such, depends entirely on maternal blood pressure. Vasoactive infusions (most often phenylephrine) are routinely used to maintain adequate MAPs in the mother, thus maintaining perfusion of the utero-placental circulation. At the end of the procedure, the volatile concentration is decreased quickly to allow for adequate uterine tone.

What Are the Fetal Anesthetic Goals?

After hysterotomy, the fetus is exposed, typically allowing for access for echocardiography and to the surgical site and one extremity for pulse oximetry and IV placement. Covering the monitored extremity with foil to prevent interference from surgical lights can optimize the pulse oximetry cable waveform. The fetal anesthesiologist also administers medications as needed to facilitate surgery, including anticholinergic agents (e.g., atropine), muscle relaxants (e.g., vecuronium), and opiates (e.g., fentanyl).

Identify the Steps for Maternal and Fetal Resuscitation

Fetal oxygenation while on uteroplacental support is expected to be 50–70%. Fetal cardiac monitoring typically involves echocardiography to assess fetal heart rate and contractility and is typically performed by a cardiologist or MFM specialist. If abnormal values are observed in any of these metrics, the maternal anesthesiologist must ensure adequate uteroplacental perfusion by optimizing maternal MAP, oxygenation, and volume status. The surgeon should concurrently assess the surgical field for compression of the umbilical cord and palpate it to confirm adequate pulse.

During an EXIT procedure, both the obstetric and pediatric anesthesiologists should be prepared for maternal or fetal distress requiring resuscitation. Maternal hemodynamics should be supported with vasopressors, adequate left uterine displacement, volume or blood replacement and 100% FiO_2. In the event of cardiopulmonary arrest, resuscitation should follow maternal cardiac arrest guidelines, ensuring 30-degree left tilt to relieve aortocaval compression, and emergent delivery of the fetus and abandonment of the EXIT procedure.

If the fetus is hypoxic or hypoperfused but the mother is stable, the fetal team should confirm adequate umbilical cord perfusion and follow the neonatal resuscitation algorithm, including administration of medications and chest compressions. If necessary, the EXIT procedure should be abandoned in favor of umbilical cord separation and continued postnatal resuscitation in the NICU.

Decreased cardiopulmonary reserve in the fetus means that instability may happen quickly, and successful resuscitation depends on excellent communication between surgical, anesthesia, and neonatal teams.

After separation of the infant and clamping the umbilical cord, uterotonics are administered, and the volatile anesthetics are discontinued in favor of an intravenous anesthetic technique. Local anesthetic and morphine are then administered through the previously placed epidural catheter.

What Postoperative Outcomes Should Be Expected in Mother and Baby?

As after all cesarean deliveries, the mother should be carefully monitored for postpartum hemorrhage and venous thromboembolism. A multimodal approach to surgical pain should be employed, including neuraxial opiates, local anesthetic via neuraxial or regional blocks (e.g., quadratus lumborum or transversus abdominis plane block), scheduled acetaminophen and nonsteroidal antiinflammatory drugs, and as needed oral or intravenous opioids.

Neonatal outcomes may be more complicated, and are usually related to the indication for the EXIT procedure. As a result of the procedure, these babies may have an artificial airway in place or require NICU support for other reasons specific to their intervention. Management of these patients should be tailored to the individual clinical scenario and led by the neonatal and pediatric surgical teams.

Case Resolution

At 37 weeks' gestation, the patient presented for surgery. After placement of two 16-gauge IVs and an arterial line, aspiration prophylaxis was administered. A lumbar epidural was placed for postoperative analgesia. The patient was brought to the operating room, and general anesthesia was induced without complications. After uterine exposure, uterine relaxation was achieved with 3.8% sevoflurane, while a phenylephrine infusion was titrated from a starting dose of 0.5 mcg/kg/min to maintain MAPs at baseline.

Hysterotomy was performed with a stapling device, and the fetus' head, neck, and left upper extremity were exposed. The fetal anesthesiologist placed a fetal pulse oximetry probe to the left hand and then administered fentanyl 10 mcg/kg, vecuronium 0.4 mg/kg and atropine 20 mcg/kg intramuscularly to the fetus. The otolaryngologist attempted direct laryngoscopy and noted an imperforate laryngeal membrane that was not amenable to endotracheal intubation. A tracheostomy was then performed with colorimetric confirmation utilizing a carbon dioxide detecting device. The fetal heart rate was maintained in a range of 120–160 throughout the procedure, and after confirmation of placement, the artificial airway was secured and the umbilical cord was clamped. Upon delivery, the neonate was passed to the neonatology team.

After delivery, the volatile concentration to the mother was rapidly decreased and oxytocin was administered via bolus followed by continuous infusion. Once surgical hemostasis was achieved, the epidural was bolused with 0.25% bupivacaine, 100 mcg fentanyl, and 3 mg preservative-free morphine, and the patient was extubated awake. The patient made adequate urine, estimated blood loss was 800 mL and no blood products were given.

On postoperative days one and two, the patient's epidural infusion was continued and she received scheduled acetaminophen and ibuprofen. On postoperative day two, the epidural was removed after a second dose of 3 mg preservative-free morphine was administered. The mother experienced no complications. The neonate remained stable in the NICU with tracheostomy in place with plans for delayed intervention by the otolaryngologists.

Suggested Reading

Braden A, Maani C, Nagy C. Anesthetic management of an ex utero intrapartum treatment procedure: a novel balanced approach. *J Clin Anesth.* 2016;31:60–3. PMID: 27185679.

Brusseau R, Mizrahi-Arnaud A. Fetal anesthesia and pain management for intrauterine therapy. *Clin Perinatol.* 2013;40(3):429–42. PMID: 23972749.

Lin EE, Moldenhauer JS, Tran KM, et al. Anesthetic management of 65 cases of ex utero intrapartum therapy: a 13-year single-center experience. *Anesth Analg.* 2016;123 (2):411–7. PMID: 27258076.

Lin EE, Tran KM. Anesthesia for fetal surgery. *Semin Pediatr Surg.* 2013 Feb;22(1):50–5. PMID: 23395146.

Sviggum HP, Kodali BS. Maternal anesthesia for fetal surgery. *Clin Perinatol.* 2013 Sep;40(3):413–27. PMID: 23972748.

Midgestational Fetal Procedures

Prenatal Repair of an Open Neural Tube Defect

Mario Patino and Arvind Chandrakantan

A 26-year-old G1P0 with a gestational age of 23 4/7 weeks presents with an open neural tube defect (NTD), namely a myelomeningocele (MMC) extending from L3 to S1. She does not have any other comorbidities. She has been seen by the maternal fetal medicine team. There is a single male fetus with an amniocentesis with a normal 46 XY karyotype. A fetal ultrasound shows some degree of hindbrain herniation compatible with a Chiari II malformation with mild hydrocephalus and normal ankle motion. The placenta is posterior with a normal amount of amniotic fluid and an estimated fetal weight of 590 grams. A psychosocial evaluation considers the patient an appropriate candidate for a prenatal repair of an NTD.

What Is an Open Neural Tube Defect and What Are Its Physiologic Effects?

Open neural tube defects (NTDs) are a group of congenital defects that occur due to failure to close the neural tube. This leads to the exposure of neural tissue to the amniotic fluid with subsequent neurodegeneration due to the persistent exposure. This exposure leads to neuronal cell death and loss of axonal connections. The most common form of open NTDs is a MMC in which the spinal cord is exposed and may be covered by the meningeal sac. This most commonly occurs in thoracolumbar, lumbar, and lumbosacral areas. The open defect leads to abnormal neurologic function at and below the level of the lesion with subsequent sensory and motor deficits such as neurogenic bowel and bladder dysfunction. More severe forms of open NTD are incompatible with life. Spinal dysraphism, such as spina bifida and tethered cord, refers to a NTD in which normal skin covers the underline of the lesion.

What Is the Incidence of NTDs and What Are the Causes?

NTDs have an approximate worldwide incidence of 1 in every 1,000 pregnancies. Although the incidence of most open NTDs is higher in females, MMC defects have an equal incidence in males and females. The causes of NTDs are multifactorial. Most of the cases are sporadic. A genetic predisposition is present in some cases with the involvement of genes that regulate folate metabolism. Environmental issues such as low folate levels or the presence of diabetes or prenatal exposure to valproic acid prenatally increases the incidence. Although some markers such as maternal alpha fetoprotein can be useful as diagnostic screening, pre-natal ultrasound during the first trimester is the gold standard to confirm the diagnosis.

What Anomalies Are Associated with NTDs

NTDs are frequently associated with other abnormalities such as skeletal, genitourinary, and gastrointestinal abnormalities. The most common associated defect with prenatal progression of a MMC is the development of a Chiari type II malformation with hindbrain herniation and hydrocephalus. This prenatal progression to a Chiari type II malformation occurs in 75% of cases and requires a VP shunt in most cases. Neurogenic bladder is also significant with 83% of patients requiring intermittent catheterization. Postnatal orthopedic repairs may also be necessary for congenital taloequinovarus (CTEV). Given the multiple medical problems, these patients require a multidisciplinary approach to management.

What Public Health Intervention Has Been Important for the Prevention of NTDs?

A worldwide primary prevention campaign has been implemented with the supplemental administration of folate to reduce the incidence of NTD. Women planning a pregnancy receive 0.4 mg of folic acid per day and women with a high risk of NTD receive 4–5 mg a day. The underlying mechanism of the preventive effect of folic acid is related to DNA replication to facilitate cell proliferation, as well as DNA methylation involving gene expression. It is estimated that even with appropriate pre-gestational administration NTDs still occur in 0.7–0.8 cases per 1,000 pregnancies.

What Are the Surgical Options for the Repair of Open NTDs?

There are three approaches to surgical management: open fetal surgery, endoscopic/fetoscopic surgery, and postnatal repair of the NTD. Parents should receive detailed information about the pros and cons of the different approaches based on the best evidence to facilitate the decision-making process. The open fetal surgery involves a transverse (Pfannenstiel) or vertical incision with the performance of a hysterotomy with fetal exposure of the defect and closure of the defect under direct visualization. The fetoscopic repair requires the exteriorization of the uterus without the performance of a hysterotomy. Instead two ports are inserted into the uterus and the amniotic fluid is partially replaced by insufflated CO_2. The postnatal repair occurs in the first 24 hours after birth to decrease the risks of infection into the central nervous system. Postnatal care requires frequent monitoring with head ultrasounds to detect worsening hydrocephalus given the high frequency of these patients requiring cerebrospinal shunting.

What Are Important Considerations During the Preanesthetic Evaluation for Patients Undergoing Prenatal Repair of an NTD?

Patient selection is critical given the potential maternal risks and the potential benefits of the procedure to the fetus. The first consideration is for maternal safety such that serious and uncompensated comorbidities preclude the performance of a fetal procedure. During the physical examination, emphasis must include the evaluation of the airway and the examination of the spine.

The description of the NTD and the surgical fetal planning has evolved. Therefore, it is important to review the studies preoperatively including fetal ultrasonography and fetal MRI. Specific points of utility to the anesthesiologist include the extension of the NTD defect, the dynamic evaluation of the motor function of the lower extremities, any associated fetal anomalies, the estimated fetal weight, the presence of a Chiari II malformation, the presence and severity of hydrocephalus, and the placenta location. Any important associated fetal anomalies or abnormal karyotype precludes fetal intervention. Another important consideration during the preoperative evaluation is a multidisciplinary approach that includes members of the fetal maternal team, a neonatologist, a neurosurgeon, a pediatric anesthesiologist with experience in fetal surgery, a pediatric surgeon, operating room nurses, and a social worker.

What Are the Advantages and Disadvantages of Proceeding with a Prenatal Repair of the NTD?

The landmark study of prenatal closure versus postnatal closure was the Management of MMC Study (MOMS). The primary outcome was the fetal or neonatal mortality and the need for the placement of cerebrospinal shunt by twelve months of age. Secondary outcomes include the evaluation of motor function and mental development in a follow up at 30 months of age. The study was prematurely discontinued due to better outcomes in the prenatal repair group. The results showed a 50% reduction in the need to perform a ventriculo-peritoneal (VP) shunt (40% vs. 82%), decreased incidence of the progression towards a Chiari II malformation at a 30-month follow up, and improvement in the neurologic function and ambulation in those undergoing prenatal closure. Although the prenatal closure provides all the advantages mentioned above, the prenatal closure group had a higher incidence of maternal complications such as preterm deliveries (mean gestational age 34.1 weeks vs. 37.3 weeks), uterine dehiscence at delivery and mandatory surgical delivery with current and subsequent pregnancies. Long-term outcomes (greater than 30 months) are still unknown. A follow up of the MOMS trial (MOMS 2) is expected in children at the ages of 6–10 years of age.

What Are the Potential Benefits of the Fetoscopic Approach?

It is important to realize that the endoscopic approach for the prenatal repair of a NTD is still experimental. It is a promising technique given the potential reduction in the short- and long-term maternal complications. Potential benefits of the fetoscopic approach include a decreased incidence of preterm deliveries and reduced newborn complications by allowing a vaginal delivery as well as reduced maternal complications associated with hysterotomy. Concerns with the fetoscopic surgery are longer surgical time, the need for further surgery after birth due to cerebrospinal fluid leak and the risk of fetal acidosis secondary to the insufflation of CO_2. Current studies have not shown indirect evidence of fetal acidosis (mainly looking at fetal heart rate as a marker of fetal distress) due to the insufflation of CO_2. An early study comparing the fetoscopic closure versus the open approach showed some concerns due to a longer operative time, higher need for postnatal reoperation rate (28% vs. 2.5%) with similar shunt rate, and perinatal mortality. A more recent report involving more experience and standardized technique reports a lower incidence of reoperation after birth due to cerebrospinal leak, greater gestational age at birth. Further prospective studies with longer follow ups are necessary to establish the role of the fetoscopic repair of NTDs and the safety of CO_2 insufflation, as well as long-term neurodevelopmental outcomes.

What General Perioperative Obstetric Anesthetic Considerations Are Necessary in Patients Undergoing a Prenatal Repair of an NTD?

Principles of anesthesia care for the obstetric patient apply during the performance of the second trimester closure of a NTD. Preinduction, this includes anti-aspiration prophylaxis with an H2 receptor antagonist and metoclopramide. Obstetric airway changes require complete airway evaluation with the use of smaller endotracheal tubes and further preparation to manage a potential difficult airway. A three minute pre-oxygenation is mandatory given the decrease in the functional residual capacity (FRC) and the increased oxygen consumption. A rapid sequence induction is performed given the risks of aspiration. Appropriate sniffing position is critical to facilitate the intubation of these patients. Intraoperative mechanical ventilation should be titrated to maintain a maternal physiologic $PaCO_2$ of 32–35 mmHg. Aortocaval compression usually starts after 20 weeks of gestation due to the mechanical effects of the uterus while lying supine with subsequent decrease in the venous return, causing hypotension and compromising the uteroplacental perfusion. Therefore, placement of a wedge to facilitate a left uterine displacement is crucial. Given the procoagulant state during pregnancy, sequential compression devices should be placed on the lower extremities.

Describe the Perioperative Care of the Patient Undergoing a Second Trimester Repair of an NTD

Intraoperative management of the patient undergoing a prenatal closure of a NTD starts with the placement of a high lumbar/low thoracic epidural catheter to manage pain upon emergence as well as to provide postoperative analgesia. Maternal cross-matched blood as well as O Rh negative irradiated leukocyte reduced blood for the fetus should be available before proceeding with the induction of anesthesia. The operating room temperature should be raised to 26.6°C to avoid maternal and fetal hypothermia. Once the surgical field is prepped and draped and all the surgical equipment is ready, general anesthesia is induced. Close monitoring and optimization of the uteroplacental perfusion requires placement of an arterial line. Appropriate large bore IV access is necessary to administer fluids and to transfuse if necessary. Judicious management of fluids is extremely important, if possible limiting the total administration of intravenous crystalloids to less than 1 liter.

In order to provide optimal conditions during the closure of a NTD (open or fetoscopic), the fetus is administered atropine (20 mcg/kg), fentanyl (5–20 mcg/kg), and vecuronium (0.2–0.4 mg/kg) intramuscularly. During the open repair of a NTD, the exposure of the fetus must be limited to preserve fetal temperature. Replacement of amniotic fluid losses during the open repair is generally done with warm lactated Ringer's solution. Fetal monitoring during the prenatal closure of a NTD is performed by echocardiography with the frequent evaluation of fetal HR, contractility, and volume status. Another useful parameter of monitoring is the umbilical artery flow since absent or reverse diastolic flow may indicate significant fetal distress. If fetal distress is detected during the prenatal closure of a NTD, a rapid sequence of events is necessary to provide in utero fetal resuscitation. Placenta abruption, maternal hemorrhage, or umbilical cord compression should be excluded. Preservation of uteroplacental perfusion must be guaranteed along with preservation of uterine relaxation. Maternal MAP is increased by 15–20% of the preoperative values, aortocaval compression syndrome is avoided, maternal normothermia maintained, and oxygen delivery maximized. If fetal distress persists, administration of IM epinephrine in doses of 1–10 mcg/kg should be considered. In rare instances fetal transfusion may be necessary. Knowing that the fetal estimated total blood volume during the second trimester is 110 mL/kg facilitates calculation of fetal blood transfusion volume. If the fetal distress persists despite all the interventions, delivery with postnatal resuscitation by a neonatology team should be considered in a viable fetus.

An important consideration is the maintenance and preservation of uterine relaxation most commonly provided with the administration of volatile anesthetics. There is a direct correlation between MAC and uterine relaxation. However, higher MAC leads to significant maternal vasodilation and myocardial depression with resultant fetal acidosis. Previous studies looking at the effects of the administration of volatile anesthetics suggest that limiting exposure to volatile anesthetics until uterine manipulation for a hysterotomy can provide better hemodynamics, better preservation of fetal myocardial function, less fetal bradycardia, and better fetal acid base status. Some authors suggest administering total intravenous anesthesia of propofol and remifentanil and switching to volatile anesthetics immediately prior to the performance of the hysterotomy. Coadjuvants and alternative options to provide muscle relaxation include nitroglycerin (bolus of 50–100 mcg followed by a continuous infusion of 0.5–1 mcg/kg/min up to 20 mcg/kg/min), magnesium sulfate (bolus of 4–6 g followed by a continuous infusion of 1–2 g/hour), and subcutaneous administration of 0.25 mg terbutaline.

For vasopressor therapy, phenylephrine has been shown to be the first line therapy given the limited transfer through the placenta with limited effect on fetal acid base status. For the preservation of uteroplacental perfusion, the maternal MAP must be equal to or greater than 65 mmHg of the blood pressure or maintenance within 10% of the preoperative values. The uteroplacental flow lacks autoregulation and is dependent on the uterine perfusion pressure.

Once the closure of a NTD is completed, the amniotic fluid is replaced, and the uterine incision is closed. In the case of fetoscopic procedures, warm lactated Ringer's solution replaces the CO_2 that was previously insufflated. Local anesthetic is administered through the epidural catheter prior to emergence. The patient is extubated under conditions of complete reversal of neuromuscular blockade, being awake, and meeting extubation criteria including appropriate pain control.

Suggested Reading

Adzick NS, Thom EA, Spong CY, et al. A randomized trial of prenatal versus postnatal repair of myelomeningocele. *N Engl J Med.* 2011 Mar 17;364(11):993–1004. PMID: 21306277.

Belfort MA, Whitehead WE, Shamshirsaz AA, et al. Fetoscopic open neural tube defect repair: development and refinement of a two-port, carbon dioxide insufflation technique. *Obstet Gynecol.* 2017;129(4):734–43. PMID: 28277363.

Blumenfeld YJ, Belfort MA. Updates in fetal spina bifida repair. *Curr Opin Obstet Gynecol.* 2018;30(2):123–9. PMID: 29489502.

Boat A, Mahmoud M, Michelfelder EC, et al. Supplementing desflurane with intravenous anesthesia reduces fetal cardiac dysfunction during open fetal surgery. *Paediatr Anaesth.* 2010 Aug;20(8):748–56. PMID: 20670239.

Copp AJ, Stanier P, Greene ND. Neural tube defects: recent advances, unsolved questions, and controversies. *Lancet Neurol.* 2013;12(8):799–810. PMID: 23790957.

Januschek E, Röhrig A, Kunze S, et al. Myelomeningocele: a single institute analysis of the years 2007 to 2015. *Childs Nerv Syst.* 2016 Jul;32 (7):1281–7. PMID: 27086130.

Joyeux L, Engels AC, Russo FM, et al. Fetoscopic versus open repair for spina bifida aperta: a systematic review of outcomes. *Fetal Diagn Ther.* 2016;39(3):161–71. PMID: 26901156.

Moldenhauer JS, Adzick NS. Fetal surgery for myelomeningocele: after the Management of Myelomeningocele Study (MOMS). *Semin Fetal Neonatal Med.* 2017;22 (6):360–6. PMID: 29031539.

Ngamprasertwong P, Michelfelder EC, Arbabi S, et al. Anesthetic techniques for fetal surgery: effects of maternal anesthesia on intraoperative fetal outcomes in a sheep model. *Anesthesiology.* 2013;118(4):796–808. PMID: 23343650.

Chapter 47 Scoliosis Surgery

Adam C. Adler and Howard Teng

> A 12-year-old female with a history of spastic quadriplegia from a perinatal hypoxemic event is scheduled to undergo surgical repair of her scoliosis. She has a history of epilepsy well controlled on levetiracetam. She requires bi-level positive airway pressure (BiPAP) 10/5 cm H_2O at night. She takes glycopyrrolate to help control excessive secretions. Her parents are concerned about postoperative pain control and ask what other medications may be used for her.

PREOPERATIVE CONSIDERATIONS

What Is Neuromuscular Scoliosis (NMS)?

Neuromuscular scoliosis is a spinal deformity associated with neuromuscular disorders such as cerebral palsy, muscular dystrophies, or paralysis. The spine deformity is caused by an imbalance of truncal muscles. It often presents at an early age and can become severe as the patient grows, often involving the entire thoracolumbar spine.

How Does NMS Differ from Idiopathic Scoliosis (IS)?

Idiopathic scoliosis has no definite known cause and is classified by age group:

- Infantile scoliosis <3 years
- Juvenile scoliosis 3–10 years
- Adolescent scoliosis >10 years – most common

Unlike NMS, idiopathic scoliosis does not continue to progress with skeletal maturity and is typically associated with mild comorbidities if at all.

What Types of Comorbidities Might a Patient with Any Scoliosis Have?

For patients with IS, the main complication is disfigurement of the torso. Some patients may also present with mild pain, although severe pain is uncommon and warrants further evaluation.

Of greater concern is the cardiopulmonary complications that can arise from scoliosis. While NMS patients are more likely to present with severe curvatures, patients with IS greater than 50 degrees may also develop cardiopulmonary difficulties. Restrictive lung disease occurs due to a decrease in vital capacity. Pulmonary hypertension due to severe restrictive lung disease and chronic hypoxia may develop in patients with extreme curvature.

Patients with NMS often have other conditions such as sleep apnea, impaired swallow and gag reflexes, impaired respiratory musculature, gastroesophageal reflux, and limited mobility. All these comorbidities may increase the risk of aspiration or infectious pneumonia.

What Is the Cobb Angle?

The Cobb angle is a measure of the curvature of the spine (Table 47.1). It is the angle formed by the perpendicular lines between the upper surface of the top vertebra and the lower surface of the bottom vertebra (Figure 47.1). An angle of greater than 10 degrees is considered abnormal and surgical intervention usually is only warranted for angles greater than 40 degrees. The correlation between the Cobb angle and patient condition is shown in Table 47.1.

Drs. Adler and Teng have contributed equally to this chapter to constitute first authorship.

INTRAOPERATIVE CONSIDERATIONS

Review the Main Surgical Stages of Scoliosis Correction Surgery and Related Anesthetic Implications

After induction of anesthesia, neuromonitoring electrodes are placed and baseline levels are obtained: the anesthetic should be stable at this point, i.e., Total intravenous anaesthesia (TIVA) started and not rapidly changing. A bite block *must* always be in place prior to neuromonitoring to protect the tongue and should be secured to avoid dislodgement. The tongue should be in the middle of the mouth free of any pressure from other lines (e.g., oral glucose tolerance (OGT)/temperature probe). Motor testing should be performed under vision to assure the tongue is not trapped by the teeth.

The patient is positioned prone and padded. All pressure points should be checked and padded appropriately. Auscultation for bilateral breath sounds should occur prior to incision. Antibiotics should be administered; however, care must be taken to avoid greater than one hour from administration to incision as the preparation is often lengthy.

Surgical exposure is associated with significant blood loss and stimulation. Surgeons will often request controlled hypotension and occasionally a single dose of neuromuscular blockage to prevent large muscle twitch with electrocautery. A short-acting neuromuscular blocker should be used and communicated with the neuromonitoring technician.

The spinous processes are removed and the pedicles exposed, also associated with progressive blood loss.

Pedicle screws are inserted bilaterally at each level to be corrected. Evoked potentials should be checked with each screw placement to ensure stability.

Table 47.1 Cobb angle measurements and associated effect on cardiopulmonary status

Cobb angle	Effect on cardiopulmonary status
<10	Normal
>25	Increased pulmonary arterial pressures seen on echocardiogram
>65	Restrictive lung disease
>100	Symptomatic lung disease

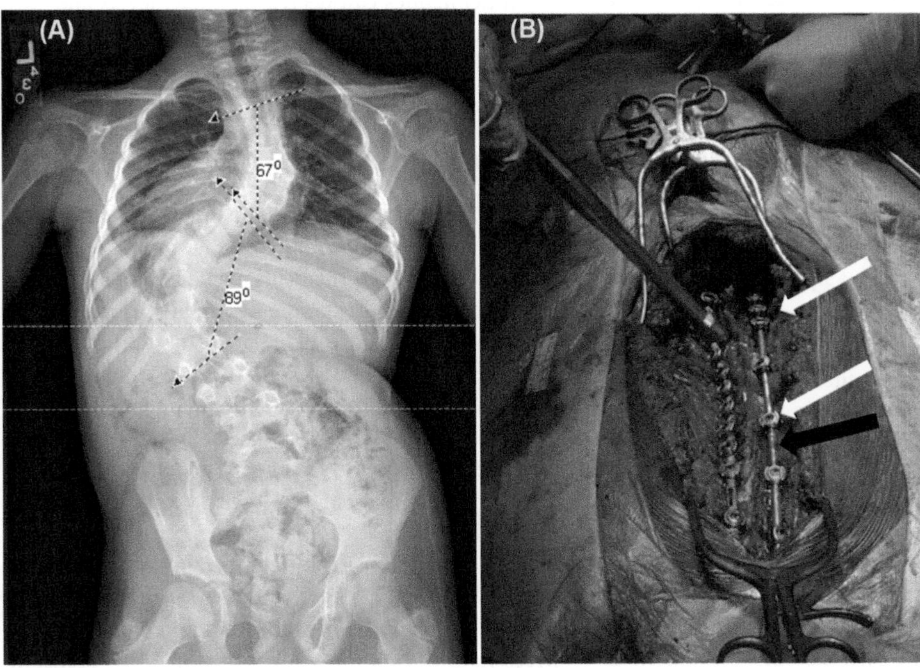

Figure 47.1 (A) Preoperative X-ray demonstrating the calculation of the Cobb angle. (B) Intraoperative image showing placement of pedicle screws (white arrows) and correction rods (black arrow) prior to curvature correction.

Vertical rods are then inserted, secured, and the curvature correction performed. Neuromonitoring should be carefully assessed for loss or reduction of signals.

Autologous and reconstituted bone matrix are packed into areas between surgical hardware and native bone to promote strong bond formation. TIVA should be adjusted planning for emergence.

Surgical closure: takes 30–60 minutes; termination of TIVA should be considered to avoid emergence delays. Long-acting liposomal bupivacaine (Exparel) may be used at the incision site to reduce postoperative pain.

What Are Anesthetic Considerations for Scoliosis Surgery with Respect to Blood Loss?

Blood loss, neuromonitoring, and positioning are the major concerns for the anesthetic management. Studies have noted that patients with adolescent idiopathic scoliosis may lose 750–1,000 mL of blood, while NMS patients experience substantially greater blood loss. Patients with Duchenne muscular dystrophy may have 2,000 to 4,000 mL of blood loss.

Large bore intravenous access and invasive monitoring are necessary, but may be more difficult in NMS patients due to severe contractures and frequent blood draws or line placements. Techniques such as hemodilution, intraoperative blood salvaging, and preoperative autologous donation can help to conserve the amount of homologous blood given.

Antifibrinolytic agents like tranexamic acid can be used to help reduce blood loss. At Texas Children's Hospital, tranexamic acid is given as a bolus at 50 mg/kg prior to incision in addition to a continuous infusion of 5 mg/kg/h.

Aminocaproic acid is another antifibrinolytic agent that may be used. Typically dosed as a bolus of 100 mg/kg followed by infusion of 1 mg/kg/h.

What Monitors/Vascular Access Should Be Considered?

Standard ASA monitors and urinary catheter should be used for all patients. Arterial line placement is generally standard for monitoring blood pressure throughout the procedure as well as measurement of hemoglobin and hematocrit.

Central lines are generally placed in patients with NMS as they are at high risk of requiring vasoactive medications. For patients with IS, central line placement is not routine.

Some institutions employ a bispectral index (BIS) monitor to identify change in trends. When neuromonitoring is performed depth of anesthesia based on EEG suppression can be discussed with the neuromonitoring staff routinely throughout the case.

Temperature should be monitored continuously with a forced air warmer placed prior to surgical draping as these patients often become hypothermic during these cases.

What Accounts for the Higher Blood Loss during Surgery with NMS Patients Compared to IS Patients?

- Usually more levels requiring instrumentation
- Requirement of pelvic alignment in addition
- Poor nutritional status
- Impaired connective tissue function
- Concomitant seizure disorders with use of antiepileptics can decrease platelet levels and factor 8 levels

Is Controlled Hypotension Safe for Spinal Surgeries?

Controlled hypotension is a common technique to prevent blood loss in various surgeries. It is best accomplished using medications that are easily titratable such as nitroprusside, esmolol, nicardipine, or remifentanil. The use of volatile anesthetics for the purposes of controlled hypotension is limited due to neuromonitoring concerns.

Controlled hypotension is usually safe in an otherwise healthy patient. A mean arterial pressure of 55–60 mmHg is often the lowest target blood pressure. Historically, extremes of hypotension were performed and are no longer recommended. Some patients, especially those with NMS, may be at risk for end-organ ischemia due to their comorbidities, necessitating caution with controlled hypotension. The risks of decreased perfusion and ischemia necessitate that normocarbia, normovolemia, and adequate hemoglobin are maintained to ensure sufficient oxygen-carrying capacity in the patient.

What Medications Are Used to Provide Controlled Hypotension Spinal Surgeries?

- Nicardipine: 0.5–5.5 mg/kg/h (total should be less than 15 mg/h)
- Esmolol: 50–150 mcg/kg/min
- Labetolol: 0.1–1 mg/kg/dose (bolus dosing)

How Will Anesthetics Affect Neurophysiologic Monitoring?

Volatile anesthetics and nitrous oxide all attenuate somatosensory evoked potential (SSEP) waveforms and thus should be maintained at a low minimum alveolar concentration (MAC) if used at all. Opioids, benzodiazepines, propofol, and dexmedetomidine all have minimal effects on SSEPs and MEPs. Ketamine can be used to augment SSEP and motor-evoked potential (MEP) amplitudes, and thus can be useful for NMS patients who have weaker waveforms at baseline. If using ketamine, it is important to maintain a steady state to ensure that changes in neuromonitoring, if present, are not related to changes in medication administration.

Wake-up tests also may be used to check for spinal cord integrity by asking the patient to move his or her hands and feet when awake. Because of the possibility of conducting a wake-up test, short-acting anesthetics such as remifentanil and desflurane are beneficial.

What Immediate Interventions Should Occur If Signal Loss Is Observed?

- Switch to 100% oxygen.
- Notify surgeon.
- If possible, reverse last surgical intervention (i.e., last pedicle screw placed).
- Increase mean arterial pressure (MAP) >80 with vasoactive medication.
- Ensure normothermia and normocarbia.
- Maintain hematocrit >30.
- Consider steroid bolus and infusion: methylprednisolone 30 mg/kg then 5.4 mg/kg/h.
- Consider wake-up test to assess function in developmentally appropriate patients.
- Consider stat MRI.

What Are the Common Anesthetics Used to Maintain Anesthesia During Spine Surgery?

Most scoliosis surgeries are done with neuromonitoring of the spinal cord tracts. Providers tend to employ total intravenous anesthesia using a combination of the following:

Hypnotic/Sedatives

- Propofol: 100–250 mcg/kg/min
- Dexmedetomidine: 0.1–1 mcg/kg/h
- Midazolam: 0.02–0.1 mg/kg/h

Analgesics

- Sufentanil: 0.2–2 mcg/kg/h
- Fentanyl: 0.5–2 mcg/kg/h
- Methadone: 0.05–0.2 mg/kg bolus at start of case
- Remifentanil: 0.2–1 mcg/kg/min
- Ketamine: 5–20 mcg/kg/min

Depth of anesthesia should be discussed with the neuromonitoring provider to allow for adjustments to the anesthetic based on the level of EEG suppression.

Some institutions allow for use of low concentrations of inhaled agents (sevoflurane or nitrous oxide).

Long-acting local anesthetic is also commonly employed (Exparel) to reduce postoperative incisional pain.

How Does Prone Positioning Affect Cardiopulmonary Status?

Prone positioning can significantly increase intraabdominal pressure. As a result, ventilation may be impaired due to reduced chest compliance. The increased intraabdominal pressure may cause compression of the inferior vena cava (IVC), and thus lead to hypotension and decreased cardiac output. Compression of the IVC can also lead to engorgement of the paravertebral and epidural veins, causing increased bleeding in the surgical field. Consequently,

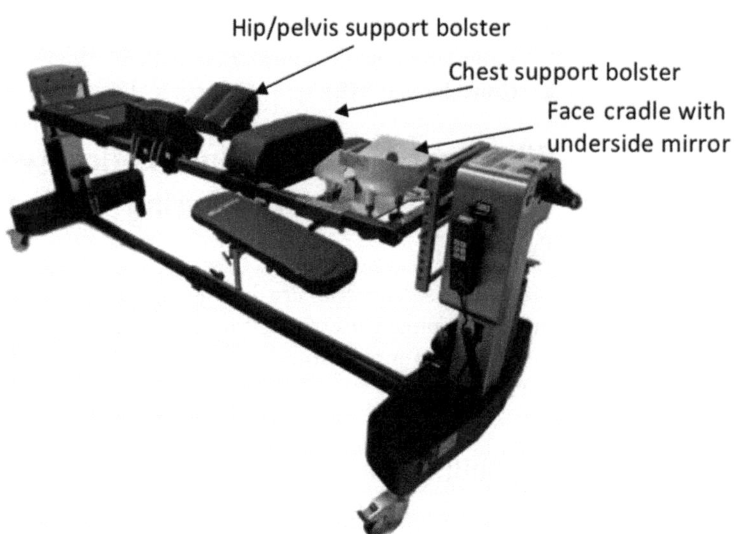

Figure 47.2 Standard spine table with key positioning features outlined

care should be taken to minimize abdominal compression by using special frames and tables (i.e., Jackson Spine table) (Figure 47.2).

What Other Considerations Are Required for Patients in the Prone Position?

Patients undergoing scoliosis surgery in the prone position are at higher risk for eye injuries. Vision loss is most frequently due to ischemic optic neuropathy. Other eye injuries include corneal abrasions, optic vein engorgements and retinal ischemia and cortical blindness. The external pressure on the face from placing the patient's head in a mask, foam pillow, or other similar devices is one of several factors that may contribute to vision loss. If the anesthetist is not careful to relieve any pressure from the eyes, ischemia may occur. Additionally, hypotension and anemia may further decrease perfusion pressure to the eyes.

As with positioning for any surgery, care must be taken to avoid pressure on peripheral nerves such as the ulnar nerve. Other areas at increased risk of external pressure injury from prone positioning include the male genitalia, breasts, feet, and the anterior superior iliac spine. A plan to close or cover the patient's incision and turn him/her supine must also be established ahead of time in case CPR is needed as the prone position affords a higher incidence of venous air embolism.

What Pharmacologic Adjuncts Can Be Used Intraoperatively?

- Ketorolac: 0.5 mg/kg up to 30 mg if hemostasis is adequate: should be discussed with the surgeon prior to administration
- Acetaminophen: 12.5–15 mg/kg IV up to 1000 mg per dose
- Diazepam: 0.1 mg/kg IV

POSTOPERATIVE CONSIDERATIONS

What Are Common Immediate Postoperative Considerations?

While rare for patients with IS, patients with NMS may require postoperative intubation. The decision to remain intubated is dependent on: preoperative respiratory status, ease of surgical procedure, degree of correction, blood loss, fluid administration, and ongoing need for transfusion or vasopressors. Scoliosis surgery itself causes a decrease in pulmonary function of up to 60 percent of baseline values during the first postoperative week and can last up to six months afterwards.

Pain can be severe after surgery and is best treated with a multimodal approach. IV opioids are often the primary analgesic and a basal infusion may be needed. Nonsteroidal antiinflammatory drugs like ketorolac are also helpful and often started on postoperative day one. However, due to concerns for impaired bone healing, the use of NSAIDs is often center-dependent. Other analgesics that may be helpful include acetaminophen, ketamine, and antiepileptics (gabapentin). Some centers use epidural catheters for the management of postoperative pain. In this method, one or two catheters are inserted by the surgeon prior to wound closure. Intraoperative methadone is frequently given, especially to patients with IS, due to its long duration of action.

Bleeding and hypotension can continue to be postoperative concerns as well. Consequently, serial labs, fluid resuscitation, and occasionally vasopressors may be needed.

Muscle spasms are a major source of morbidity and pain postoperatively, especially in patients with NMS that are unable to ambulate. Muscle relaxants (e.g., diazepam) should be considered, as early as in PACU. Untreated muscle spasms, especially in children with NMS, are often confused with incision pain and are less well managed by opioids.

What Are Common Postoperative Considerations in the Days Following Scoliosis Surgery?

Patients with IS should be considered for enhanced early recovery pathway.

Attention to aggressive pulmonary toilet, especially for nonambulatory patients, is crucial to avoid pulmonary morbidity:

Early ambulation and physical therapy.

Removal of indwelling lines as early as tolerated.

Advance diet as tolerated.

Encourage use of non-opioid analgesics as well as bowel regiment.

Compression boots for DVT prophylaxis.

Suggested Reading

DePasse JM, Palumbo MA, Haque M, et al. Complications associated with prone positioning in elective spinal surgery. *World J Orthop*. 2015:6: 351–9. PMID: 25893178.

Gornitzky AL, Flynn JM, Muhly WT, et al. A rapid recovery pathway for adolescent idiopathic scoliosis that improves pain control and reduces time to inpatient recovery after posterior spinal fusion. *Spine Deform*. 2016 Jul;4(4):288–95. PMID: 27927519.

Halawi MJ, Lark RK, Fitch RD. Neuromuscular scoliosis: current concepts. *Orthopedics*. 2015:38: e452–6. PMID: 26091215.

Muhly WT, Sankar WN, Ryan K, et al. Rapid recovery pathway after spinal fusion for idiopathic scoliosis. *Pediatrics*. 2016;137(4). pii: e20151568. PMID: 27009035.

Shapiro F, Sethna N. Blood loss in pediatric spine surgery. *Eur Spine J*. 2004;13 Suppl 1:S6–17. PMID: 15316883.

Chapter

48

Pectus Excavatum

The Nuss Procedure

Adam C. Adler

A 16-year-old female with a history of pectus excavatum (CT: Haller index 3.5) without cardiopulmonary dysfunction presents for cosmetic repair of her pectus deformity. She and her parents are most concerned about postoperative pain control.

What Is Pectus Excavatum?

Pectus excavatum is a congenital deformity consisting of abnormal sternum development that leads to a characteristic caved-in appearance of the anterior chest. The severity of the disease varies greatly from a simple cosmetic deformity to one with significant cardiopulmonary compromise. In addition to the physiologic effects, the deformity itself can cause significant psychosocial and emotional disturbances, particularly during adolescence. Pectus excavatum occurs in roughly 1:300–1,000 live births, with a 4:1 male predominance. Often there is progression of the deformity during puberty.

What Are the Indications for Surgical Correction of Pectus Excavatum?

The indications for surgical repair must include at least two of the following:

- Presence of symptoms most commonly including: shortness of breath with exercise, lack of endurance, and chest pain.
- Physical exam shows that there is a moderate to severe pectus excavatum deformity which may be symmetric or asymmetric.
- The chest wall imaging shows severe pectus excavatum deformity defined as a Haller index > 3.2 or correction index >10%.
- The chest imaging shows cardiac and/or pulmonary compression or displacement.
- Pulmonary function studies demonstrating a restrictive or obstructive pattern.
- Cardiology evaluation elucidates cardiac compression or displacement, rhythm disturbance, and/or mitral valve prolapse.
- Significant body image and/or psychosocial impairment.

What Is the Haller Index?

The Haller index is a measure of severity of compression. It is calculated using dimensions from an axial CT by: transverse diameter of the chest from the inside of the ribcage and the anteroposterior diameter from the inside of the sternum to the vertebral body (at the shortest distance) (Figure 48.1). A normal Haller index is <2.5.

Describe the Surgical Repair of Pectus Excavatum?

The modified Ravitch and Nuss procedures represent the two most widely used procedures for pectus repair. The older Ravitch procedure requires significant exposure of the sternum and resection of abnormal cartilage followed by placement of a metal strut that is later removed. This procedure has nearly been abandoned with the creation of the less invasive Nuss procedure, which provides a minimally invasive alternative that does not require osteotomy or cartilage removal.

The Nuss procedure involves two small incisions, one on each side of the lateral chest wall. A thoracoscope is inserted and the chest is insufflated using CO_2 allowing for an introducer to be tunneled under the sternum by direct vision. The bar is pulled through under vision to avoid injury to the heart using umbilical tape as a guide. The bar ends are curved appropriately followed by a 180° rotation of the bar. The bar ends are affixed to the chest wall to avoid dislodgement (Figure 48.2). The created pneumothorax is evacuated by placing chest tubes with the distal ends under water followed by application of intrathoracic positive pressure to remove all air bubbles.

What Are the Anesthetic Concerns during Pectus Excavatum Repair?

The anesthetic concerns include cardiovascular injury when the introducer and Nuss Bar are placed over the heart, and pain control in the postoperative period. The provider should be vigilant during bar placement for occurrence of arrhythmia and/or hypotension due to external cardiac compression. Rare case reports have documented damage to the right ventricle and cardiac tamponade.

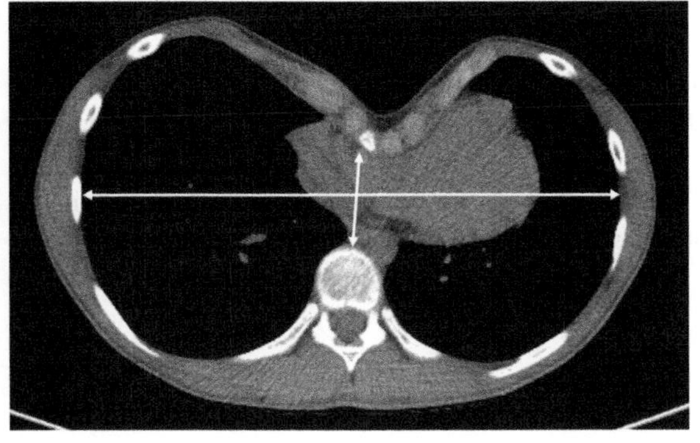

Figure 48.1 Axial CT identifying the Haller index of a patient with pectus excavatum.

Residual pneumothoraces are possible following evacuation of the insufflated CO_2 and should be considered in cases of PACU respiratory compromise.

What Is the Plan for Postoperative Analgesia after Pectus Excavatum Repair?

Anesthesiologists should prepare patients by setting reasonable expectations for their pain after surgery. The extrusion of the chest wall is accompanied by severe pain and a balance must exist between analgesia and respiratory suppression from opioids. Multimodal pain control may include a thoracic epidural, paravertebral block (and catheter), erector spinae plane block and/or intercostal nerve blocks or ablations. An opioid-based patient-controlled analgesia (PCA) is often used either in addition to or in lieu of regional techniques.

Other adjuncts are shown in Table 48.1.

Use of incentive spirometry should be encouraged to avoid atelectasis and postoperative pneumonia. Bowel regimens should be considered for all patients using opioids to avoid significant opioid-induced constipation.

What Are the Complications of the Nuss Procedure?

Early complications include residual pneumothorax, surgical site infection, pneumonia, pleural effusion, pericarditis, and hemothorax. Late complications include bar displacement/dislodgement, over-correction, late wound infection, bar allergy, and need for re-correction.

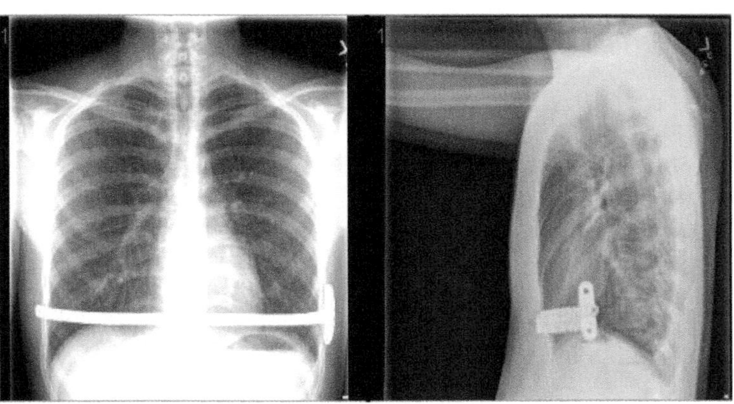

Figure 48.2 Posterioranterior (PA) and lateral chest X-rays demonstrating postoperative placement of a single Nuss bar

Table 48.1 Analgesic agents with commonly used doses for the Nuss procedure by peri- and postoperative courses.

	Perioperatively	Postoperatively
Diazepam	0.1 mg/kg IV	0.1 mg/kg q6hrs
Gabapentin	10 mg/kg PO preoperatively	5 mg/kg PO q8hrs
Methadone	0.1–0.2 mg/kg once	N/A
Ketorolac	0.5 mg/kg IV once Max 30mg/dose	0.5 mg/kg q6hrs Max 30 mg/dose
Acetaminophen	15 mg/kg IV q6hrs	30 mg/kg PO q6hrs

Commonly used bars contain nickel and should not be used in patients with known nickel allergy. Some centers perform nickel allergy testing prior to implantation and use titanium bars in cases where allergy is present. Most patients have the bar removed after two to four years with 98.3% achieving good results after removal.

What Concerns Are Relevant for Removal of Nuss Bar Procedures?

While significantly less complex, removal of the bar involves some of the same risks as during insertion. General endotracheal anesthesia should be performed allowing for positive pressure ventilation and insufflation, should a pneumothorax occur. The ECG should be monitored for arrhythmia when the bar passes over the pericardium. Ventricular damage may occur rarely. A chest X-ray should be done in the PACU to exclude pneumothoraces. Not uncommonly, significant bony formation over the bar and anchoring can make this procedure difficult as the bar becomes affixed to the chest wall requiring greater manipulation which can result in more postoperative pain.

Suggested Reading

Keller BA, Kabagambe SK, Becker JC, et al. Intercostal nerve cryoablation versus thoracic epidural catheters for postoperative analgesia following pectus excavatum repair: Preliminary outcomes in twenty-six cryoablation patients. *J Pediatr Surg.* 2016;51(12):2033–8. PMID: 27745867.

Loftus PD, Elder CT, Russell KW, et al. Paravertebral regional blocks decrease length of stay following surgery for pectus excavatum in children. *J Pediatr Surg.* 2016;51 (1):149–53. PMID: 26577910.

Nuss D, Obermeyer RJ, Kelly RE. Nuss bar procedure: past, present and future. *Ann Cardiothorac Surg.* 2016;5(5):422–33. PMID: 27747175.

Chapter 49 Vertical Expandable Prosthetic Titanium Rib Insertion

Paulus Steyn

A two-year-old boy is scheduled for placement of a vertical expandable prosthetic titanium rib (VEPTR) system for progressive thoracic insufficiency syndrome in the setting of unilateral thoracic hypoplasia. His past medical history includes a staged repair of a tracheoesophageal fistula and a protracted hospital stay in the newborn period, including a tracheostomy that remained in place until about 1 year of age. His current medications include metoprolol and preoperative vancomycin. His current vital signs are: blood pressure 86/52 mmHg; heart rate 110/min and regular; respiratory rate 37/min; temperature 36.5°C; SpO_2 93% on room air. Physical exam reveals an alert and anxious child with normal facial structures. He has a tracheostomy scar. He is not flaring, but he is using his left-sided accessory muscles of breathing. He has right-sided neck torticollis but his airway exam is otherwise unremarkable.

Chest radiograph demonstrates scoliosis with a curve of 100 degrees in the thoracic spine and left sided lung volumes four times smaller than the right side (Figure 49.1).

What Is Thoracic Insufficiency Syndrome?

Thoracic insufficiency syndrome results from any condition that alters thoracic development and results in decreased lung growth. The normal thorax has two important functions: to maintain a constant and normal lung volume and to effortlessly change this volume. Lung volume depends on thoracic spine height and an equally broad and wide enough rib cage. Ventilation (lung volume exchange) depends on normal bilateral diaphragm excursion, rib orientation (recall the bucket handle mechanism) and functioning of the secondary muscles of respiration. The components of the normal thorax consist of the spine, sternum, ribs, secondary muscles of respiration, and diaphragm.

Lung development depends on normal thoracic growth, which entails a coordinated increase in thoracic spine height, and symmetrical enlargement of the rib cage that requires both rib growth and the correct orientation of the ribs. The thoracic spine lengthens by about 1.5 cm/year for the first five years of life, then slows down to about 0.5 cm/year until it experiences another growth spurt of 1.2 cm/year from 11–15 years of age. In the first two years of life, the rib cage is square shaped, the ribs are orientated horizontally and grow in length. Between two and 10 years of age it courses downward and forms an oval-shaped thoracic cross-section. There is a rapid increase in rib growth after the age of 10 years until the child reaches maturity; the final cross-section of the thorax is rectangle shaped.

The diagnosis of thoracic insufficiency is made when the patient has physiologic signs of respiratory impairment, a decrease in chest wall mobility, and worsening lung volumes on imaging. If obtained, pulmonary function tests demonstrate a restrictive pattern with a smaller than predicted vital capacity.

What Conditions Are Associated with Thoracic Insufficiency Syndrome?

Causes of thoracic insufficiency syndrome can be divided into disorders that affect stable lung volumes and disorders that affect normal ventilation.

Disorders that affect stable lung volume include scoliosis with fused or missing ribs, scoliosis with a windswept deformity, Jeune syndrome (asphyxiating thoracic dysplasia, a rare genetic disorder marked by a narrow/small thorax and progressive kidney failure), and spondylocostal dysplasia (previously known as Jarcho–Levin syndrome), a rare congenital disorder that presents with at least 10 consecutive vertebrae that are fused, missing, or partially formed. *Spondylocostal dysplasia* is also marked by ribs that are broadened, fused, growing in bizarre directions, or altogether missing.

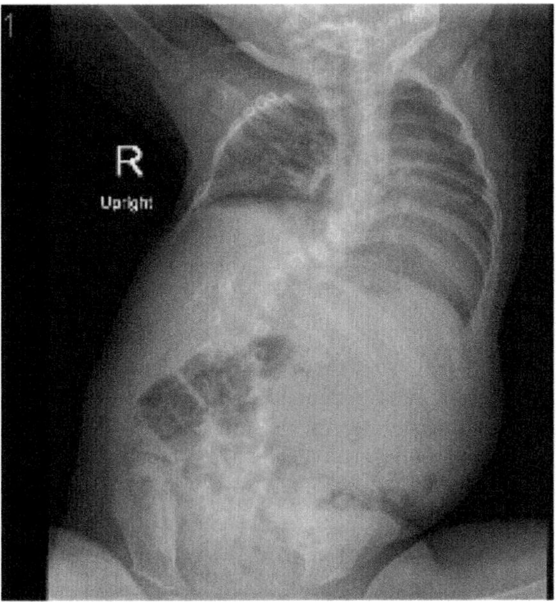

Figure 49.1 AP chest X-ray demonstrating poorly formed and concave vestigial ribs. Reproduced with permission from Springer Nature from Campbell, R.M., VEPTR: past experience and the future of VEPTR principles. *Eur Spine J* 2013;22 Suppl 2:S106–17

Disorders that affect normal ventilation (movement of lung volume) include: congenital diaphragmatic hernia and hemidiaphragmatic paralysis (think phrenic nerve injury from lateral hyperextension of the neck at birth).

Note that standard scoliosis is not typically considered a cause of thoracic insufficiency syndrome.

What Is a VEPTR Procedure?

The Vertical Expandable Prosthetic Titanium Rib (VEPTR) is a device designed to address the complex disorders that cause progressive thoracic insufficiency syndrome in a three-dimensional manner. It is used to stabilize and progressively expand the thorax. Depending on the exact condition it is placed in conjunction with a wedge/expansion thoracotomy, but can also act as the sole device used to stabilize and expand a hemithorax such as in cases where absent ribs cause flail chest. The goals of a VEPTR system are to improve thoracic volume and function by correcting scoliosis and establishing symmetry of the thorax. The idea is to maintain these corrections as the patient grows using successive expansions every four to six months (Figure 49.2).

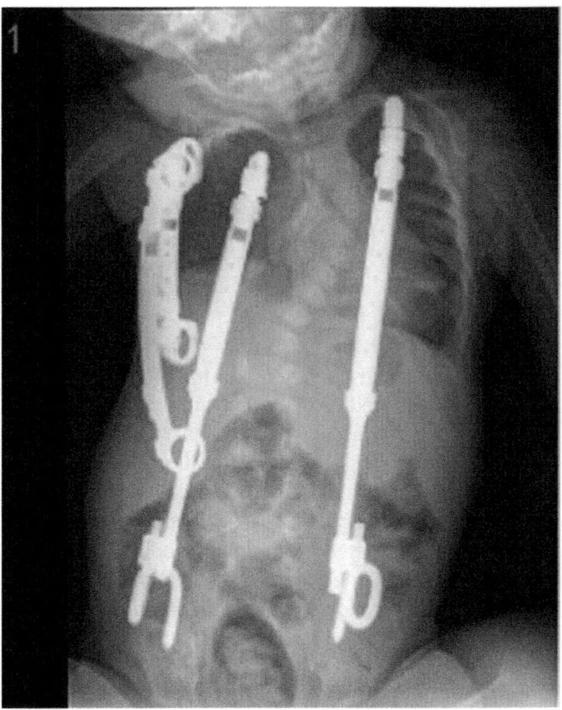

Figure 49.2 Postoperative AP chest X-ray demonstrating VEPTR placement. Reproduced with permission from Springer Nature from Campbell, R.M., VEPTR: past experience and the future of VEPTR principles. *Eur Spine J* 2013;22 Suppl 2:S106–17

What Are the Indications for a VEPTR?

The VEPTR device is indicated to treat patients with conditions that cause thoracic insufficiency syndrome. They include conditions that cause progressive multidimensional defects of the thorax that are present from birth (congenital), such as scoliosis with absent ribs and flail chest, neurogenic scoliosis (rib abnormalities not necessarily present), and scoliosis with fused ribs, congenital conditions that cause hypoplastic chest wall defects such as Jeune Syndrome or spondylocostal dysplasia (Jarcho–Levin Syndrome), or acquired chest wall defects that may arise from trauma or tumor resections.

What Are Common Surgical Complications of the VEPTR Device?

Described complications include wound infection, skin breakdown, and brachial plexus injuries. The device can migrate or break, which will entail surgical repair.

Is There Anything Else You Want to Know before Proceeding with This Case?

A thorough medical assessment will reveal associated cardiac and genitourinary conditions. Recall that patients with congenital defects of the vertebrae may also have anal atresia, tracheoesophageal fistulas, cardiac anomalies, radial atresia, and renal abnormalities (VACTERL syndromes). Echocardiography is important for assessing cardiac status. MRI can delineate spinal cord deformities and preexisting areas of spinal stenosis. The patient may have chronic hypoxia with compensatory metabolic alkalosis and polycythemia. A preoperative CT scan or MRI is helpful as a blueprint to map out chest wall deformities and assess lung volumes and the extent of thoracic insufficiency.

What Are the Important Anesthetic Implications?

Since the spinal cord will be manipulated and/or stressed, in our practice we routinely monitor somatosensory and motor evoked potentials, facilitated by a total intravenous general anesthetic with propofol and the anesthesiologist's opioid of choice. Intraoperative changes in neurophysiological signals warrant optimization of hemoglobin level and blood pressure, and immediate investigation of a surgical cause.

For the child that receives their first VEPTR device or presents for an expansion, we typically place one or two intravenous lines following inhalational induction using sevoflurane. Because of their underlying condition, and the relatively high frequency of their need for procedures, it is common for these children to be quite challenging to obtain IV access. Therefore, we usually employ ultrasound guidance, often with the aid of our radiology colleagues. Many of these children will already have had placement of an indwelling peripheral or central venous access. Unless dictated by the severity of their underlying condition, direct arterial monitoring is usually not necessary. Original insertion of the VEPTR will occasionally warrant red cell transfusion for intraoperative or preexisting anemia.

Intraoperative hypothermia is common, due to prolonged exposure during induction, IV placement, and surgical positioning. Therefore, all modalities should be taken to prevent hypothermia, including adjusting the OR temperature, use of a forced air warming blanket, and IV fluid warming device. A urinary catheter will only be necessary for procedures expected to last longer than three to four hours.

The surgical procedure is performed in the prone position. Therefore, adequate attention is paid to optimization of position and airway stabilization. All patients for VEPTR receive an endotracheal tube unless they have a preexisting tracheostomy. The anesthesia provider must have flexible endotracheal tube extensions, a soft bite block, and different sized prone pillows immediately available.

What Are Important Postoperative Concerns?

The most important postoperative concern is pain. Many of these children do not have appropriate age-related or cognitive development to use patient controlled analgesic devices; therefore, extra attention is warranted to optimize pain control with opioids and additional adjuvants. Ideally, the institution's pain team should be consulted on these children during the initial VEPTR placement.

Suggested Reading

Campbell RM Jr. VEPTR: past experience and the future of VEPTR principles. *Eur Spine J.* 2013;22 Suppl 2:S106–17. PMID: 23354777.

Harris JA, Mayer OH, Shah SA, et al. A comprehensive review of thoracic deformity parameters in scoliosis. *Eur Spine J.* 2014;23(12):2594–602. PMID: 25238798.

Pediatric Epidural Anesthesia

Adam C. Adler

A one-week-old child born at 38 weeks is coming to the operating room to undergo a laparotomy for repair of duodenal atresia. The mother inquires about the potential for regional anesthesia techniques and how they differ between adults and children.

How Would You Place an Epidural Catheter in a Small Child?

Epidural catheters can be placed via an interlaminar (lumbar/thoracic) or caudal approach after induction of general anesthesia. For interlaminar placement, the child is typically placed in lateral position with hips and knees flexed and spine arched to open the interlaminar space. Loss of resistance to saline as opposed to air is considered to be safer in neonates and infants, as even a small volume of intravascular air can cause a clinically significant air embolus in an infant or small child.

What Is the Depth to the Epidural Space in Children?

The epidural space is extremely superficial in small children, with several guidelines used to estimate the distance.

The mean depth to the epidural space is 1 cm in neonates, ranging from 0.3 to 1.5 cm.

Between 6 months and 10 years of age, the epidural space is estimated to be 1 mm/kg body weight of depth.

For a caudal approach, an 18-gauge intravenous catheter is first inserted into the caudal space via the usual technique and a wire-reinforced epidural catheter is threaded into the desired space/level. The level of the catheter tip can be confirmed via ultrasound, and/or fluoroscopy.

Should a Test Dose Be Performed in Children under General Anesthesia?

Regardless of technique, careful aspiration for blood followed by a test dose using local anesthetic and epinephrine should be considered to exclude inadvertent subarachnoid or intravascular injection. Typically, a test dose is conducted with 0.5 mcg/kg of epinephrine or 0.1–0.2 mL/kg of lidocaine 1:200,000 solution.

The most suggestive sign of intravascular injection (100% sensitivity) is an EKG T-wave amplitude increase of >25%. Other signs include a systolic blood pressure increase of >15 mmHg or heart rate increase of >10 beats per minute with a sensitivity of 95% and 71% respectively.

What Are the Risks and Benefits of Awake versus Asleep Epidural Placement in Pediatric Patients?

Epidurals have been placed safely in pediatric patients under general anesthesia for many years. Risks of the asleep patient include limited feedback of potential neurologic symptoms, whereas risks of the awake patient include limited patient cooperation and movement. The Pediatric Regional Anesthesia Network (PRAN) studies have shown similar or even lower rates of complications in blocks performed on sedated children as compared to those who were awake. Current recommendations suggest performing regional anesthesia in pediatric patients under general anesthesia or deep sedation.

Identify Some Major Differences in Epidural Placement between Neonates and Adults

- Toxicity in children, especially neonates may manifest by agitation, restlessness, and myoclonic activity and may be hard to differentiate.

- Neonates have a lower threshold for local anesthetic toxicity due to decreased protein binding of local anesthetics.
- The spinal cord and thecal sac end at L1 and S1 respectively in neonates while in adults these locations are at L3 and S3.
- The distance to the epidural space is shallower in children.
- In neonates, the ligaments and bone are less calcified resulting in less tactile feedback and more likely intraosseous injection.
- Neonates have a larger CSF volume/kg (4 cc/kg) than older children and adults (2 cc/kg).
- Neonates have a faster CSF production and absorption when compared to adults.

What Are the Common Local Anesthetic Solutions Used for Epidural Analgesia in Children?

Bupivacaine 0.1–0.125% or ropivacaine 0.1% in normal saline are the most commonly used local anesthetics for postoperative analgesia.

Epidural solutions are dosed based on the local anesthetic component.

Typical dosing regimens include: 0.1–0.4 mg/kg/h of local anesthetics with or without the addition of analgesic adjuncts.

Neonatal epidurals are often managed using 3% chloroprocaine by continuous infusion. Dosing includes a bolus of 1.5–2.0 mL/kg followed by a continuous infusion of 1.5–2.0 mL/kg/h. Chloroprocaine is often used in neonates due to its relative safety in this group as well as ability for fast plasma esterase degradation in the event of toxicity.

What Are Commonly Used Additives to Epidural Solutions?

- Clonidine 0.2 mcg/kg/h
- Fentanyl 1 mcg/kg/h
- Hydromorphone 1 mcg/kg/h
- Morphine 2.5 mcg/kg/h

Identify Some Contraindications to Pediatric Epidural Placement

- Parental refusal
- Overlying skin infection
- Sepsis
- Coagulopathy
- Spinal deformities (spina bifida)
- Baclofen pumps
- Prior spinal instrumentation

Suggested Reading

Kozek-Langenecker SA, Marhofer P, Jonas K, et al. Cardiovascular criteria for epidural test dosing in sevoflurane- and halothane-anesthetized children. *Anesth Analg.* 2000;90(3):579–83. PMID: 10702441.

Kraemer FW, Rose JB. Pharmacologic management of acute pediatric pain. *Anesthesiol Clin.* 2009;27(2):241–68. PMID: 19703675.

Polaner DM, Taenzer AH, Walker BJ, et al. Pediatric Regional Anesthesia Network (PRAN): a multi-institutional study of the use and incidence of complications of pediatric regional anesthesia. *Anesth Analg.* 2012;115(6):1353–64. PMID: 22696610.

Chapter

51

Upper Extremity Nerve Blocks

Arvind Chandrakantan and Nihar V. Patel

> A six-year-old previously healthy boy with diffuse right shoulder pain presents with osteosarcoma of the right scapula. The orthopedic surgeon has scheduled him for a right scapular resection of tumor. What are the options to provide regional anesthesia for this patient?

INTERSCALENE BLOCK

What Are the Options for Pain Control Postoperatively?

Surgical operations of the shoulder involve a significant amount of postoperative pain. A few options to treat the pain postoperatively include intravenous pain medications, with opiates being the foundation of a standard pain control regimen. In addition, NSAIDs and acetaminophen are frequently employed in a multimodal regimen. Administration of the opioid is most commonly done with patient-controlled analgesia (PCA). Opioid PCAs have been used extensively in children as young as eight years old with great efficacy and pain control. Children less than eight years of age may have difficulty using PCA. An alternative option would be an interscalene brachial plexus nerve block or catheter placement to manage postoperative pain control.

The brachial plexus innervates nearly the entire upper extremity. The plexus arises from the ventral rami of spinal nerves C5-T1 with occasional contribution from C4 and T2. The plexus transitions as it divides into the arm from five roots to three trunks to six divisions to three cords and five major branches. Each of the upper extremity nerve blocks targets a particular portion of the brachial plexus in its division (Figure 51.1).

What Are the Indications for an Interscalene Brachial Plexus Block?

An interscalene brachial plexus block is ideal for any operation involving the shoulder and upper extremity. It involves the blockade of the brachial plexus at the level of the superior (C5/C6), middle (C7), and inferior trunks (C8) in the interscalene groove between the anterior and middle scalene muscles. Since the suprascapular nerve arises off the brachial plexus just after the interscalene groove but prior to the supraclavicular position, a supraclavicular nerve block cannot reliably provide analgesia to operations involving the shoulder. There is a degree of ulnar sparing that occurs making the use of an interscalene block for procedures below the elbow less optimal than a supraclavicular, infraclavicular or axillary brachial plexus block. The block can be done as a single shot or with placement of a catheter to allow for continuous nerve blockade postoperatively to provide analgesia as well as facilitate initial rehabilitation and physical therapy.

What Are the Contraindications to Performing an Interscalene Block?

The standard contraindications for any regional block apply: patient refusal is an absolute contraindication. Relative contraindications include infection at planned injection site, preexisting neurologic deficits, local anesthetic allergy, coagulopathy, as well as impaired respiratory reserve such as contralateral phrenic nerve palsy, diaphragmatic impairment, or chronic obstructive pulmonary disease (COPD).

What Are the Complications and Side Effects Associated with an Interscalene Block?

The complications of an interscalene block include pneumothorax, epidural or subarachnoid injection,

---

Drs. Patel and Chandrakantan have contributed equally to this chapter to constitute first authorship.

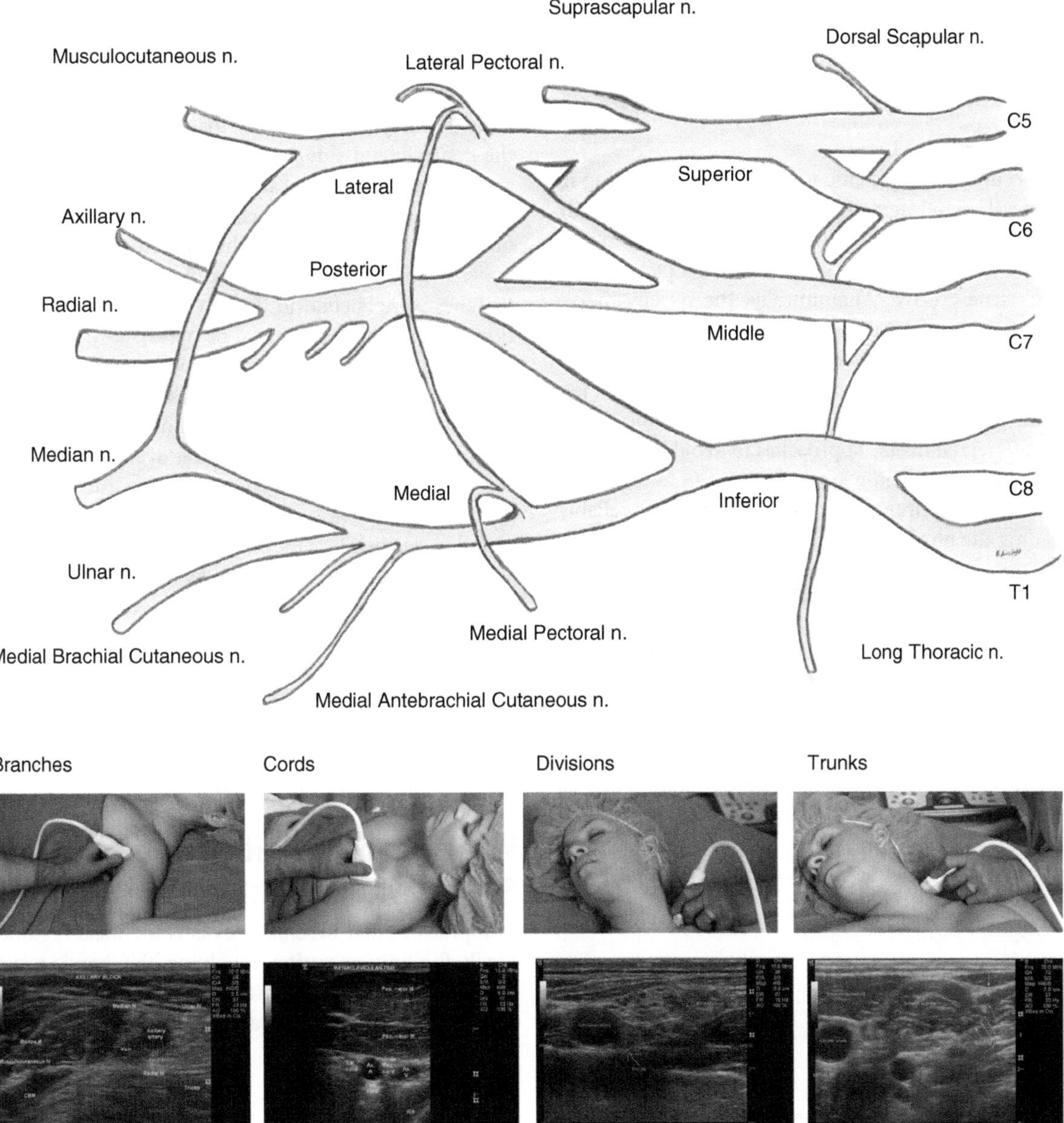

Figure 51.1 From left to right, the axillary, infraclavicular, supraclavicular, and interscalene blocks are highlighted with the division of the brachial plexus targeted. Reproduced with permission from Arbona FL, Khabiri B, Norton JA (eds.) 2011. *Ultrasound-Guided Regional Anesthesia: A Practical Approach to Peripheral Nerve Blocks and Perineural Catheters*. Cambridge, UK: Cambridge University Press

permanent neurological injury, and vagal and/or recurrent laryngeal nerve blockade. With the increased utilization and ability to visualize target structures, the rate of complications has fallen precipitously. Common side effects of an interscalene block include a Horner's syndrome from blockade of the cervical sympathetic nerves as well as phrenic nerve blockade. Both nerves are in close proximity to the interscalene brachial plexus and have higher incidences with increased volumes of injection for nerve blockade.

What Is the Incidence of Phrenic Nerve Blockade When Performing an Interscalene Block? How Can That Be Avoided?

The occurrence of phrenic nerve blockade resulting in ipsilateral diaphragmatic paralysis was traditionally stated to be 100% owing to the close proximity of the phrenic nerve to the interscalene brachial plexus in its interscalene groove. Anatomically, the phrenic nerve lies in an anterolateral position on the anterior scalene muscle surface. However, there is considerable variability in the anatomic position. With use of ultrasound, decreased volume of local anesthetic, and differential needle approaches to avoid the phrenic nerve, there has been a small decrease (<20%) in the incidence of phrenic nerve blockade, but reliably avoiding the phrenic nerve has proven elusive.

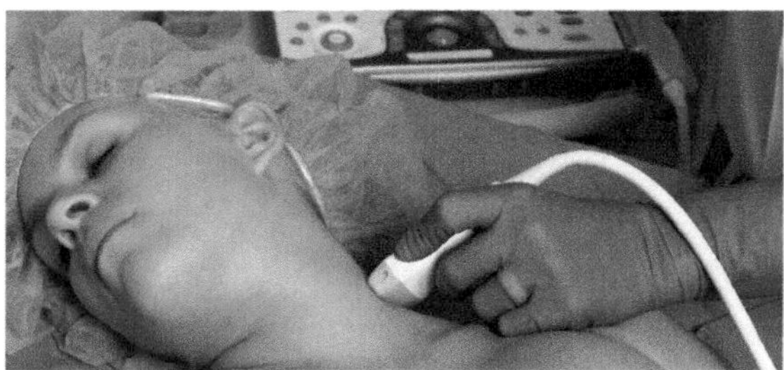

Figure 51.2 Patient and probe positioning for in-plane interscalene nerve block. Reproduced with permission from Arbona FL, Khabiri B, Norton JA (eds.) 2011. *Ultrasound-Guided Regional Anesthesia: A Practical Approach to Peripheral Nerve Blocks and Perineural Catheters.* Cambridge, UK: Cambridge University Press

How Is an Interscalene Block Performed?

With the traditional nerve stimulation technique, the patient was positioned with the head turned toward the contralateral side to be blocked. The interscalene groove was identified at the level of C6 (cricoid cartilage) posterolateral to the clavicular head of the sternocleidomastoid between the anterior and middle scalene muscles. The needle would be advanced until twitches were elicited in the brachial plexus distribution (deltoid, biceps, triceps, or hand).

The predominant method of performing an interscalene block currently is with ultrasound guidance (Figures 51.2–51.4). For smaller children, a linear ultrasound transducer with the smallest available footprint allows for optimal visualization of target structures with adequate surface area for needle approach. The ultrasound image below is the desired image to acquire.

Local anesthetic would be deposited in aliquoted fashion with frequent aspiration to avoid intravascular or intrathecal injection. Typical dosing for a single-shot block would be 0.2–0.4 cc/kg of ropivacaine 0.2%–0.5% or bupivacaine 0.25%–0.5%. If a catheter is placed for postoperative pain control, a typical infusion rate is 0.1–0.2 mL/kg/h of ropivacaine 0.1–0.2% or bupivacaine 0.1–0.25%.

What Are the Indications for a Supraclavicular Brachial Plexus Block?

A supraclavicular brachial plexus is the ideal regional block for any operation involving the hand, wrist, forearm, elbow, and distal humerus. This block should cover tourniquet pain.

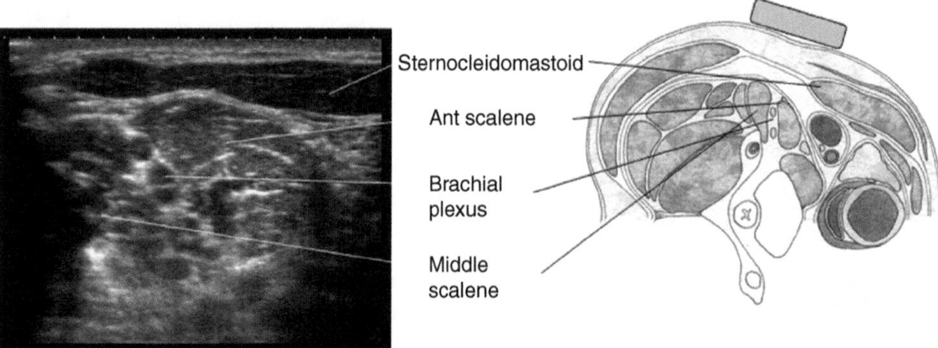

Figure 51.3 Interscalene anatomy. Reproduced with permission from Arthurs G, Nicholls B (eds.) 2016. *Ultrasound in Anesthesia, Critical Care, and Pain Management*. Cambridge, UK: Cambridge University Press

What Are the Complications and Side Effects Associated with a Supraclavicular Block?

Phrenic nerve paralysis is fairly common with a supraclavicular block and should be performed with caution in children with respiratory issues (poor reserve, contralateral pneumothorax, diaphragmatic paralysis).

Pneumothorax, while rare, is a known complication following supraclavicular block.

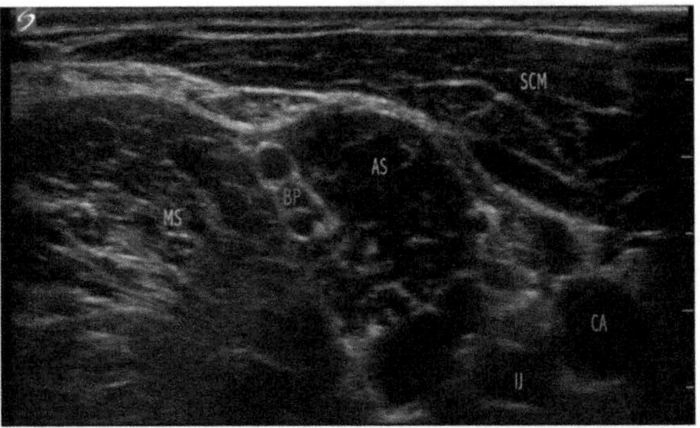

Figure 51.4 Ultrasound anatomy of interscalene nerve block. CA, Carotid Artery; IJ; Internal Jugular Vein; SCM, Sternocleidomastoid; AS, Anterior Scalene; MS, Middle Scalene; BP, Brachial Plexus

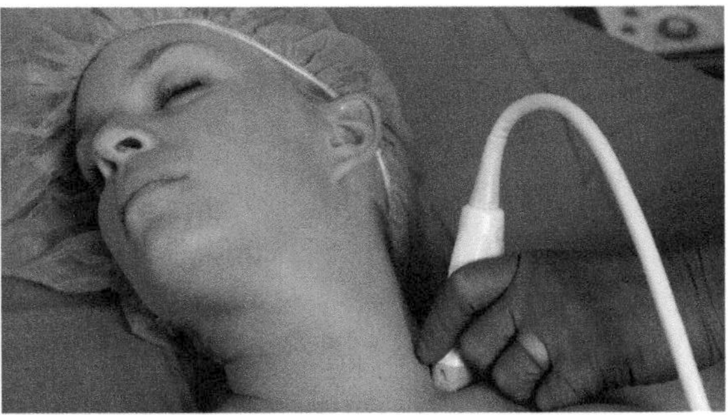

Figure 51.5 Probe positioning for supraclavicular block. Reproduced with permission from Arbona FL, Khabiri B, Norton JA (eds.) 2011. *Ultrasound-Guided Regional Anesthesia: A Practical Approach to Peripheral Nerve Blocks and Perineural Catheters*. Cambridge, UK: Cambridge University Press

How Is a Supraclavicular Block Performed?

Scanning should be performed above the clavicle. Superficial to the first rib and the subclavian artery is the location where the brachial plexus trunks divide into divisions and where the block is performed. The patient is positioned supine with the head turned to the contralateral side. The probe positioning can be seen in Figures 51.5–51.7.

INFRACLAVICULAR BLOCK

> A nine-year-old male is scheduled for urgent reimplantation of his right index finger after partial amputation from a woodcutting accident. He has no other past medical history of note. The anesthesiologist has a detailed discussion with the family about regional blocks, specifically infraclavicular catheter placement.

What Are the Indications for an Infraclavicular Block? What Are the Landmarks of Note?

The indications for an infraclavicular block include elbow, forearm, and hand surgery. The supraclavicular and infraclavicular blocks are essentially interchangeable based on the patient's anatomy. As the names imply, the approach for the supraclavicular block is above the clavicle, while the infraclavicular block is below the

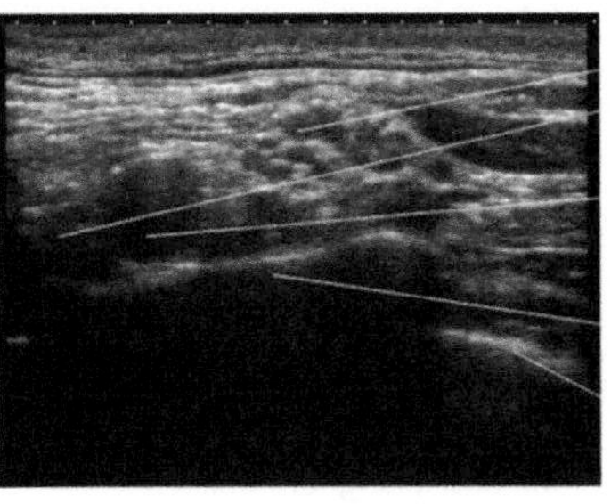

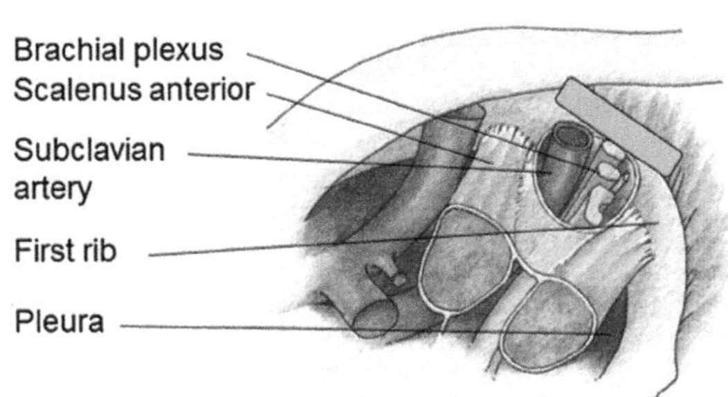

Figure 51.6 Supraclavicular block anatomy. Reproduced with permission from Arthurs G, Nicholls B (eds.) 2016. *Ultrasound in Anesthesia, Critical Care, and Pain Management*. Cambridge, UK: Cambridge University Press

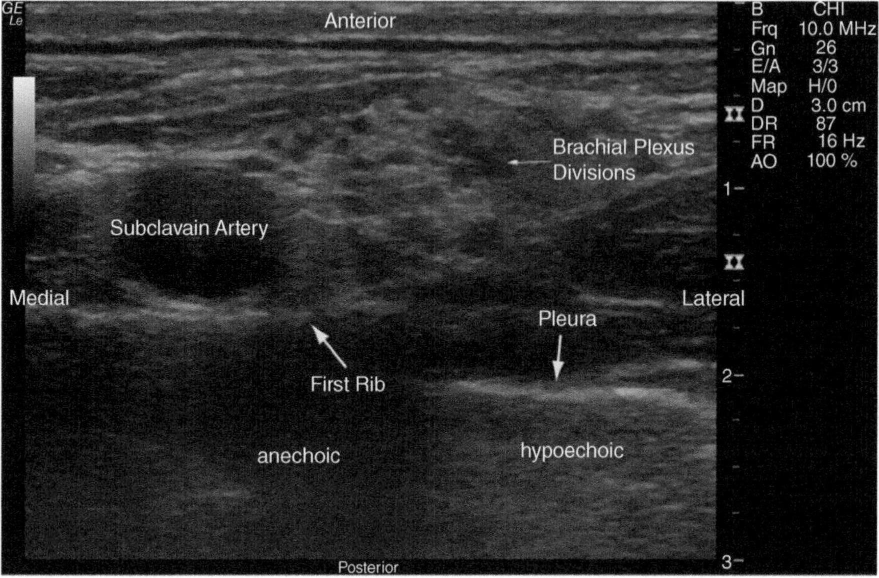

Figure 51.7 Left ultrasound guided supraclavicular block. Reproduced with permission from Arbona FL, Khabiri B, Norton JA (eds.) 2011. *Ultrasound-Guided Regional Anesthesia: A Practical Approach to Peripheral Nerve Blocks and Perineural Catheters*. Cambridge, UK: Cambridge University Press

clavicle. The boundaries for block placement for the infraclavicular block are: medially by the ribs, laterally by the coracoid process, superiorly by the clavicle, and anteriorly by the pectoralis minor muscle. The apex of the lung is also very close to the needle placement side, so the use of ultrasound is now the standard of care.

What Are the Contraindications to Infraclavicular Catheter Placement?

There are very few true contraindications to catheter placement. A lot of the patient factors (anxiety, movement) are not present in the pediatric population as the majority of blocks are performed on anesthetized patients. However, given the proximity to the great vessels, caution should be exercised in patients with coagulopathy/documented local anesthetic allergies. Caution should also be exercised in patients who have preexisting neurological deficits in the limb under consideration.

Is There a Benefit of Ultrasound Over Nerve Stimulation Techniques for Catheter Placement?

There is clear and compelling data from multiple studies that utilization of ultrasound decreases the number of needle passes and time to block placement, and increases block efficacy. This effect seems to be more pronounced in younger children. Whether the addition of nerve stimulation to ultrasound adds more benefit is unclear. In the authors' experience, when the nerve bundles are clearly visualized it probably does not add more value to simultaneously use nerve stimulation.

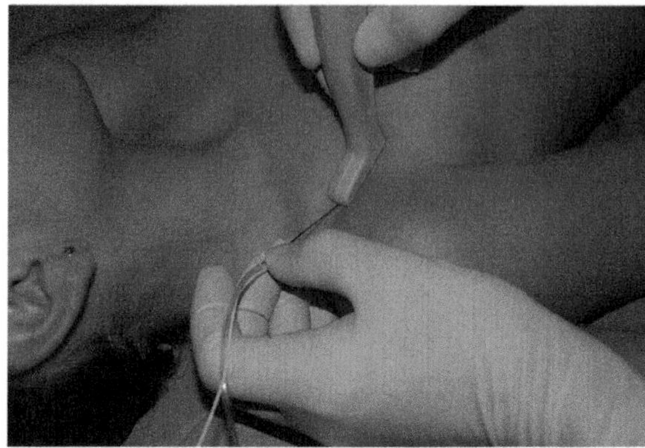

Figure 51.8 Patient and probe positioning for in-plane infraclavicular nerve block. Reproduced with permission from Mannion S, Iohom G, Dadure C, Reisbig MD, Ganesh A (eds.) 2015. *Ultrasound-Guided Regional Anesthesia in Children*. Cambridge, UK: Cambridge University Press

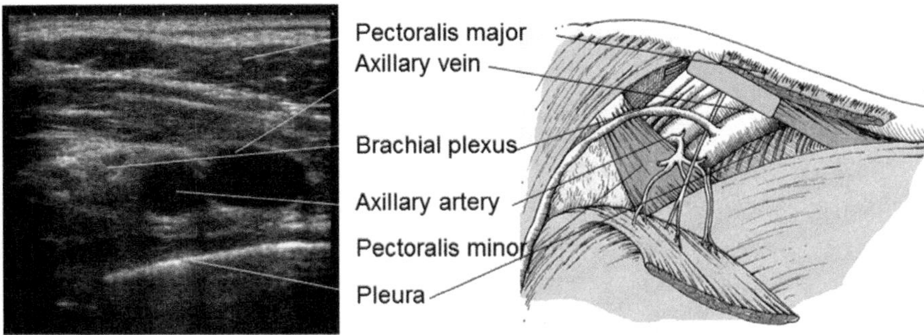

Figure 51.9 Infraclavicular anatomy. Reproduced with permission from Arthurs G, Nicholls B (eds.) 2016. *Ultrasound in Anesthesia, Critical Care, and Pain Management*. Cambridge, UK: Cambridge University Press

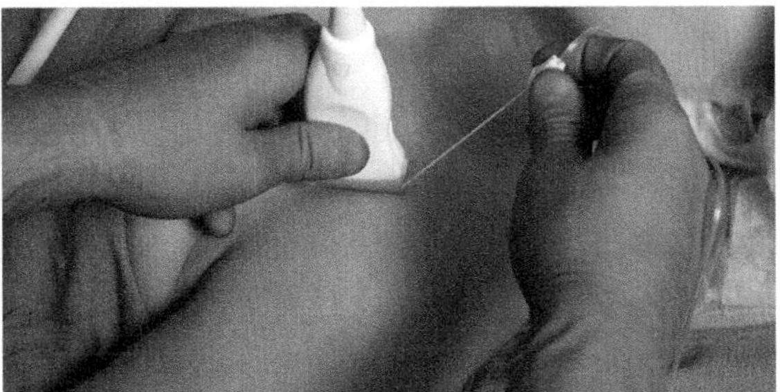

Figure 51.10 Probe and needle position for performance of in-plane infraclavicular block. Reproduced with permission from Arbona FL, Khabiri B, Norton JA (eds.) 2011. *Ultrasound-Guided Regional Anesthesia: A Practical Approach to Peripheral Nerve Blocks and Perineural Catheters*. Cambridge, UK: Cambridge University Press

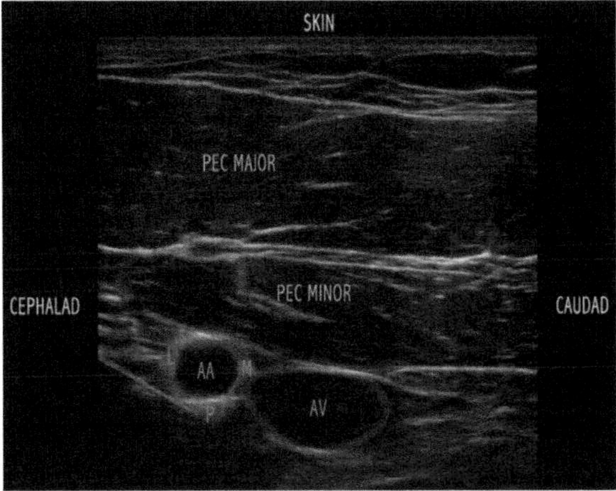

Figure 51.11 Ultrasound anatomy of the infraclavicular block. AA, Axillary Artery; AV, Axillary Vein; L: Lateral Cord; M, Medial Cord; P, Posterior Cord

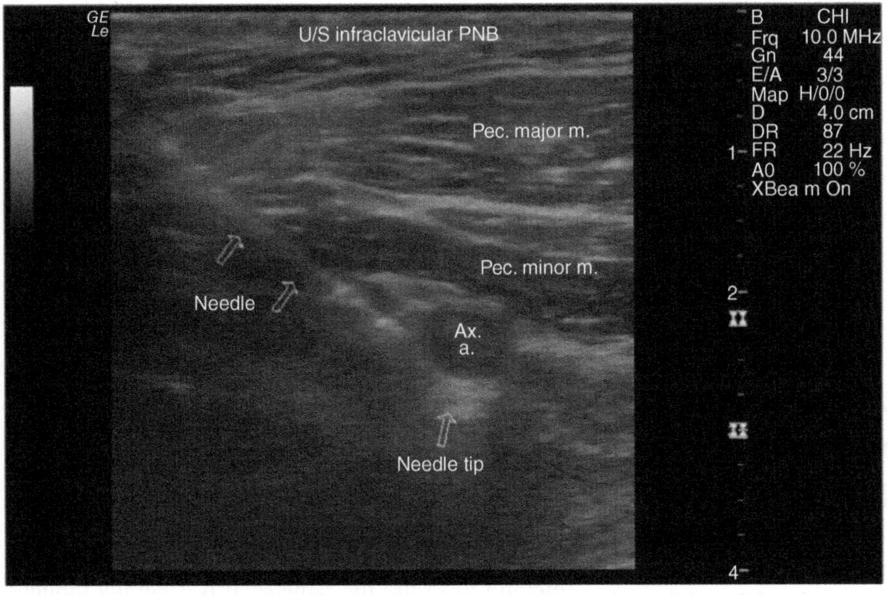

Figure 51.12 In-plane approach to the infraclavicular nerve block. Reproduced with permission from Arbona FL, Khabiri B, Norton JA (eds.) 2011. *Ultrasound-Guided Regional Anesthesia: A Practical Approach to Peripheral Nerve Blocks and Perineural Catheters*. Cambridge, UK: Cambridge University Press

Table 51.1 Summary of the brachial plexus terminal branches and their function. Reproduced with permission from Arbona FL, Khabiri B, Norton JA (eds.) 2011. *Ultrasound-Guided Regional Anesthesia: A Practical Approach to Peripheral Nerve Blocks and Perineural Catheters.* Cambridge, UK: Cambridge University Press.

Brachial plexus terminal branch	Cutaneous sensation	Joint sensation	Motor action
Axillary nerve (C5, C6)	Over deltoid muscle	Glenohumeral	Abduction of arm
		Acromioclavicular	Flexion of arm
			Extension of arm
			Lateral rotation of arm
Radial nerve (C5–T1)	Posterior arm and forearm	Elbow	Extension of arm
	Dorsum of hand	Radius–ulna	Extension and supination of forearm
	Dorsum of first three fingers and lateral half of fourth finger to DIP	Wrist	Extension of wrist, fingers, and thumb
			Abduction of thumb
Median nerve (C5–T1)	Thenar eminence	Elbow	Pronation and flexion of forearm
	Palmar surface of first three fingers and lateral half of fourth finger	Radius–ulna	Flexion of the wrist, fingers, and thumb
	Dorsum of first three fingers and lateral half of fourth finger distal to DIP	Wrist	Abduction of thumb
		Fingers	Opposition of the thumb
Musculocutaneous nerve (C5–C7)	Lateral aspect of forearm	Elbow	Flexion of arm
		Proximal radius–ulna	Flexion and supination of forearm
Ulnar nerve (C8–T1)	Hypothenar eminence	All in hand except thumb and ulna-carpal	Flexion of wrist and fingers, especially fourth and fifth
	Dorso-medial surface of hand		Adduction and flexion of thumb
	Dorsal and palmar surface of fifth finger and medial half of fourth finger		Opposition of fifth finger
			Spreading and closing of fingers

What Medications/Dosages Are Used for the Continuous Catheter? What Is the Best Way to Secure the Catheter?

There is no de facto drug, concentration, or regimen established for infraclavicular blockade. Single shot blocks are typically dosed at 0.2–0.5 mL/kg of ropivacaine 0.2–0.5% or bupivacaine 0.25–0.5% with strict adherence to toxic dose limits. For continuous catheter infusions, typical dosing is 0.1–0.2 mL/kg/h of either ropivacaine 0.1–0.2% or bupivacaine 0.1–0.2%.

While the evidence is weak to declare a best method to secure the catheter, it is generally thought that anchoring the catheter through the pec major and pec minor muscles and tunneling the catheter subcutaneously will provide for greater security.

What Are the Expected Post Op Considerations for Continuous Perineural Catheter Placement?

Catheter dislodgement is common but ensuing complications are quite rare. This should be suspected when the patient has a block that is wearing off despite adequate infusion rates and local anesthetic concentration. Occasionally, the catheter can be repositioned under ultrasound alone, however due to its inherent flexibility this is rarely successful. Often, catheter malposition or poor blockade requires insertion of a new catheter under the same conditions as noted previously. Clinicians should also be wary of the presenting symptoms of LAST, which is covered elsewhere in this book.

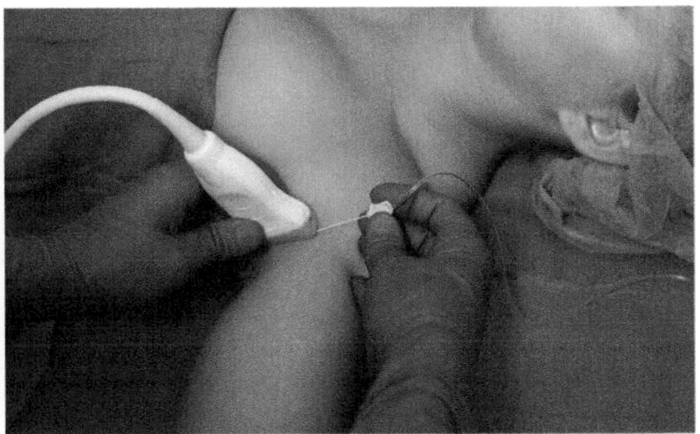

Figure 51.13 Probe and needle positioning for axillary nerve block. Reproduced with permission from Arbona FL, Khabiri B, Norton JA (eds.) 2011. *Ultrasound-Guided Regional Anesthesia: A Practical Approach to Peripheral Nerve Blocks and Perineural Catheters.* Cambridge, UK: Cambridge University Press

AXILLARY NERVE BLOCK

What Are the Indications for an Axillary Nerve Block?

The axillary nerve block targets terminal branches of the five major nerves of the brachial plexus.

The axillary nerve block is suitable for surgical procedures involving the distal arm. Targeting individual nerves is appropriate for highly specific surgical procedures for which other nerves need not be blocked.

0.1–0.3 mL/kg of local anesthetic is typically sufficient to provide coverage (Table 51.1, Figures 51.13–51.14).

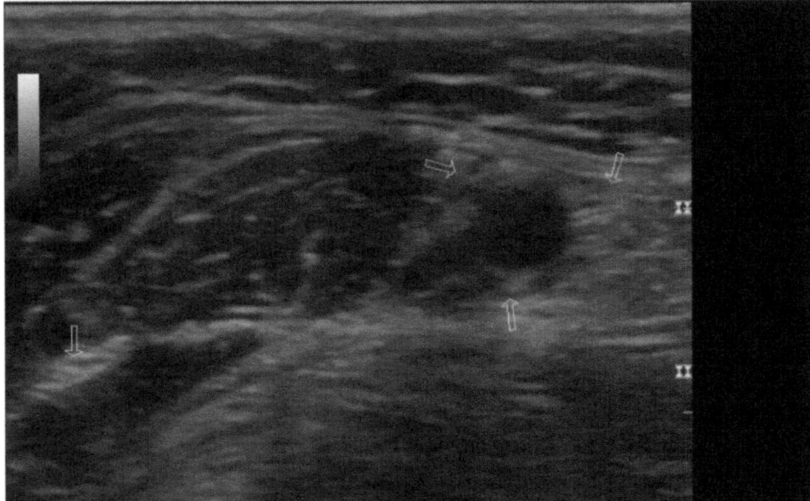

Figure 51.14 Caption: ultrasound anatomy of the axillary nerve block. CBM: coracobrachialis muscle. Reproduced with permission from Arbona FL, Khabiri B, Norton JA (eds.) 2011. *Ultrasound-Guided Regional Anesthesia: A Practical Approach to Peripheral Nerve Blocks and Perineural Catheters.* Cambridge, UK: Cambridge University Press

Suggested Reading

Gorlin A, Warren L. Ultrasound guided interscalene blocks. *J Ultrasound Med.* 2012;31:979–83. PMID: 22733845.

Tsui BCH. Interscalene brachial plexus blockade. In Tsui B and Suresh S (eds.) 2016. *Pediatric Atlas of Ultrasound- and Nerve Stimulation-Guided Regional Anesthesia.* New York, NY: pages 267–81.

Tsui BCH. Infraclavicular block. In Tsui BH (ed.) 2007. *Atlas of Ultrasound and Nerve Stimulation Guided Regional Anesthesia.* New York, NY. pages 87–98.

Chapter 52

Lower Extremity Nerve Blocks

Nihar V. Patel

A family vacationing in the mountains experienced a motor vehicle accident (MVA) involving their six-year-old daughter and four-year-old son. Both were taken to the local hospital for treatment of non-life-threatening orthopedic injuries sustained in the MVA.

The six-year-old girl was complaining of bilateral leg pain for which X-rays demonstrated a right-sided femoral neck fracture.

Her orthopedic surgeon wishes to repair her fracture with surgical pinning and asks if there is a regional block that can be performed to assist in her postoperative pain relief.

What Is the Innervation to the Lower Extremity?

The entire lower extremity is innervated by the lumbar and sacral plexus and their corresponding terminal nerves. The lumbar plexus arises from the L1–L4 spinal nerves (with some patients adding T12) and innervates mostly the ventral aspect of the lower extremity while the sacral plexus arising from S1–S4 innervates mostly the dorsal aspect. Figures 52.1–52.3 and Table 52.1 demonstrate the lower extremity innervation.

What Are the Regional Anesthesia Options for This Procedure?

Femoral neck fractures are high enough on the femur that the typical injection site of a femoral nerve block at the inguinal crease will not provide blockade at the surgical site. A proximal femoral nerve block in combination with a lateral femoral cutaneous nerve block can be performed to cover the sensory area overlying the surgical site. Historically, the three-in-one femoral nerve block, where a large volume femoral nerve block injection in combination with applied distal pressure would cause the local anesthetic to spread proximally in a retrograde fashion and block the femoral, obturator, and lateral femoral cutaneous nerves, was thought to accomplish anesthesia of proximal femur/hip. Several studies have questioned the reliability of that technique. A fascia iliaca block could reliably block the lateral femoral cutaneous nerve as well as femoral nerve providing good coverage to the fracture. A lumbar plexus block where the femoral, lateral femoral cutaneous, and obturator nerves are blocked at their proximal plexus would also provide coverage. Lastly, a lumbar epidural block would likely provide excellent coverage at the expense of obtaining a bilateral block, and unnecessarily involving the unaffected side, and other possible side effects such as loss of motor control, and urinary retention.

How Is a Lumbar Plexus Block Performed?

Lumbar plexus blockade was traditionally done using anatomical landmarks to locate the plexus whose depth could be deep with vital organs in close proximity. With the patient in lateral position, a line was drawn connecting the iliac crest laterally and the spinous processes in the midline (at approximately the level of L3–L4). A spot is marked approximately 4–5 cm lateral to the midline on that line where the needle would be inserted in a perpendicular fashion. With a nerve stimulator set at 1.5 mA, a quadriceps twitch should be elicited. Once done, the current should be reduced to obtain stimulation between 0.5 and 1.0 mA.

The current standard of care is to use ultrasound to perform a lumbar plexus block as vital organs and adjacent structures can be visualized and avoided, such as the kidney, peritoneum, and intervertebral foramen. The most common views to visualize the lumbar plexus are the paramedian sagittal (Trident sign), the paramedian transverse oblique (Wave sign).

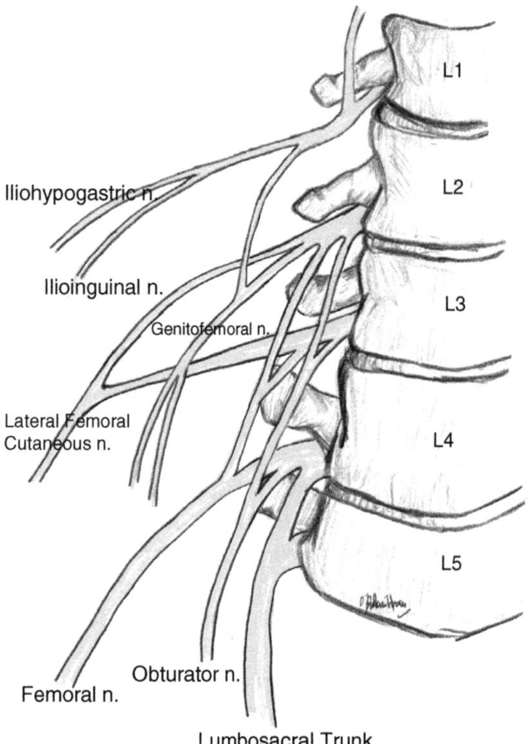

Figure 52.1 Lumbar plexus nerve distribution. Reproduced with permission from Arbona FL, Khabiri B, Norton JA (eds.) 2011. *Ultrasound-Guided Regional Anesthesia: A Practical Approach to Peripheral Nerve Blocks and Perineural Catheters*. Cambridge, UK: Cambridge University Press

and the transverse (Shamrock sign) scan. In the paramedian scan, the probe is placed longitudinally adjacent to the spinous processes (Figures 52.4–52.6). The resultant spinous processes can then be identified, including the desired L3 and L4 spinous processes. The view that results appears like a "trident" with the psoas muscle in between the transverse processes (spears of the trident). The lumbar plexus lies in the posterior third of the body of the psoas muscles which will appear to be the most superficial third of the muscle in this view.

In the paramedian transverse view, the ultrasound probe is placed transversely in the paramedian posterior regional at the level of L3/4. The desired view is termed the "wave sign" as the hyperechoic periosteum of the vertebral body, facet joint, and spinous process appear similar to a wave.

Lastly, the transverse scan with probe placement on the iliac crest produces an image where the three muscle bellies of the erector spinae, psoas, and quadratus lumborum muscles surround the L4 transverse process to mimic a "Shamrock." The lumbar plexus lies in the posterior third of the psoas adjacent to the transverse process. This approach allows for full in-plane view of the needle as it approximates the plexus.

What Are the Local Anesthetic Dosing Options for a Lumbar Plexus Block?

The lumbar plexus block is a large-volume block with no widely accepted universal dosing regimen. Generally speaking, 0.2–0.5 cc/kg of 0.25% bupivacaine or 0.2% ropivacaine can be used depending on the desired block duration. Careful attention should be paid to not exceed the maximum toxic dose of local anesthetic.

> Case continued: In addition to the child's right lower extremity injury, left leg X-rays of the daughter showed a mid-shaft fracture of the femur.

What Are the Regional Anesthesia Options for This Portion of the Surgery?

Given that the innervation of the femur is the femoral nerve, the options for regional anesthesia include the aforementioned lumbar plexus block, femoral nerve block, fascia iliaca block, and if the fracture is low lying enough, an adductor canal block. All three blocks reliably block the femoral nerve.

How Is a Femoral Block Performed?

A femoral block is performed utilizing the knowledge that the femoral nerve lies adjacent and lateral to the femoral artery and vein in the orientation lateral to medial (vein being medial) (Figure 52.7). In the nerve stimulator technique, the inguinal ligament is identified, and the femoral artery is palpated just distal to the inguinal crease. The needle with nerve stimulator should be inserted just lateral to the artery and a twitch of the quadriceps muscle should be elicited at current of 1 mA initially and then dialed down to 0.5 mA or below.

Ultrasound guidance is now more commonplace as the triad of the femoral vein, femoral artery, and femoral nerve can be directly visualized under the fascial iliaca in a medial to lateral fashion, respectively. The optimal image is as shown in Figures 52.8–52.9.

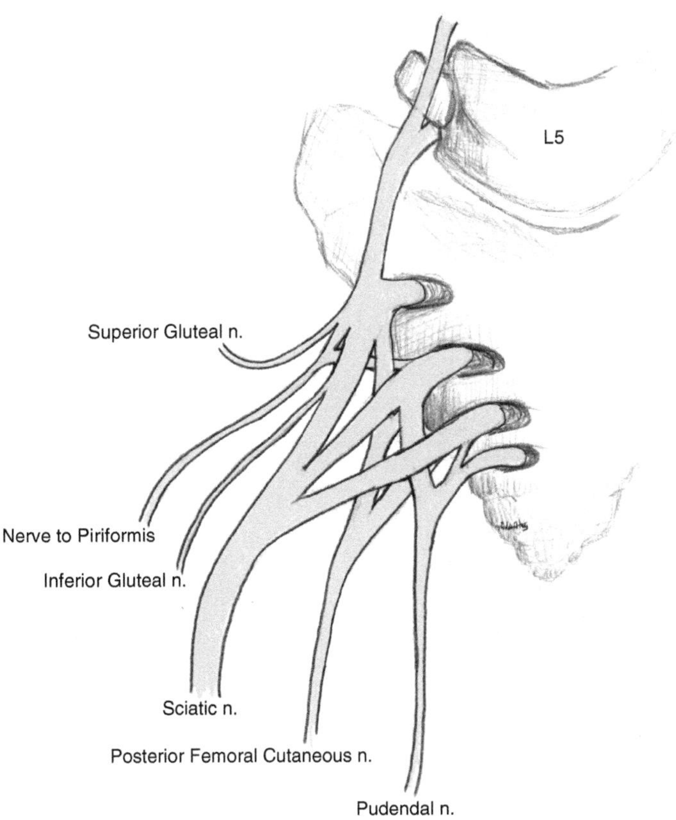

Figure 52.2 Sacral plexus nerve distribution. Reproduced with permission from Arbona FL, Khabiri B, Norton JA (eds.) 2011. *Ultrasound-Guided Regional Anesthesia: A Practical Approach to Peripheral Nerve Blocks and Perineural Catheters*. Cambridge, UK: Cambridge University Press

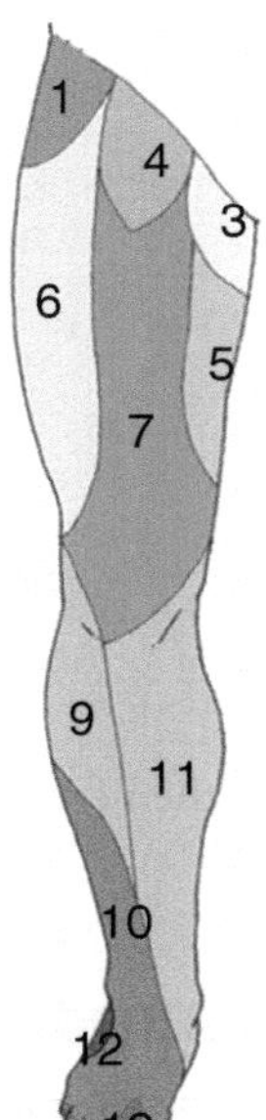

1. Thoracic T12 nerve
2. Iliohypogastric
3. Ilioinguinal
4. Genitofemoral
5. Obturator
6. Lateral cutaneous nerve of thigh
7. Anterior cutaneous nerve of thigh
8. Posterior cutaneous nerve of thigh
9. Lateral cutaneous nerve of calf
10. Superficial peroneal nerve
11. Saphenous nerve
12. Sural
13. Deep peroneal nerve
14. Plantar
15. Calcaneal nerve

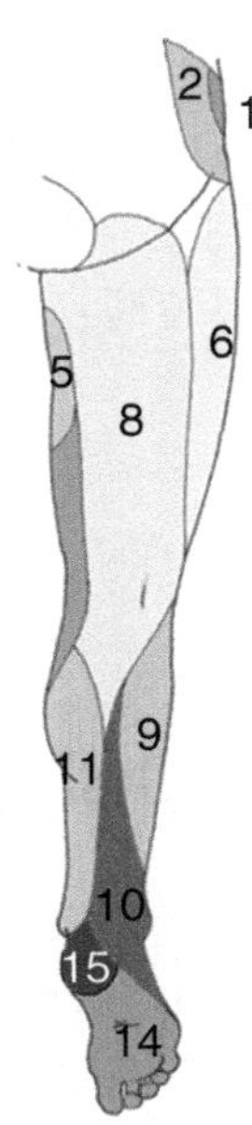

Figure 52.3 Cutaneous innervation of the lower extremity. Reproduced with permission from Arthurs G, Nicholls B (eds.) 2016. *Ultrasound in Anesthesia, Critical Care, and Pain Management*. Cambridge, UK: Cambridge University Press

Table 52.1 Summary of the lumbo-sacral plexus terminal nerve functions. Reproduced with permission from Arbona FL, Khabiri B, Norton JA (eds.) 2011. *Ultrasound-Guided Regional Anesthesia: A Practical Approach to Peripheral Nerve Blocks and Perineural Catheters*. Cambridge, UK: Cambridge University Press.

Lumbo-sacral plexus terminal branch	Cutaneous sensation	Joint sensation	Motor action
Iliohypogastric nerve (L1, +/–T12)	Inferior abdomen Anterior hip	None	Abdominal muscles (transverse abdominus and obliques)
Ilioinguinal nerve (L1)	Medial, proximal thigh Anterior scrotum/labia majora	None	Abdominal muscles (transverse abdominus and obliques)
Genitofemoral nerve (L1, L2)	Over femoral triangle Fascia and skin of scrotum/ labia majora	None	Elevation of scrotum (cremaster muscle)
Obturator nerve (L2–L4)	Medial aspect of thigh Medial aspect of knee	Anteromedial hip, flexion of thigh	Adduction of thigh Extension of thigh
Femoral nerve (L2–L4)	Anterior thigh Medial leg and ankle, +/– medial foot	Anterior hip, knee	Flexion and lateral rotation of thigh, extension of leg Flexion of leg
Lateral femoral cutaneous nerve (L2, L3)	Lateral thigh	None	None
Pudendal nerve (S2–S4)	Much of external genitalia	None	Muscles of perineum
Posterior cutaneous nerve of thigh (S1–S3)	Posterior thigh Posterior leg	None	None
Sciatic nerve (L4–S3)	See below for terminal branches	Posterior and posteromedial hip, Posterior knee, ankle, foot	Flexion of thigh, adduction of thigh Flexion of leg See below for terminal branches
Superficial peroneal nerve (L4–S2)	Lateral leg Dorsal foot	None	Eversion of foot Plantarflexion of foot
Deep peroneal nerve (L4–S2)	Webspace between first and second toes	Ankle	Inversion of foot Dorsiflexion of foot Extension of toes
Tibial nerve (L4–S3)	Plantar surface of foot	Ankle Foot	Flexion of leg, plantarflexion of foot, flexion of toes Adduction and abduction of toes
Sural nerve (S1)	Lateral foot and fifth toe	Lateral ankle	None

What Are the Local Anesthetic Dosing Options for a Femoral Block?

Local anesthetic for a femoral block is typically dosed based on expected duration of blockade. 0.2 to 0.5 cc/kg of 0.25% bupivacaine or 0.2% ropivacaine are typical. Studies have shown that lower doses can be used with the ultrasound technique versus the nerve-stimulator-based landmark techniques.

How Is a Fascia Iliaca Block Performed?

A fascia iliaca block involves blockade of the lateral femoral cutaneous nerve by depositing local anesthetic

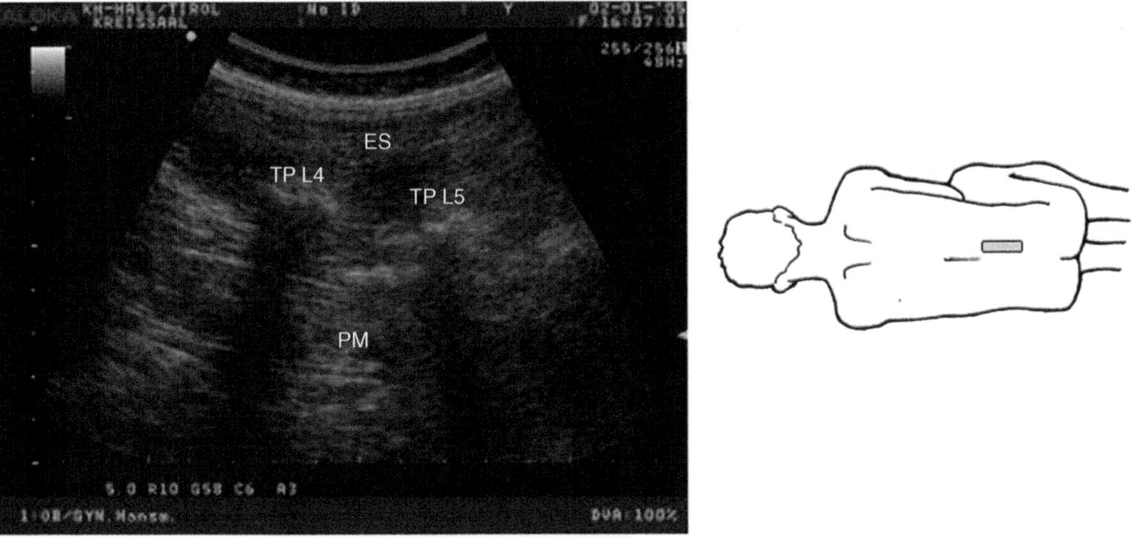

Figure 52.4 Lumbar plexus paravertebral region longitudinal view. TP, transverse process; ES, erector spinae; PM, psoas major. Reproduced with permission from Arthurs G, Nicholls B (eds.) 2016. *Ultrasound in Anesthesia, Critical Care, and Pain Management*. Cambridge, UK: Cambridge University Press

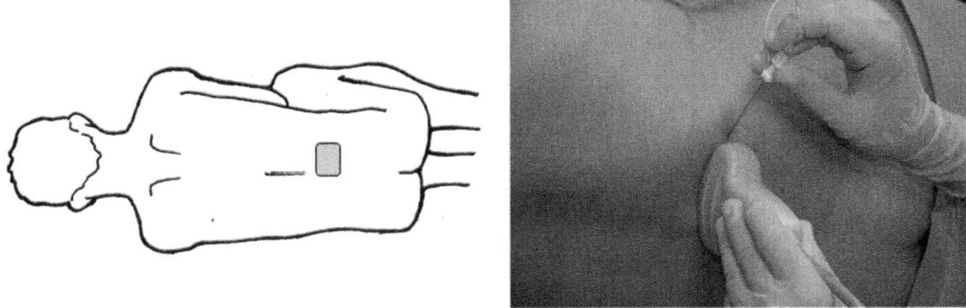

Figure 52.5 Lumbar plexus block with patient and probe positioning. Reproduced with permission from Arthurs G, Nicholls B (eds.) 2016. *Ultrasound in Anesthesia, Critical Care, and Pain Management*. Cambridge, UK: Cambridge University Press

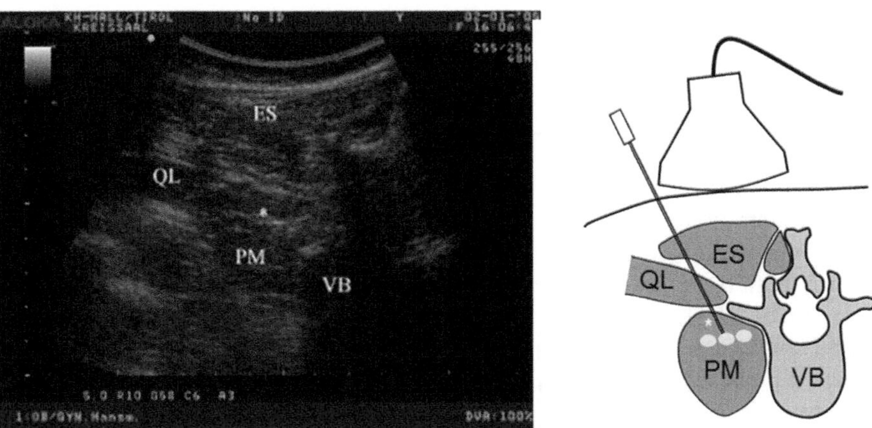

Figure 52.6 Cross-sectional view of lumbar plexus with "shamrock" sign. ES, erector spinae; PM, psoas major; QL, quadratus lumborum; VB, vertebral body. Reproduced with permission from Arthurs G, Nicholls B (eds.) 2016. *Ultrasound in Anesthesia, Critical Care, and Pain Management*. Cambridge, UK: Cambridge University Press

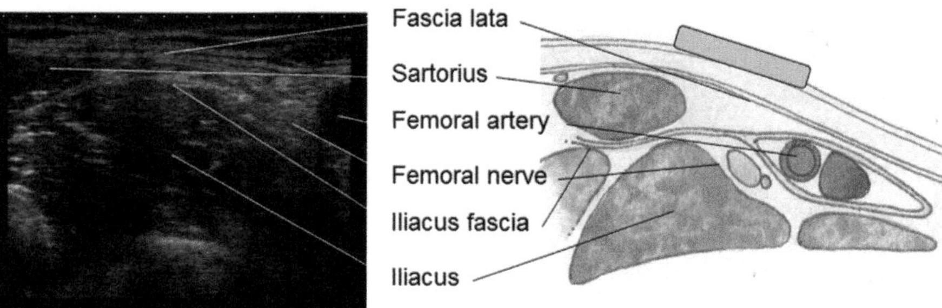

Figure 52.7 Femoral nerve anatomy. Reproduced with permission from Arthurs G, Nicholls B (eds.) 2016. *Ultrasound in Anesthesia, Critical Care, and Pain Management*. Cambridge, UK: Cambridge University Press

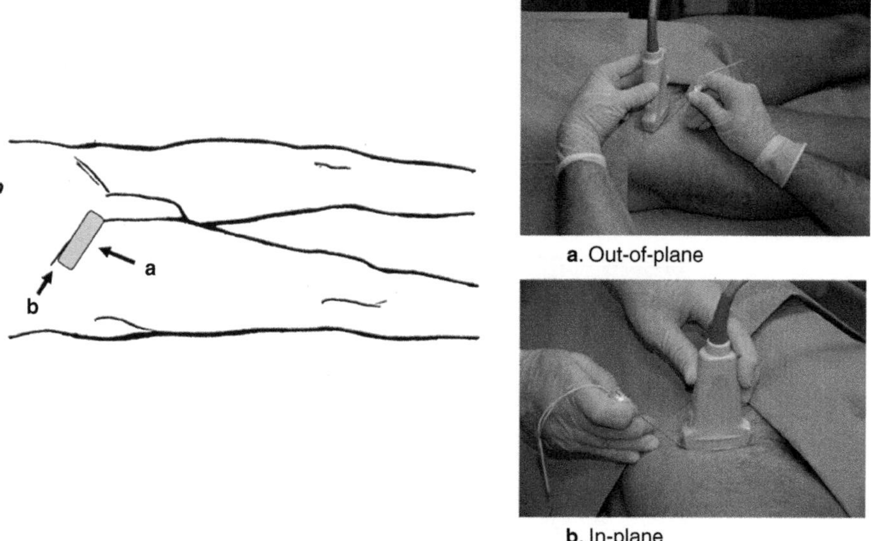

Figure 52.8 Patient and probe positioning for femoral nerve block. Reproduced with permission from Arthurs G, Nicholls B (eds.) 2016. *Ultrasound in Anesthesia, Critical Care, and Pain Management*. Cambridge, UK: Cambridge University Press

below the fascia iliaca lateral to where a femoral nerve block would be performed. With injection at that site, one can block the lateral femoral cutaneous as well as femoral nerve and, less reliably, the obturator nerve.

In the landmark-based technique, one draws a line from the anterior superior iliac spine (ASIS) to the pubic tubercle and divides the line into thirds (Figure 52.10). At one-third from the ASIS, one advances a needle perpendicularly until two pops are felt, which deposits the local anesthetic. The two pops correspond to the fascia lata and fascia iliaca.

In the ultrasound technique, the probe is placed in a transverse position, angled slightly caudad as shown in Figure 52.11. The resulting ultrasound image will show the fascia iliaca as it overlies the iliacus muscle and ileum (Figure 52.11). The local anesthetic is deposited immediately below the fascia iliaca but not in the belly of the iliacus muscle.

Case continued: Her four-year-old brother was complaining of left lower leg pain and sustained an open tibial-fibular fracture above the ankle which was posted for open-reduction/internal fixation.

Given the Injury, What Would Be the Regional Anesthesia Options for This Procedure?

With both bones of the lower extremity fractured and a need for complete, circumferential analgesia of the left lower leg, one can see that both the terminal branches of the sciatic and femoral nerve (saphenous) need to be blocked to provide 100% analgesia to the lower extremity. Since the injury is at the distal aspect of the extremity, proximal nerve blocks, such as lumbar plexus or sacral/subgluteal sciatic, would be poor choices as they would cause motor weakness of the entirety of the extremity. Instead, a targeted approach of the nerves innervating the structures below the knee would be most prudent. Namely, an adductor canal nerve block to block the saphenous nerve combined with a mid-thigh or popliteal sciatic nerve block.

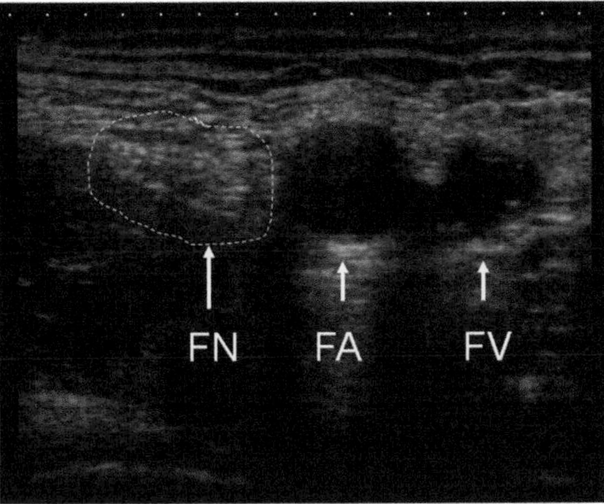

Figure 52.9 Cross-sectional anatomy of the femoral anatomy. FN, femoral nerve; FA, femoral artery; FV, femoral vein. Reproduced with permission from Arthurs G, Nicholls B (eds.) 2016. *Ultrasound in Anesthesia, Critical Care, and Pain Management*. Cambridge, UK: Cambridge University Press

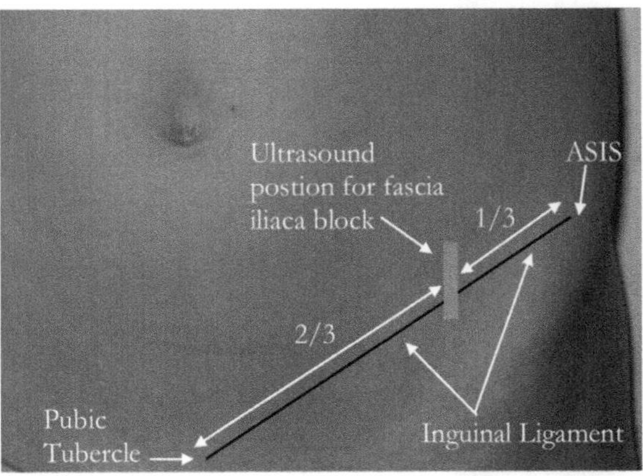

Figure 52.10 Anatomic placement of the ultrasound probe (grey box) one-third the distance from the anterior superior iliac spine (ASIS) and two-thirds the distance from the pubic tubercle along the inguinal ligament

What Is the Difference between a Femoral Block and an Adductor Canal Block? Which Would Be Preferable in This Instance?

The femoral nerve block is used to block the femoral nerve at a relatively proximal position from its emergence from the lumbar plexus, causing blockade of all the quadriceps muscles in addition to blockade of the majority of the femur. The adductor canal, on the other hand, blocks the terminal branch of the femoral nerve, the saphenous nerve, which is a purely sensory nerve of the medial aspect of the leg below the knee. There is no associated motor block with the blockade of the saphenous nerve. Since this patient has an injury below the knee, there is no discernable advantage to blocking the femoral nerve and causing quadriceps weakness in this patient.

How Would You Perform the Adductor Canal Block with Ultrasound?

With the patient supine and leg slightly abducted and externally rotated, an ultrasound probe is placed in a transverse orientation at a distance slightly past mid-thigh (Figure 52.12). The target structure that is

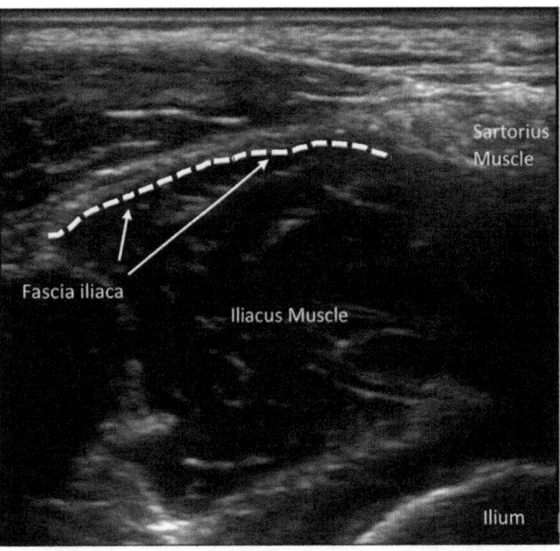

Figure 52.11 Ultrasound anatomy of the fascia iliaca plane

sought out is the adductor (or Hunter's) canal where the femoral artery immediately under the sartorius muscle lies in close proximity to the saphenous nerve (Figure 52.13).

Local anesthetic dosing volumes are similar to that of femoral nerve blocks, with 0.2–0.5 cc/kg of 0.25% bupivacaine or 0.2% ropivacaine used.

How Would You Perform the Sciatic Nerve Block?

The sciatic nerve, the largest peripheral nerve in the human body, can be blocked at one of many locations along its path: sacral, subgluteal, midthigh, or popliteal. In the case of our patient, a popliteal nerve block or midthigh sciatic would make the most sense as they would spare motor weakness of the hamstring muscles that would result from the sacral or subgluteal sciatic block.

The popliteal sciatic block can be performed in either the supine or prone position (Figures 52.14–52.17). Since the patient would be induced in a supine fashion, it is the practice of the author to perform the sciatic block in the supine position by elevating the leg with either towels or a table stand. With the leg elevated, the ultrasound probe can be placed on the underside of the leg to scan the leg from a posterior position as shown in

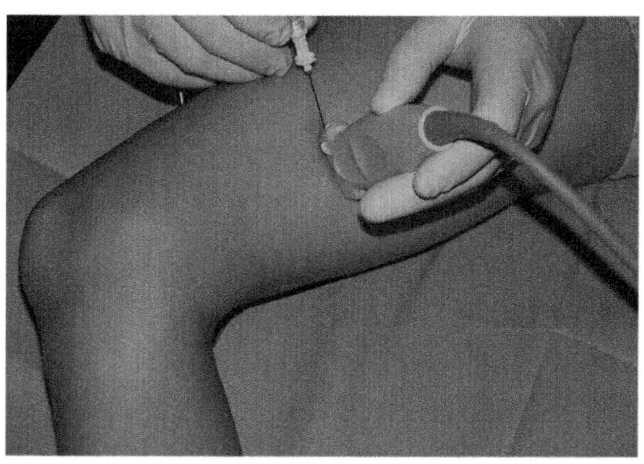

Figure 52.12 Probe and needle position for saphenous nerve block/adductor canal block. Reproduced with permission from Mannion S, Iohom G, Dadure C, Reisbig MD, Ganesh A (eds.) 2015. *Ultrasound-Guided Regional Anesthesia in Children*. Cambridge, UK: Cambridge University Press

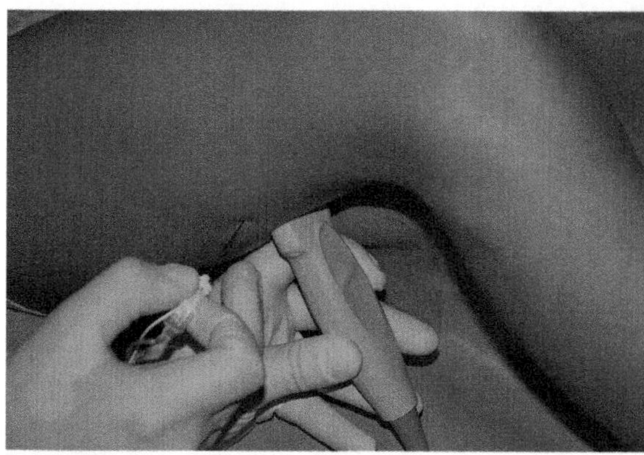

Figure 52.14 Ultrasound and needle positioning for distal sciatic nerve block with the patient in the supine position. Reproduced with permission from Mannion S, Iohom G, Dadure C, Reisbig MD, Ganesh A (eds.) 2015. *Ultrasound-Guided Regional Anesthesia in Children*. Cambridge, UK: Cambridge University Press

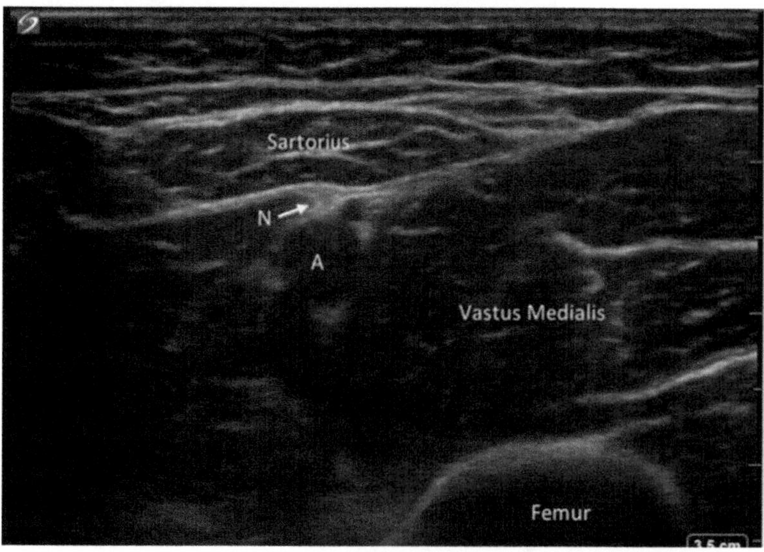

Figure 52.13 Ultrasound image of adductor canal block. A, femoral artery; N, saphenous nerve.

Figures 52.15–52.17. The resulting image will demonstrate the popliteal artery and vein in close proximity to the branches of the sciatic nerve: the common peroneal and the tibial nerve. The nerves can be blocked separately at that site or the probe can be moved more proximal until the nerves coalesce to become the sciatic, approximately 6–10 cm above the popliteal crease.

Upon completing the surgery with successful nerve blockade, you are called to the PACU to address a patient who underwent open reduction and internal fixation (ORIF) of 4 metatarsal bones who is in severe pain.

How Can You Perform an Ankle Block?

The ankle block is a basic landmark-based block that can be easily performed by novice regional anesthesiologists. After thorough sterile prep and drape with towels, the medial and lateral malleoli are identified,

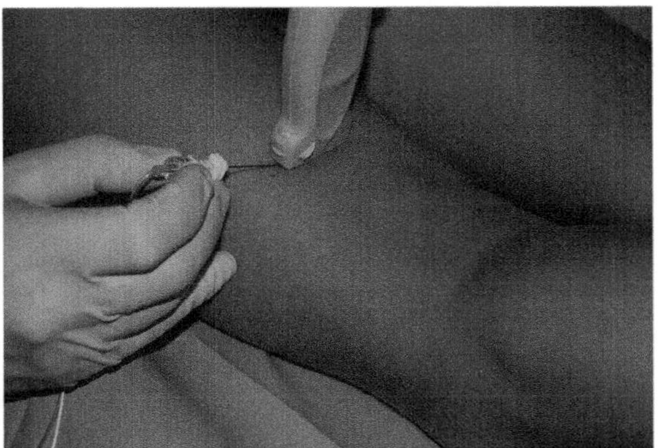

Figure 52.15 Ultrasound and needle positioning for distal sciatic nerve block with the patient in the prone position. Reproduced with permission from Mannion S, Iohom G, Dadure C, Reisbig MD, Ganesh A (eds.) 2015. *Ultrasound-Guided Regional Anesthesia in Children*. Cambridge, UK: Cambridge University Press

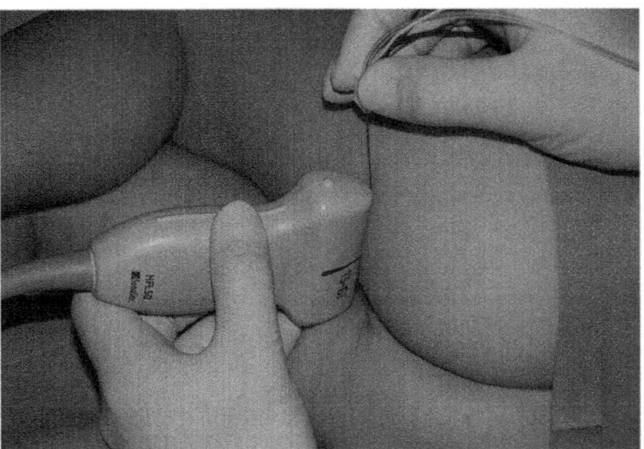

Figure 52.17 Ultrasound and needle positioning for proximal sciatic nerve block (subgluteal) with the patient in the lateral position. Reproduced with permission from Mannion S, Iohom G, Dadure C, Reisbig MD, Ganesh A (eds.) 2015. *Ultrasound-Guided Regional Anesthesia in Children*. Cambridge, UK: Cambridge University Press

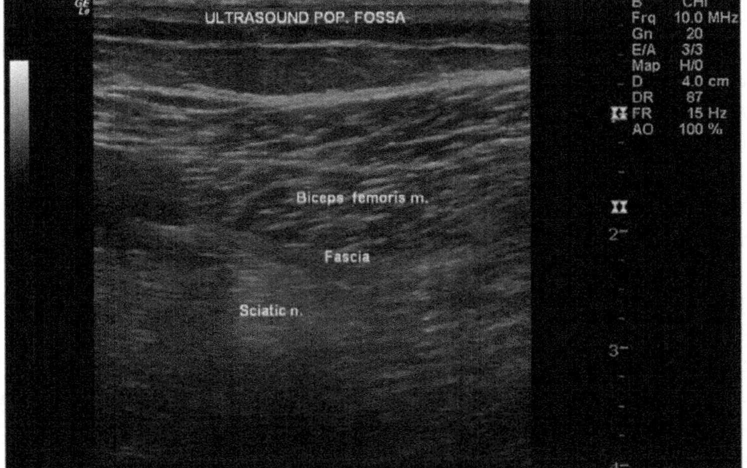

Figure 52.16 Ultrasound image if sciatic nerve block at the level of the prepopliteal space. Reproduced with permission from Arbona FL, Khabiri B, Norton JA (eds.) 2011. *Ultrasound-Guided Regional Anesthesia: A Practical Approach to Peripheral Nerve Blocks and Perineural Catheters*. Cambridge, UK: Cambridge University Press

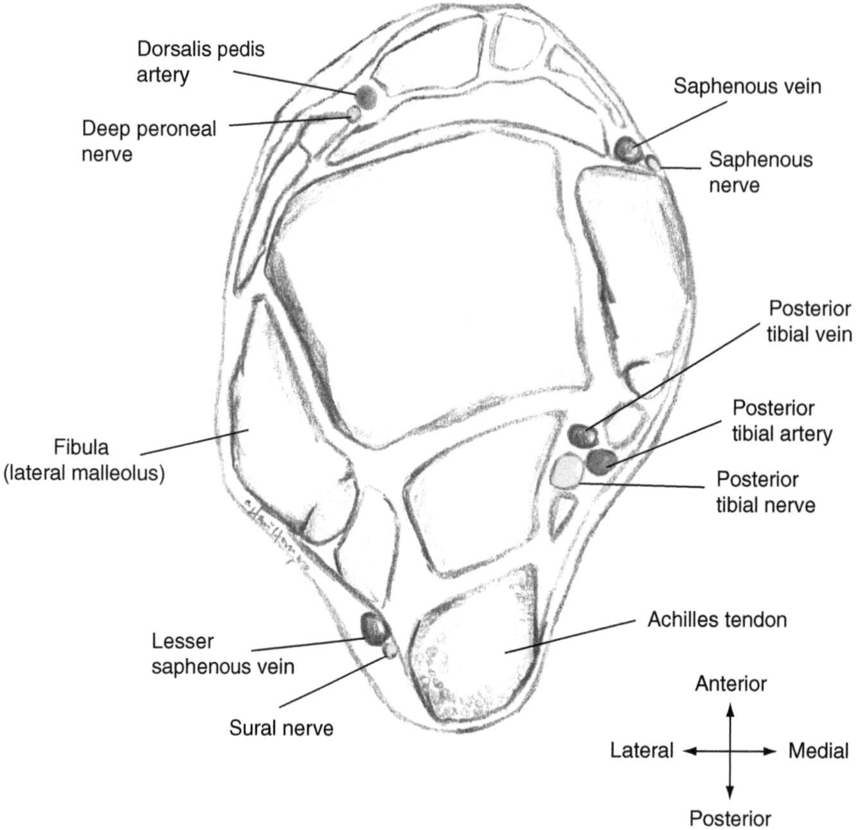

Figure 52.18 Cross-section drawing of ankle anatomy. Reproduced with permission from Arbona FL, Khabiri B, Norton JA (eds.) 2011. *Ultrasound-Guided Regional Anesthesia: A Practical Approach to Peripheral Nerve Blocks and Perineural Catheters.* Cambridge, UK: Cambridge University Press

and a line is drawn connecting them. Approximately mid-length along that line, lateral to the extensor halluces longus tendon lies the deep peroneal nerve. A 25–27G needle can be inserted immediately perpendicular to that spot until contact is made with periosteum. Withdraw the needle 1 mm and aspirate and inject one-fifth of your local anesthetic. Then take your needle and withdraw to beneath the surface of the skin and aim for the medial malleolus subcutaneously with your needle and upon withdrawing towards the needle entry site (adjacent to extensor halluces longus tendon) inject one-fifth of the local anesthetic creating a skin wheel. This will block the saphenous nerve. Repeat the same subcutaneous injection towards the lateral malleolus and block the superficial peroneal nerve with one-fifth of your local anesthetic. Next, palpate the fossa immediately posterior to the medial malleolus where the tibial artery can be felt pulsating. Insert the needle into the fossa, taking care to avoid the artery or vein (by aspirating) and contact the periosteum. Withdraw the needle 1 mm and inject one-fifth of your local anesthetic to block the posterior tibial nerve. Lastly, palpate the lateral malleolus and locate the fossa immediately posterior. Insert your needle until periosteum is contacted. Withdraw your needle 1 mm and inject the remaining one-fifth of your local anesthetic solution. This circumferential ring block at the level of the malleoli provides complete blockade of the foot distal to the ankle block (Figure 52.18).

What Is the Typical Dosing of Ankle Block?

0.1 cc/kg of 0.25% bupivacaine or 0.2% ropivacaine can be used to dose the ankle block. Epinephrine should *not* be added to the local anesthetic.

Suggested Reading

Arbona FL, Khabiri B, Norton JA. *Ultrasound-Guided Regional Anesthesia*. Cambridge: Cambridge University Press; 2011.

Hadzic A. *Textbook of Regional Anesthesia and Acute Pain Management*. 2nd Edition. New York, NY: McGraw-Hill Education; 2017.

Mannion S, Iohom G, Dadure C, Reisbig MD, Ganesh A. *Ultrasound-Guided Regional Anesthesia in Children*. Cambridge: Cambridge University Press; 2015.

Tsui B, Suresh S. *Pediatric Atlas of Ultrasound and Nerve-Stimulation-Guided Regional Anesthesia*. New York, NY: Springer; 2016.

Chapter 53 Truncal Blocks

Monica Chen

A three-year-old, former 33-week premature infant with a history of an omphalocele presents with a ventral hernia. She is now scheduled for repair. Her laboratory testing is unremarkable. The surgeon is requesting a regional block for this procedure and wants to discuss the options.

What Are the Boundaries of the Anterior Abdominal Wall?

The anterior abdominal wall extends from the costal margin of the seventh to tenth ribs and xiphoid process to the iliac crests, inguinal ligament, and pubic crest/symphysis. The lateral borders are demarcated by the bilateral mid-axillary lines.

What Muscles Make Up the Anterior Abdominal Wall?

The anterior abdominal wall is made up of three concentric muscle layers. From superficial to deep, they are the external oblique muscle, internal oblique muscle, and the transversus abdominis muscle.

The rectus abdominis muscle is a pair of vertical muscles that run down the midline of the anterior abdominal wall.

Some individuals may also have a second midline muscle known as the pyramidalis.

How Is the Anterior Abdominal Wall Innervated?

The anterior abdominal wall is innervated by the T_6–T_{12} thoracoabdominal nerves. These nerves originate from the T_6–T_{12} spinal nerves and traverse across the neurovascular transversus abdominis plane that lies between the internal oblique muscle and the transversus abdominis muscle (Figure 53.1).

The ilioinguinal and iliohypogastric nerves arise from the L1 spinal nerve. These nerves emerge from the lateral border of the psoas muscles and travel superior and parallel to the iliac crest. They both eventually pierce the transversus abdominis muscles, though there is variability in the location at which they enter the transversus abdominis plane.

How Is the Rectus Sheath Formed?

The rectus sheath encompasses the rectus abdominis muscle anteriorly and posteriorly. The anterior rectus sheath is formed from the aponeurosis of the external oblique and the internal oblique muscles. The posterior rectus sheath is formed from the aponeurosis of the internal oblique and transversus abdominis muscles.

What Changes Occur in the Rectus Sheath below the Arcuate Line?

The lower limit of the posterior rectus sheath is the arcuate line. Inferior to this point, the aponeurosis of the external oblique, internal oblique, and transversus abdominis muscles all pass anterior to the rectus abdominis muscles.

What Are the Major Muscles That Comprise the Posterior Abdominal Wall?

The muscles of the posterior abdominal wall include the latissimus dorsi muscle, erector spinae muscle, quadratus lumborum muscle, and the psoas major.

The erector spinae muscle is comprised of three paraspinal muscles: the iliocostalis muscle, the longissimus muscle, and the spinalis muscle.

What Is the Significance of the Thoracolumbar Fascia?

The thoracolumbar fascia encloses the deep muscles of the back. It is comprised of three layers: anterior,

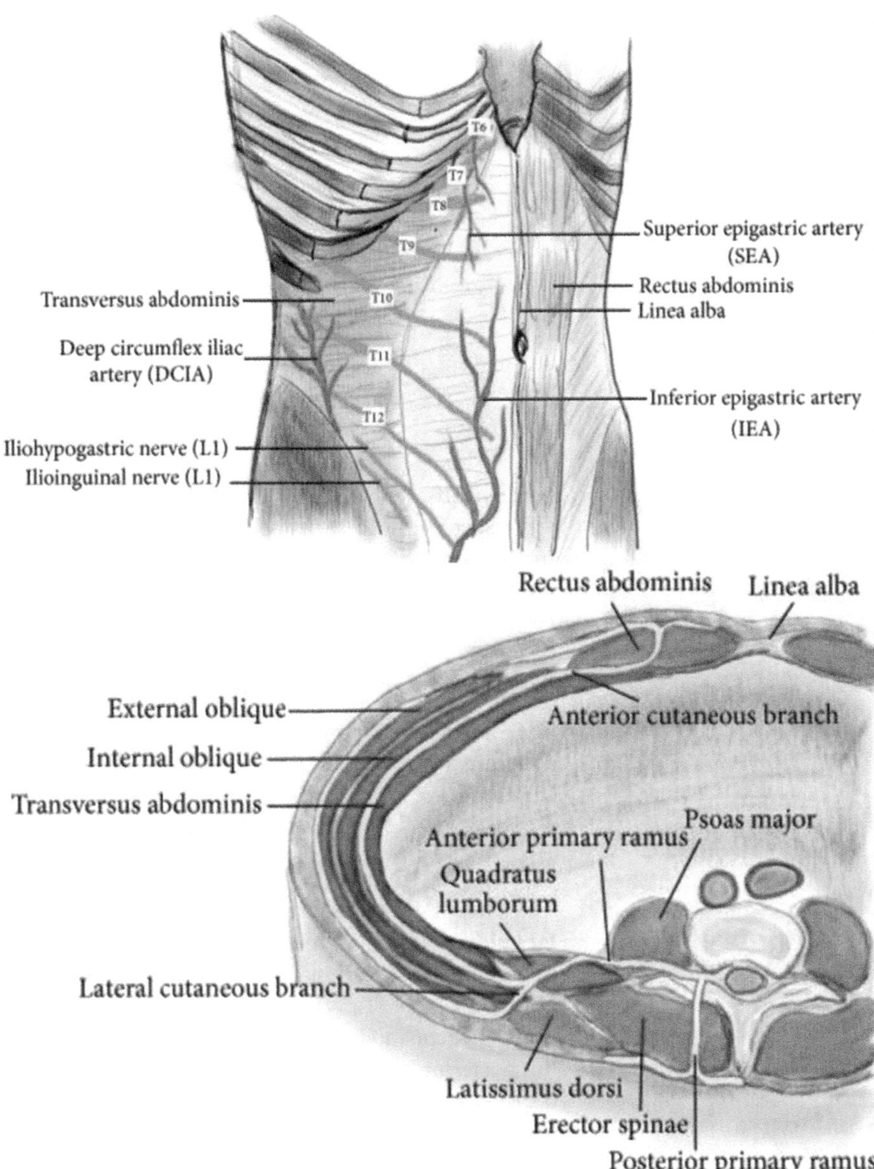

Figure 53.1 Anatomy of the anterior abdominal wall. Reproduced from Tsai H-C, Yoshida T, Chuang T-Y, et al. Transversus abdominis plane block: An updated review of anatomy and techniques. *BioMed Research International*, 2017, Article ID 8284363, under CC BY 4.0 license https://creativecommons.org/licenses/by/4.0/

middle, and posterior. The anterior layer is often referred to as the "transversalis fascia" and lies on the anterior surface of the quadratus lumborum muscle. It is thought that the thoracolumbar fascia may serve as a conduit for local anesthetic spread when performing the quadratus lumborum block.

What Are Commonly Performed Truncal Blocks?

- Transversus abdominis plane block
- Rectus sheath block
- Ilioinguinal-iliohypogastric block

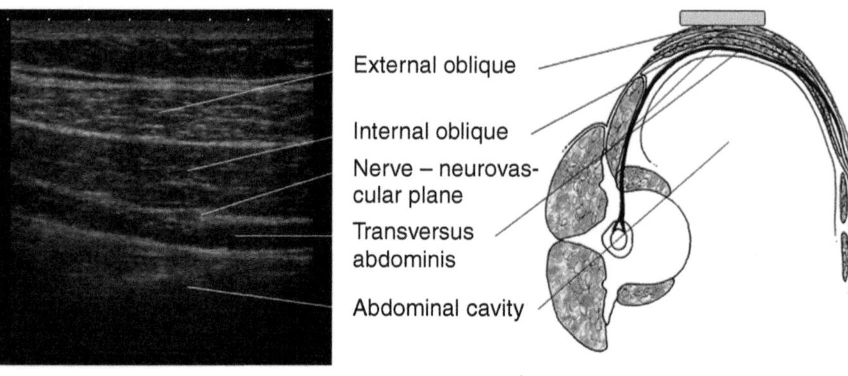

Figure 53.2 Abdominal wall anatomy. Reproduced with permission from Arthurs G, Nicholls B (eds.) 2016. *Ultrasound in Anesthesia, Critical Care, and Pain Management*. Cambridge, UK: Cambridge University Press

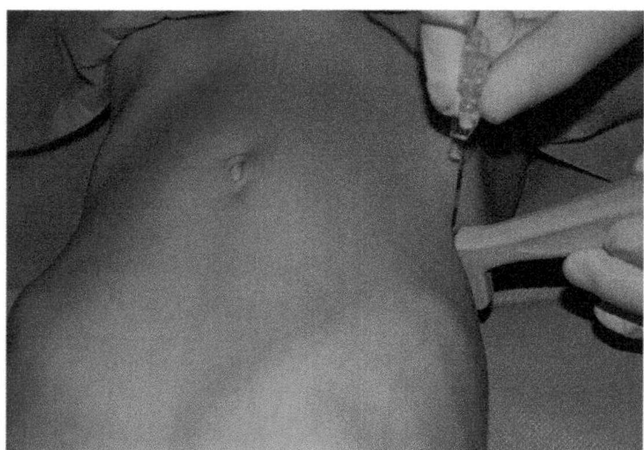

Figure 53.3 Ultrasound probe and needle position for transversus abdominis plane block. Reproduced with permission from Mannion S, Iohom G, Dadure C, Reisbig MD, Ganesh A (eds.) 2015. *Ultrasound-Guided Regional Anesthesia in Children*. Cambridge, UK: Cambridge University Press

- Paravertebral block
- Quadratus lumborum block
- Erector spinae block

What Is a Transversus Abdominis Plane Block?

A transversus abdominis plane (TAP) block provides somatic analgesia for the anterior abdominal wall by targeting the thoracoabdominal nerves (T_6–L_1). There are multiple approaches to performing the TAP block including the subcostal, oblique-subcostal, and lateral techniques. The lateral technique is used more commonly and is the easiest to perform. The patient is placed in the supine position for all approaches. The probe is held in the transverse position (i.e., parallel to the costal margin and iliac crest) and lies anywhere between the midaxillary to midclavicular line. The needle is inserted lateral to the probe, with the ultimate target for local anesthetic deposition being the transversus abdominis plane – which lies deep to internal oblique muscle and superficial to the transversus abdominis muscle (Figures 53.2–53.4).

What Are the Indications for a TAP Block?

The TAP block provides somatic analgesia for abdominal surgeries including laparoscopic surgeries, laparotomies, and caesarean sections.

What Is the Rectus Sheath Block?

The rectus sheath block provides somatic analgesia for midline incisions in the anterior abdominal wall by targeting the terminal branches of the thoracoabdominal nerves (T_{9-11}). These nerves lie in the plane deep to rectus abdominis muscles and superficial to the posterior rectus sheath. The probe is held in the transverse orientation – superior to the umbilicus and lateral to the linea alba (Figures 53.5–53.7).

In What Surgeries Would a Rectus Sheath Block Be Useful?

Rectus sheath blocks are commonly used for surgeries that involve midline incisions. These include umbilical hernia repairs, pyloromyotomies, and laparoscopic procedures with midline port insertions.

What Is the Ilioinguinal-Iliohypogastric Block?

The ilioinguinal and iliohypogastric nerves arise from L_1. They may occasionally also have contributions

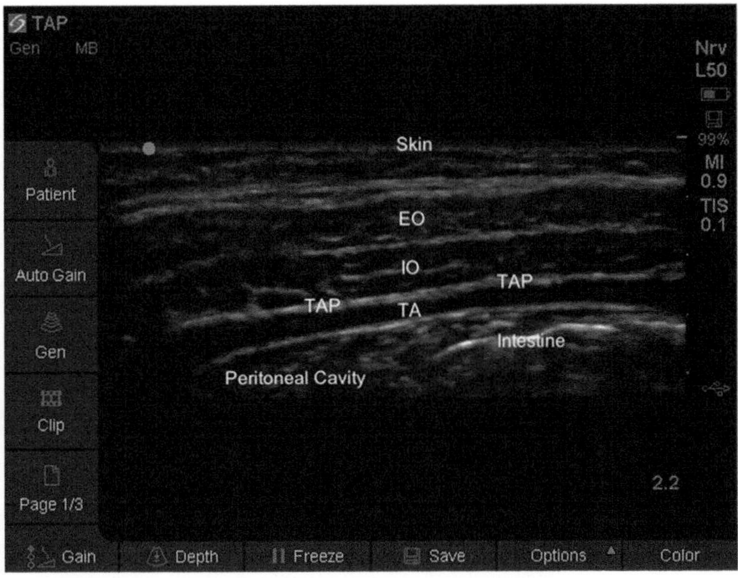

Figure 53.4 Ultrasound image of transversus abdominis plane block. Reproduced with permission from Mannion S, Iohom G, Dadure C, Reisbig MD, Ganesh A (eds.) 2015. *Ultrasound-Guided Regional Anesthesia in Children*. Cambridge, UK: Cambridge University Press

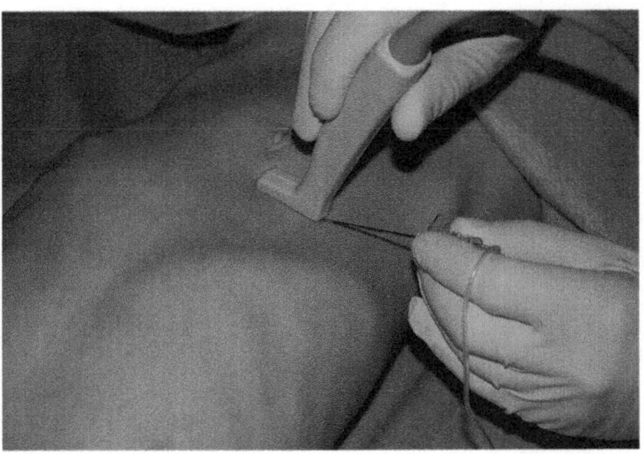

Figure 53.5 Ultrasound probe and needle position for rectus sheath block. Reproduced with permission from Mannion S, Iohom G, Dadure C, Reisbig MD, Ganesh A (eds.) 2015. *Ultrasound-Guided Regional Anesthesia in Children*. Cambridge, UK: Cambridge University Press

from T_{12}, L_2, and L_3. The ultrasound-guided ilioinguinal-iliohypogastric block targets these nerves as they lie in transversus abdominis plane. The probe is placed posterior and superior to the ASIS, parallel to the line between the ASIS and umbilicus. Here the external oblique, internal oblique, and transversus abdominis muscles can be visualized. Additionally, the acoustic shadow of the ASIS can be seen as well. The nerves are not always consistently visualized in this window, but injection of local anesthetic into the TAP plane at this level will provide for somatic analgesia at the level of the inguinal fossa (Figures 53.8 and 53.9).

What Surgeries Would Use an Ilioinguinal-Iliohypogastric Block?

Ilioinguinal-iliohypogastric blocks are classically used in inguinal hernia repairs and urology surgeries (e.g., orchiopexy).

What Is the Paravertebral Vertebral Space?

The paravertebral space is a potential space that extends from the cervical spine down to the lumbosacral spine. At the thoracic level, this triangular-shaped space is demarcated anteriorly by the parietal pleural, posteriorly by the costotransverse ligament, and medially by the posterolateral border of the vertebral body and intervertebral discs. The paravertebral space contains thoracic spinal nerves, the sympathetic chain, intercostal vessels, and fatty tissue.

What Is the Paravertebral Nerve Block?

The paravertebral nerve block is frequently used for perioperative analgesia associated with chest wall surgeries, rib fractures, and renal surgeries. The key landmark in the paravertebral nerve block is the costotransverse ligament, which forms the posterior border of the paravertebral space (Figures 53.11–53.12). Using a linear probe, the costotransverse ligament can be found using in-plane or out-of-plane approaches, though the out-of-plane

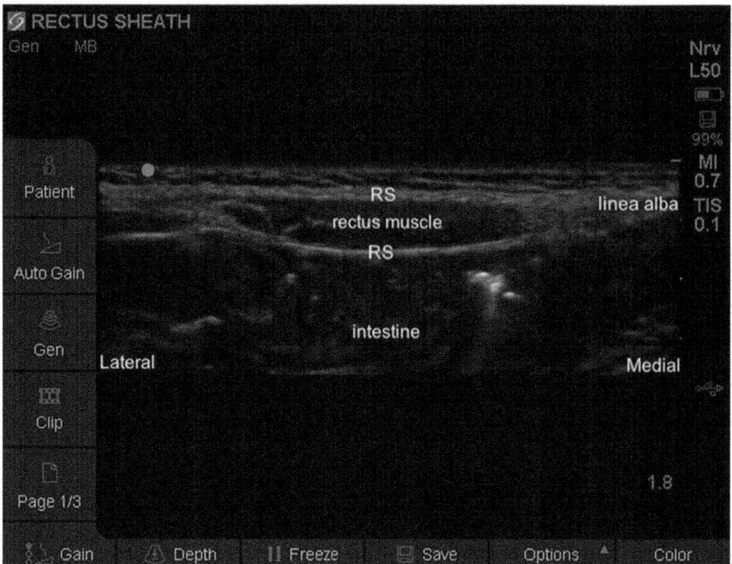

Figure 53.6 Ultrasound image of rectus sheath anatomy. RA, rectus sheath. Reproduced with permission from Mannion S, Iohom G, Dadure C, Reisbig MD, Ganesh A (eds.) 2015. *Ultrasound-Guided Regional Anesthesia in Children*. Cambridge, UK: Cambridge University Press

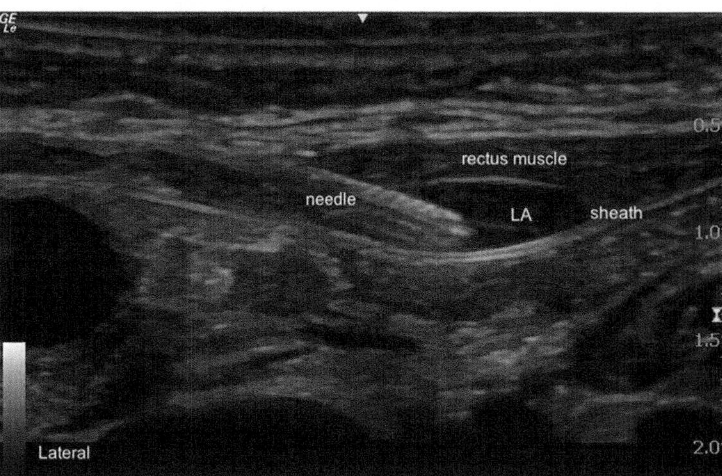

Figure 53.7 Ultrasound image of rectus sheath block. LA, local anesthetic. Reproduced with permission from Mannion S, Iohom G, Dadure C, Reisbig MD, Ganesh A (eds.) 2015. *Ultrasound-Guided Regional Anesthesia in Children*. Cambridge, UK: Cambridge University Press

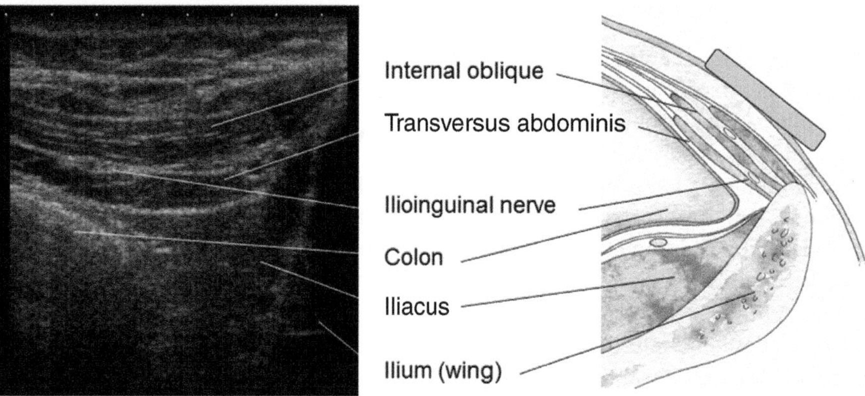

Figure 53.8 Ilioinguinal nerve anatomy. Reproduced with permission from Arthurs G, Nicholls B (eds.) 2016. *Ultrasound in Anesthesia, Critical Care, and Pain Management*. Cambridge, UK: Cambridge University Press

approach is favored. The ultrasound probe is positioned along the mid-scapular line at the desired level. The layers of intercostal muscles are identified, and in between the transverse process is the hyperechoic costotransverse ligament. Local anesthetic is injected between the costotransverse ligament with subsequent downward displacement of the pleura.

What Is a Quadratus Lumborum Block?

The ultrasound-guided quadratus lumborum (QL) block deposits local anesthetic in or around the quadratus lumborum muscle (Figure 53.13). The block was first described as a "posterior TAP block," however, emphasis has since been placed on the QL muscle as the sonographic landmark and the role of the thoracolumbar fascia in the spread of local anesthetic.

There are four main approaches to the QL block, with names based on the location of the needle relative to the QL muscle.

- Lateral QL block
- Posterior QL block
- Anterior QL block
- Intramuscular QL block

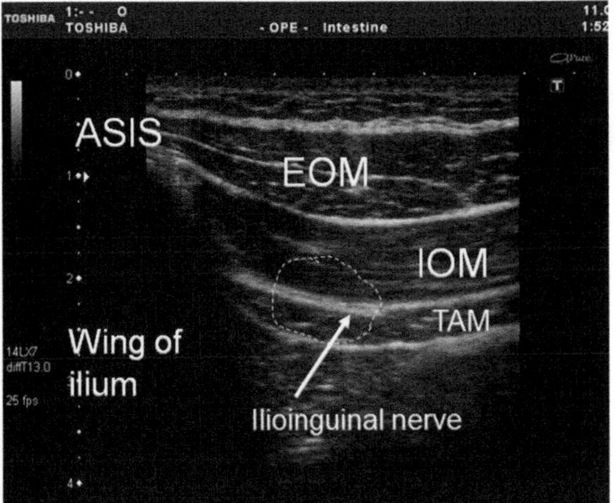

Figure 53.9 Ultrasound Ilioinguinal nerve block. ASIS, anterior superior iliac spine; EOM, external oblique muscle; IOM, internal oblique muscle; TAM, transversus abdominal muscle. Reproduced with permission from Arthurs G, Nicholls B (eds.) 2016. *Ultrasound in Anesthesia, Critical Care, and Pain Management*. Cambridge, UK: Cambridge University Press

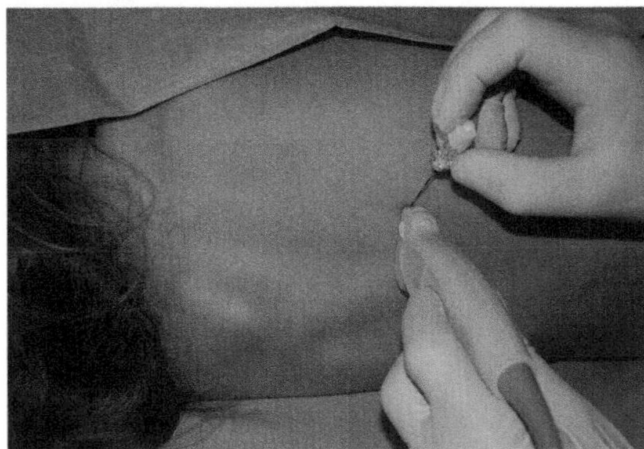

Figure 53.11 Ultrasound probe and needle position for lateral paravertebral nerve block. Reproduced with permission from Mannion S, Iohom G, Dadure C, Reisbig MD, Ganesh A (eds.) 2015. *Ultrasound-Guided Regional Anesthesia in Children*. Cambridge, UK: Cambridge University Press

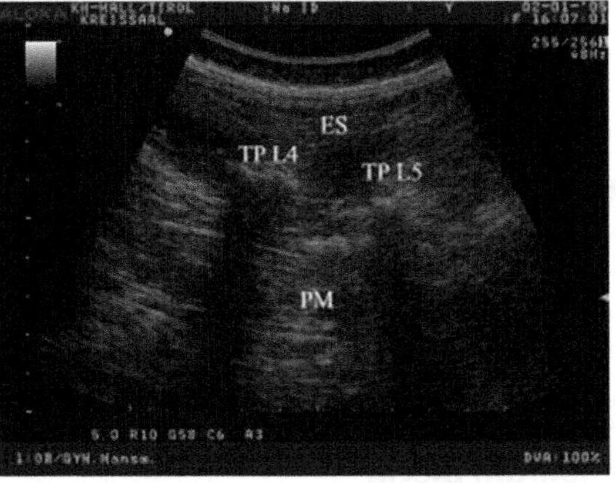

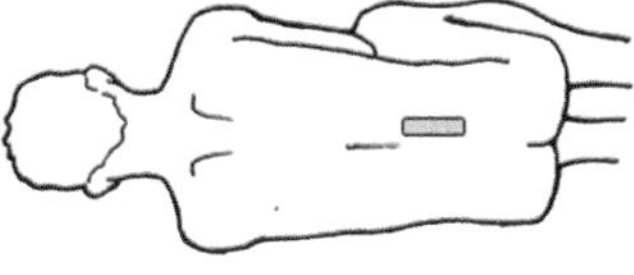

Figure 53.10 Ultrasound Ilioinguinal nerve block. ASIS, anterior superior iliac spine; EOM, external oblique muscle; IOM, internal oblique muscle; TAM, transversus abdominal muscle. Reproduced with permission from Arthurs G, Nicholls B (eds.) 2016. *Ultrasound in Anesthesia, Critical Care, and Pain Management*. Cambridge, UK: Cambridge University Press

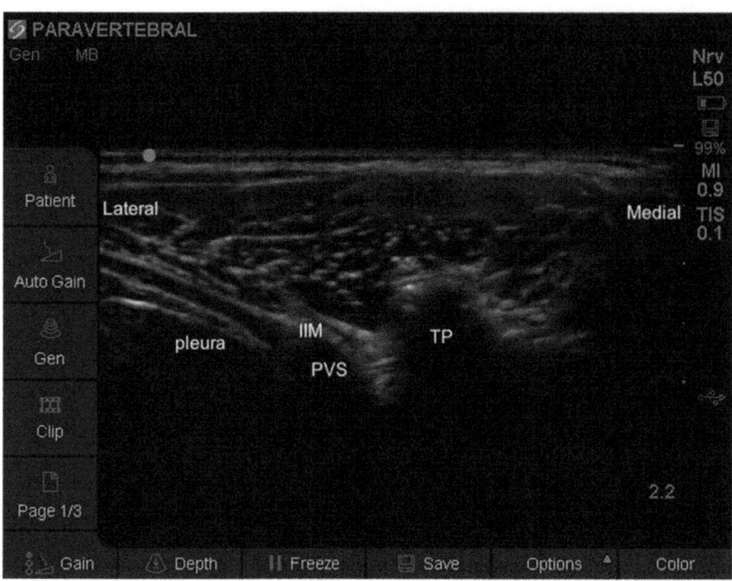

Figure 53.12 Ultrasound-guided lateral paravertebral nerve block. PVS, paravertebral space; IIM, internal intercostal membrane; TP, transverse process. Reproduced with permission from Mannion S, Iohom G, Dadure C, Reisbig MD, Ganesh A (eds.) 2015. *Ultrasound-Guided Regional Anesthesia in Children*. Cambridge, UK: Cambridge University Press

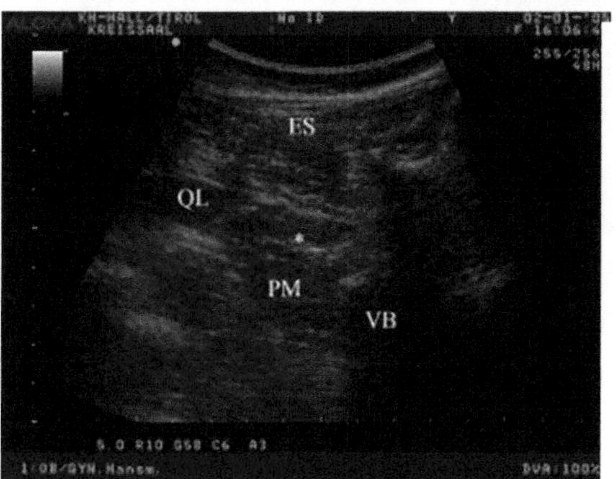

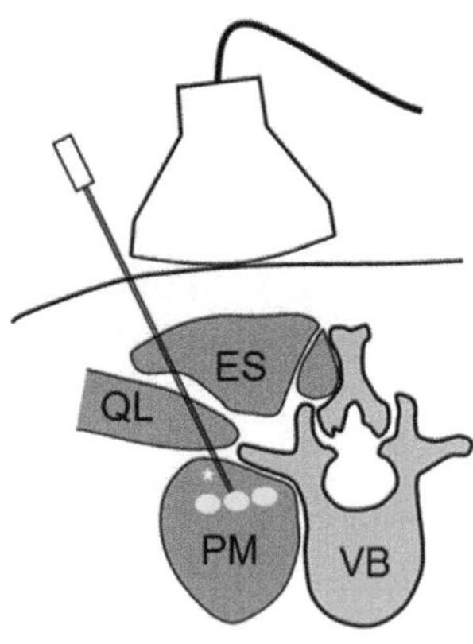

Figure 53.13 Cross-sectional view of lumbar plexus with "shamrock" sign. ES, erector spinae; PM, psoas major; QL, quadratus lumborum; VB, vertebral body. Reproduced with permission from Arthurs G, Nicholls B (eds.) 2016. *Ultrasound in Anesthesia, Critical Care, and Pain Management*. Cambridge, UK: Cambridge University Press

The lateral QL block is also known as the QL 1 block. The posterior QL block is also known as the QL 2 block. The anterior QL block is also known as the transmuscular or QL 3 block.

How Does the QL Block Work?

There is currently no consensus on the mechanism of local anesthetic spread for QL blocks. A common theory is that the thoracolumbar fascia likely acts as a conduit for spread of local anesthetic into the paravertebral space – which encompasses the sympathetic trunk and the ventral and dorsal rami of the spinal nerves.

Are there Advantages to the Quadratus Lumborum Block over the TAP Block?

With potential spread into the paravertebral space, the QL block may provide both somatic and visceral analgesia. In contrast, the TAP block provides only somatic analgesia.

What Are the Indications for a Quadratus Lumborum Block?

The QL block has been used for exploratory laparotomy, bowel resections, laparoscopic/open

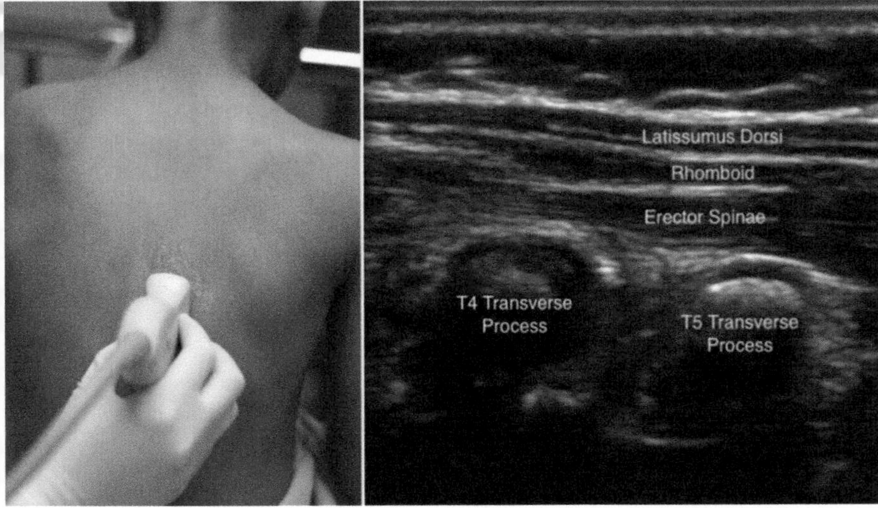

Figure 53.14 Probe positioning for erector spinae plane block (left). Ultrasound image of erector spinae plane block (right)

appendectomies, laparoscopic/open cholecystectomies, hysterectomies, cesarean sections, nephrectomies, and renal transplant surgeries.

The block has also been used in urologic surgeries, inguinal hernia repairs, iliac crest bone grafts, and hip surgeries.

What Is an Erector Spinae Muscle Block?

First described in 2016, the erector spinae block is an interfascial plane block that has been utilized in thoracic surgery, breast surgery, abdominal surgery, and hip surgery. The ultrasound probe is placed in the longitudinal position in the sitting or lateral position. The transverse process at the target level is identified and the needle is advanced in the cephalad to caudad through the trapezius, rhomboid major, and erector spinae muscles. The needle subsequently contacts the transverse process and local anesthetic is subsequently injected deep to the erector spinae muscle (Figure 53.14).

How Does the Erector Spinae Block Work?

Unlike the paravertebral block, the erector spinae plane block does directly penetrate the costotransverse ligament. The mechanism of action is thought to be diffusion of local anesthetic into the paravertebral space.

What Complications May Be Associated with Truncal Blocks?

- Intraperitoneal injection.
- Vascular trauma and/or injection.
- Pneumothorax.
- Pleural puncture.
- Epidural spread of local anesthetic.

What Is the ASRA/ESRA Recommended Dose of Truncal Blocks?

In 2018, ASRA/ESRA published recommendations for dosing ultrasound-guided blocks in pediatric patients. For fascial plane blocks, they recommend using 0.25–0.75 mg/kg of bupivacaine or ropivacaine.

What Are the Approaches to the Pectoralis Block?

From superficial to deep, the anterior chest wall comprises of the pectoralis major, pectoralis minor, and the serratus anterior muscle. The lateral pectoral nerve originates from the lateral cord of the brachial plexus and provides sensory innervation to the head of the pectoralis major. The medial pectoral nerve originates from the medial cord of the brachial plexus and innervates the pectoralis major and pectoralis minor.

The Pecs blocks are frequently used in breast surgery and have been reliably performed with ultrasound guidance. They are both interfascial plane blocks.

The Pecs-1 targets lateral and medial pectoral nerves. A linear probe is placed in the midclavicular line, and local anesthetic is deposited between the pectoralis major and pectoralis minor.

The Pecs-2 block targets the intercostal nerves and the long thoracic nerve. A linear probe is placed sagittally along the anterior axillary line and local anesthetic is deposited between the lateral edge of the pectoralis minor and the serratus anterior muscle.

Summary of Ultrasound-Guided Truncal Blocks

Table 53.1 Summary of the commonly performed truncal blocks

Block	Probe placement	Transducer orientation	Plane of injection	Clinical indications
Tap block	Midaxillary line, parallel to subcostal margin and iliac crest	Transverse	Between internal oblique and transversus abdominis	Somatic analgesia for incisions in upper and lower anterior abdominal wall
Rectus sheath block	Lateral to linea alba, superior to iliac crest	Transverse	Between rectus abdominis and posterior rectus sheath	Somatic analgesia for midline incisions in anterior abdominal wall
Ilioinguinal-iliohypogastric block	Posterior and superior to ASIS, parallel to line between ASIS and umbilicus	Transverse/ oblique	Medial to acoustic shadow of ASIS, between internal oblique and transversus abdominis	Somatic analgesia for incisions in the right or left iliac fossa of the abdomen
Pecs-1 block	Infraclavicular, in the midclavicular line	Transverse	Between the pectoralis major and pectoralis minor	Somatic analgesia for chest wall
Pecs-2 block	Anterior axillary line, over 3rd or 4th rib	Sagittal	Pectoralis minor and serratus anterior	Somatic analgesia for chest wall
Quadratus lumborum block	Parallel to the iliac crest, toward posterior axillary line	Transverse	Lateral, anterior, or posterior to QL muscle	Analgesia for abdominal wall
Paravertebral block	Lateral to spinous processes	Sagittal	Between the costotransverse ligament and pleura	Analgesia for thoracic and abdominal surgeries
Erector spinae block	Lateral to spinous processes	Sagittal	Between erector spinae and transverse process	Analgesia for thoracic surgeries

Suggested Reading

Abrahams M, Derby R, Horn JL. Update on ultrasound for truncal blocks: a review of the evidence. *Reg Anesth Pain Med.* 2016;41 (2):275–88. PMID: 26866299.

Chelly JE. Paravertebral blocks. *Anesthesiol Clin.* 2012 Mar;30 (1):75–90. PMID: 22405434.

Chin KJ, McDonnell JG, Carvalho B, et al. Essentials of our current understanding: abdominal wall blocks. *Reg Anesth Pain Med.* 2017;42(2):133–83. PMID: 28085788.

Elsharkawy H. Quadratus lumborum blocks. *Adv Anesth.* 2017;35 (1):145–57. PMID: 29103570.

Forero M, Adhikary SD, Lopez H, et al. The erector spinae plane block: a novel analgesic technique in thoracic neuropathic pain. *Reg Anesth Pain Med.* 2016;41(5):621–7. PMID: 27501016.

Suresh S, Ecoffey C, Bosenberg A, et al. The European Society of Regional Anaesthesia and Pain Therapy/American Society of Regional Anesthesia and Pain Medicine Recommendations on Local Anesthetics and Adjuvants Dosage in Pediatric Regional Anesthesia. *Reg Anesth Pain Med.* 2018;43(2):211–16. PMID: 29319604.

Suresh S, De Oliveira GS Jr. Local anaesthetic dosage of peripheral nerve blocks in children: analysis of 40 121 blocks from the Pediatric Regional Anesthesia Network database. *Br J Anaesth.* 2018;120(2):317–22. PMID: 29406181.

Tsai HC, Yoshida T, Chuang TY, et al. Transversus abdominis plane block: an updated review of anatomy and techniques. *Biomed Res Int.* 2017;2017:8284363. PMID: 29226150.

Local Anesthetic Systemic Toxicity (LAST)

Arvind Chandrakantan and Aysha Hasan

A nine-year-old, 35 kg boy presents for an open reduction and internal fixation of a right lateral condyle fracture. The patient has a past medical history of headaches presenting with nausea and vomiting. The main provoking factor is anxiety. The alleviating factors for the headaches are bed rest and caffeine. The parents provide consent for general anesthesia with regional anesthesia for pain management. He complains of a headache that seems to improve after intravenous midazolam is given. He is positioned for an ultrasound-guided supraclavicular block. Following negative aspiration, 10 mL of 0.5% ropivacaine is injected. He is resting comfortably in the holding area. After 30 minutes, the patient complains that his headache has returned and he begins to feel nauseous. He begins stuttering and cannot formulate sentences and begins to seize prior to entering the operating room.

What Is the Differential Diagnosis?

It is important to differentiate this patient's migraine from local anesthetic toxicity. The patient began having headaches that seemed to reflect his past medical history of having terrible migraines. Although the needle aspiration was negative upon placement of the supraclavicular block and a significant amount of time had passed prior to the onset of symptoms, local anesthetic toxicity cannot be ruled out. The patient has a past medical history that confounds the diagnosis even under direct ultrasound guidance and visualization.

What Is Local Anesthetic Systemic Toxicity (LAST) and When Does It Occur?

LAST can occur in any patient at any location of local anesthetic placement. Pregnant patients, young patients, and patients with preexisting hypoxia and/or respiratory acidosis are at highest risk for developing LAST. LAST most commonly occurs during an intravascular injection of local anesthetic. However, even the correct placement of anesthetic can cause systemic toxicity. Factors that affect LAST include: concurrent medications, patient risk factors, location and technique of the block, total anesthetic dose, timeliness of detection, and adequacy of treatment.

What Is the Incidence of LAST?

The location of the block is a significant risk factor for patients developing LAST. Supraclavicular and interscalene blocks have shown an incidence of 79 of 10,000 patients developing LAST symptoms in one institution. LAST is more likely to occur in infants compared to adults because of the infant's low protein binding and low intrinsic clearance of local anesthetics. As most infants and children have blocks performed under general anesthesia, the central nervous system manifestations of LAST, such as seizures, are not seen as commonly.

What Are the Signs/Symptoms of LAST?

LAST has a classical presentation of central nervous system (CNS) disturbance. Auditory changes, circumoral numbness, metallic taste, agitation, and seizures are common presentations. This can progress to abrupt onset of psychiatric symptoms, drowsiness, respiratory arrest, and coma. Cardiac manifestations do not commonly occur prior to CNS manifestations. Typical cardiac manifestations are: hypertension, tachycardia, and ventricular arrhythmias. This can progress to bradycardia, conduction block, asystole, and cardiac arrest. Intravascular injections will cause a quicker onset of symptoms. However, onset of symptoms can occur from five minutes post injection to hours post injection. The danger of LAST occurring hours post anesthetic injection is that typically the patient is in a non-monitored area or perhaps even home. Forty percent of LAST symptoms have atypical presentation, such as delayed onset or cardiac issues prior to CNS manifestations.

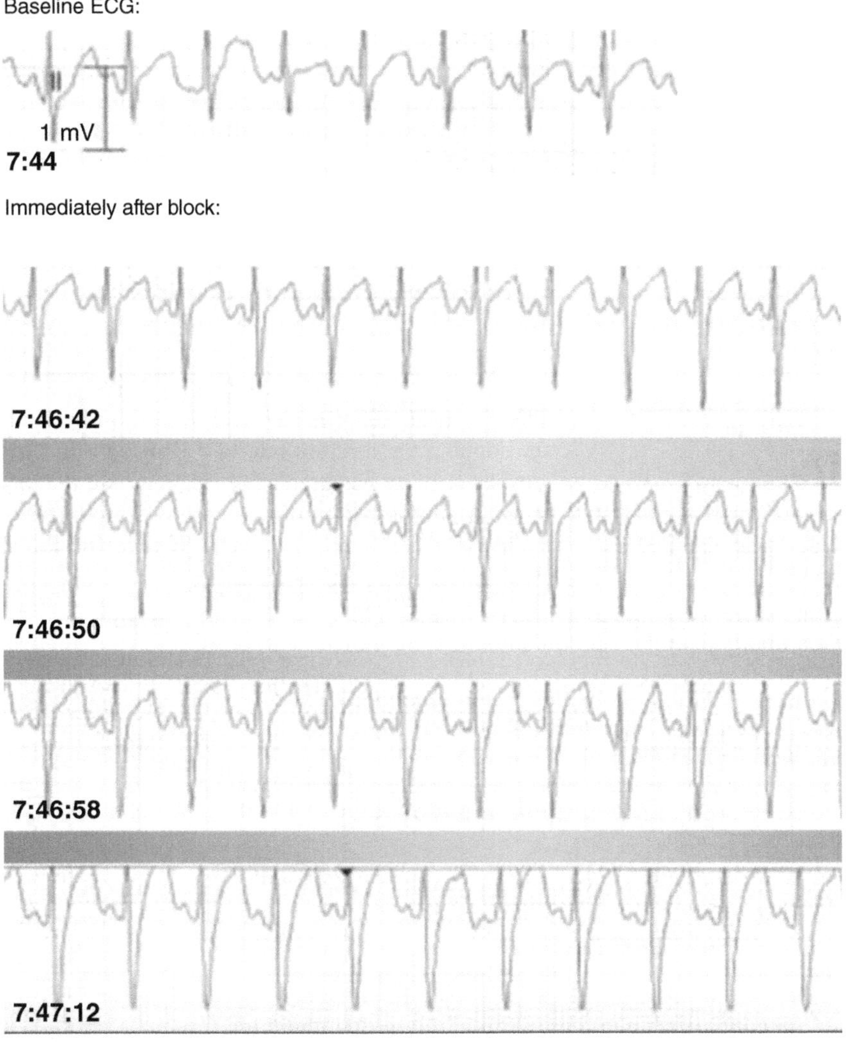

Figure 54.1 Electrocardiography changes associated with intravascular injection of local anesthetic. Images courtesy of Kathleen Chen, MD

However, under anesthesia (e.g., caudal blocks) cardiac manifestations are often the first indication of LAST, and it is important to observe and document ECG changes after local anesthetic administration.

Immediately after Performing a Caudal Block on an Anesthetized Child, the ECG Appearance Changes as Follows. What Are the ECG Manifestations of LAST?

A "peaked T wave" or T wave amplitude increase as well as widening of the QRS complex is seen in this ECG (Figure 54.1). This should raise suspicion for LAST, especially in the anesthetized patient. Peaked T waves has been described after a test dose of local anesthetic with epinephrine but local anesthetic alone in toxic doses has also been reported to cause the same ECG changes. A study of bupivacaine infusion in pigs has shown that slower injection of bupivacaine can identify T wave elevation sooner compared to a fast injection of toxic doses. This supports the idea of incremental injection of local anesthetic during administration.

How Do You Prevent LAST?

- Use the lowest effective dose for local anesthetic delivery

- Inject small amounts incrementally and aspirate frequently
- Use epinephrine (0.5 mcg/kg) in local anesthetic injection. T wave elevations or a systolic blood pressure greater than or equal to 15 mmHg in systolic blood pressure is an indicator of possible vascular involvement with potential for toxicity.
- Although ultrasound guidance would seemingly help decrease LAST, its use hasn't appreciably lowered the incidence of this complication
- Patients under four months of age, >70 years of age, and those with cardiac ischemic disease should receive lower doses

How Do You Treat LAST?

Control of the airway is of utmost priority and has been shown to prevent hypoxia and acidosis, and halt seizures and cardiac manifestations.

To treat for seizures, administer a benzodiazepine. It is prudent to avoid propofol, if possible, in patients with LAST, especially if the patient displays cardiac manifestations. Alert the nearest facility to have cardio-pulmonary bypass available. Begin advanced cardiac life support/basic life support (ACLS/BLS) with avoidance of local anesthetics, vasopressin, calcium channel blockers, and beta-blockers. Reduce epinephrine dosage to less than 1 mcg/kg because larger doses of epinephrine can impair resuscitation in patients with LAST. Administer lipid emulsion therapy with 1.5 mg/kg IV over one minute, followed by a lipid emulsion infusion of 0.25 mg/kg/min. Repeat the bolus once or twice for persistent cardiopulmonary failure and double the infusion rate to 0.5 mg/kg/min. After cardiac stability has been achieved, continue the infusion for another 10 minutes. Continue to monitor the patient for a prolonged amount of time for further cardiopulmonary depression and recurrence.

Suggested Reading

Neal JM, Bernards CM, Butterworth JF 4th, et al. ASRA practice advisory on local anesthetic systemic toxicity. *Reg Anesth Pain Med.* 2010;35 (2):152–61. PMID: 20216033.

Weinberg GL. Lipid emulsion infusion: resuscitation for local anesthetic and other drug overdose. *Anesthesiology.* 2012;117:180–7. PMID: 22627464.

Weinberg GL. Treatment of local anesthetic systemic toxicity (LAST). *Reg Anesth Pain Med.* 2010;35:188–93. PMID: 20216036.

Chapter 55

Acute Postoperative Pain Management

Zoel A. Quiñónez and Jamie W. Sinton

As the acute pain attending physician, you are asked to develop a perioperative pain management plan for a 13-year-old, 51 kg boy, who presents for a thoracotomy for re-repair of a coarctation of the aorta that was initially repaired two years ago. At baseline, the patient reports left chest pain along the previous incision and occasional muscle tightness along the left chest. He states that he does not have any prescribed analgesics for the pain, but rates it as a 2/10 burning pain at rest, increasing to 5/10 intermittently, associated with muscle tightness that he cannot assign a numeric score to. There are no identifiable inciting or alleviating factors. When you probe further, he states that he has taken codeine that was left over from a dental procedure, and occasionally takes hydrocodone that he gets from family members. He is otherwise healthy. His blood pressure is 122/67 on his right arm and 74/40 on his right leg.

How Is Pain Classified?

Pain is generally an adaptive response to tissue injury, but can become its own maladaptive disease state. As such, pain may be classified as either adaptive or maladaptive.

Nociceptive and inflammatory pain are two types of adaptive pain responsible for detecting tissue damage and aiding in healing and prevention of continued tissue injury, respectively. Nociception involves the perception of hot, cold, or sharp sensations in response to chemical, thermal, or mechanical injury.

Inflammatory pain is an immune-mediated response to injury from infection or tissue trauma. The infiltration of immune cells and inflammatory mediators encourages healing, but the discomfort associated with this infiltration dissuades the person from exposing the tissue to continued injury.

Neuropathic pain and dysfunctional pain (sometimes referenced with the misnomer "functional pain") are maladaptive pain states that include ongoing pain without an ongoing noxious stimulus. When present, inflammation is usually absent or minimal; although in maladaptive pain, it occurs as a result of altered neural processing, rather than the cause of the pain itself.

What Mechanisms Underlie Each Type of Pain?

Nociception occurs via receptors termed *nociceptors*. They are free nerve endings that are present through most tissues of the body and respond to noxious stimuli. Mechanical stimuli are carried towards the central nervous system via the faster A∂ fibers, and chemical and thermal stimuli are carried via the slower C fibers. Pain perception can then be modulated by descending pathways that affect the perception of pain by the central nervous system.

Inflammatory pain occurs through an interplay of tissue injury and a cascade of inflammatory mediators to produce the associated redness, swelling, and hyperalgesia. Ions, bradykinins, and other mediators are released from damaged cells. These, along with cytokines, prostaglandins, neurotrophic growth factors, and neurogenic factors, such as the neuropeptides substance P and calcitonin gene-related peptide (CGRP), act as either sensitizing agents that increase the sensation of pain, or act to directly stimulate nociceptors and cause pain spontaneously.

Neuropathic pain generally occurs with direct injury to nerves, either peripherally or centrally. Patients will describe neuropathic pain in a variety of ways that range from dysesthesia (hyperalgesia and allodynia) to paresthesia (tingling, numbness). Itching and burning are commonly described by patients.

Dysfunctional pain encompasses a variety of pain syndromes including fibromyalgia, "functional abdominal pain," irritable bowel syndrome, headaches, and other syndromes where there is substantial pain without

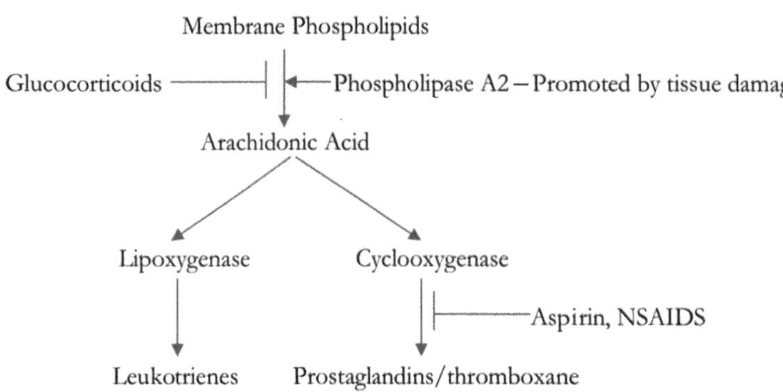

Figure 55.1 The arachidonic acid pathway. Illustration by Adam C. Adler, MD

an ongoing noxious stimulus. The term "Amplified Pain Syndrome" is sometimes used to describe this collection of pathologic pain syndromes defined by a predisposition of the body to a heightened pain experience in the absence of a known noxious stimulus.

What Nonopioid Strategies Are Used to Treat the Different Pain Types?

Generally, an appropriate strategy for perioperative pain control includes a multimodal approach that consists of pharmacologic and nonpharmacologic techniques that target various levels of the pain pathway.

Regional and neuraxial anesthesia are safe and effective for the management of postoperative pain in children that targets either the dorsal root ganglia or peripheral nerves, and should be performed whenever possible, particularly for children with chronic pain. This may include caudal/epidural blocks, paravertebral blocks, plexus blocks (brachial, lumbar), or peripheral nerve blocks. Continuous catheters have been demonstrated to be safe, and to improve pain recovery in children, and should be used when children undergo procedures associated with significant and prolonged pain.

Antinociceptive agents include nonsteroidal antiinflammatory medications (NSAIDs), such as ibuprofen and ketorolac, acetaminophen, and glucocorticoids (e.g., dexamethasone) (Figure 55.1). Nonsteroidal antiinflammatory agents prevent the synthesis of prostaglandins via inhibition of cyclooxygenase in the central nervous system and the periphery in addition to their antiplatelet and antiinflammatory effects. Acetaminophen works similarly to NSAIDs, but without the antiplatelet and antiinflammatory effects. Both of these types of medications may have an additive analgesic effect. Dexamethasone has been shown to improve pain control, reduce opiate requirements, and prolong the effect of regional anesthetic techniques.

Neuropathic agents include gabapentinoids, such as gabapentin and pregabalin, the voltage-gated sodium channel blocker lidocaine, alpha-2 agonists, such as dexmedetomidine and clonidine, as well as the NMDA-antagonist ketamine.

Gabapentin reduces calcium currents by decreasing spontaneous firing at voltage-gated calcium channels in the central nervous system. While its ability to prevent neuropathic pain is debatable, gabapentin is effective in the treatment of various forms of neuropathic pain. For this reason, it is commonly used as an adjunct in surgeries with a higher likelihood of neurologic injury, such as spinal fusion surgeries, and can be given prophylactically in patients with a neuropathy who present for surgery.

Dexmedetomidine and clonidine act at alpha-2 receptors in the substantia gelatinosa of the dorsal horn of the spine, and work to inhibit the perception of somatic pain via inhibitory pathways. Generally administered systemically as part of a multimodal approach to analgesia, clonidine can be administered as part of a regional or neuraxial technique to strengthen or prolong the analgesia provided. Particularly useful in children is the fact that both clonidine and dexmedetomidine can serve as useful premedication when administered orally or intra-nasally.

Ketamine is a noncompetitive NMDA antagonist that has been shown to prevent hyperalgesia and decrease perioperative pain intensity. This seems to happen through its prevention of sensitization to pain via NMDA antagonism in the central nervous system. It also works to decrease release of glutamate, an excitatory neurotransmitter involved in pain sensation, at nerve terminals.

The evidence for its opiate-sparing effect is mixed, partly due to the heterogeneity of available studies; but it does seem to decrease opiate requirements in patients with chronic pain.

Lidocaine works at the level of neurons to block sodium channels and increase the depolarization threshold. This mechanism underlies its ability to decrease the propagation of pain signals, as well as its antiarrhythmic property to increase the threshold for spontaneous electrical activity and signal propagation within the cardiac conduction tissue. Studies have shown efficacy in the treatment of pain in adults and children. One concern specific to pediatrics is the potential for accumulation of monoethylglycineexylidide (MEGX), a lidocaine metabolite with a longer half-life. MEGX poses the greatest risk to neonates and children with renal dysfunction.

Other agents, such as the tricyclic antidepressants (TCA) and selective serotonin norepinephrine reuptake inhibitors (SNRI) (amitriptyline and duloxetine), as well as mixed-mechanism analgesic tramadol (opiate + SNRI) fit into the category of neuropathic agents.

What Are the Dosing Guidelines for Common Opiate-Based Analgesics?

While opiate conversion tables are common, they are limited because they are based on the equivalence of a single dose of medication. Accumulation of drug, as well as drug metabolites, is not accounted for. This would seem particularly relevant when comparing short-acting opioids, like remifentanil and fentanyl, to longer-acting opioids, like morphine and hydromorphone. Additionally, medications such as fentanyl may have a short duration of action when administered as a single dose, yet have a relatively prolonged context-sensitive half-life when compared to other opioids with a single dose short duration of action. Thus, while opiate conversion tables serve as a useful guide for opiate administration, they should be approached cautiously, and with an understanding of their limitations.

How Do You Assess Pain in Children in the Postoperative Period?

Pain scales represent a popular topic with regards to assessment of recovery in children, but provide only a portion of pain assessment (e.g., PQRST assessment). As a whole, pain scales measure pain intensity, which represents a small part of a postoperative recovery assessment that should focus on functional benchmarks, such as nutritional intake, ambulation, bowel movements, activities of daily living, etc. Nonetheless, these scales allow us to track pain recovery and to track response to interventions.

Self-reported pain is preferred and should be sought when developmentally appropriate. This is not possible in many young children, and guidelines focus on the use of an appropriate pain scale. Several barriers exist, though, when it comes to pain intensity assessment in children. First, a multitude of scales exist, but many lack validation. Second, even when validated scales are used, inconsistency exists in the use of a developmentally appropriate scale.

In neuro-developmentally intact children, the Face, Legs, Activity, Cry, and Consolability Pain Assessment Tool (FLACC) or the COMFORT Scale can be used from the newborn period through seven years of life. The Faces Pain Scale (FPS-R) can be used from 4 years old onwards, as can the FLACC and COMFORT scales. And from the age of seven, children should be able to properly use either the Visual Analogue Scale (VAS), Numeric Rating Scale (NRS), or the FPS-R.

What May Be the Consequence to the Suboptimal Treatment of Postoperative Pain?

While no direct link has been established, particularly in children, prolonged pain or higher pain scores postoperatively have been linked to persistent postsurgical pain (PPSP). It is difficult to establish whether a common predisposition leads to both higher postoperative pain and persistent pain, or if the inadequate treatment of pain leads to a protracted pain trajectory, but nonetheless the association exists.

For both thoracotomies and orthopedic surgeries, higher pain scores in the first 24 hours were associated with PPSP. A similar association was found for scoliosis and pectus surgeries.

How Do You Assess Pain in Children with Cognitive Impairment?

Children with cognitive impairment suffer a greater pain burden, and yet their pain is more likely to be underappreciated. As with neurodevelopmentally intact children, the assessment of pain should focus on the patient's comfort and a recovery towards baseline function. Additional barriers exist in the assessment of pain in these patients. For instance, pain behavior may differ in children with cognitive impairment, part of which may be due to physical limitations that are present along with this cognitive impairment. For example, someone using the FLACC scale may underestimate pain in the setting of flaccid paralysis of the lower extremities.

Strategies exist to account for these confounding factors. Several scales with varying degrees of clinical utility have been created for the assessment of pain in nonverbal children and those with varying degrees of cognitive impairment. The Noncommunicating Child's Pain Checklist – Postoperative Version (NCCPC-PV), the Individualized Numeric Rating Scale (INRS), the Pediatric Pain Profile (PPP), and the revised Face, Leg, Activity, Cry, and Consolability scale (r-FLACC) represent commonly reported scales. As parents have the greatest knowledge of their own child's pain behaviors, parental input becomes important in defining pain categories for several of these scales (INRS, PPP, r-FLACC). The r-FLACC is the most studied of these scales, and may have the most clinical utility, in part due to a shorter observation time when compared to some scales, optional parental input, and provider familiarity with the commonly used FLACC scale.

Is There a Role for Patient-Controlled Analgesics Postoperatively?

Patient-controlled analgesics (PCAs), whether with intravenous or nerve catheter-based delivery methods, have an established place in the postoperative care of adult patients. Adolescents prefer to be in control of their analgesic management and PCAs can be effectively administered to them as well. Further, "as needed" pain medication doses are often interpreted by nursing staff as "as little as possible"; therefore, parent/nurse-controlled analgesia (PNCA) is more effective than PRN or "as needed" dosing.

PCAs are safe in young children. PNCA is safe in children under age six years. Patient-controlled PCAs allow the child to direct their pain control and may reduce anxiety surrounding pain by providing more autonomy.

Patients with PCAs, especially nurse/parent-controlled PCAs, should be monitored continuously. Suggested PCA doses can be found in Chapter 1.

How Do You Evaluate a Patient on a Patient-Controlled Analgesia Pump?

For each patient, the individual pain plan should be reviewed in addition to the recent PCA usage.

If the patient has pain but there is little usage of the PCA, it must be understood why (i.e., side effects, dose not working, anxiety associated with usage).

If the pain is not relieved with the use of the PCA bolus, consideration for increasing the dose may be warranted. If the pain returns prior to the next dose being available, the interval between bolus doses may require adjustment.

If the pain is not well controlled with sole use of a PCA, addition of adjuncts to the pain regimen should be considered.

What Are Common Side Effects of Postoperative Pain Therapies?

Opioid analgesic side effects such as nausea, vomiting, constipation, pruritus, and analgesic tolerance are to be expected following major surgery in which opioids are used as the primary analgesic. Additionally, opioid-induced hyperalgesia (OIH) is of particular interest in this patient as his pain has persisted, he has continued to use opioids, and he is undergoing a second painful procedure.

OIH can be separated from tolerance to opioids by a change in pain sensitivity as both can occur in patients who received opioids acutely or chronically. While not available in our patient, cold pressor testing can be used to determine pain sensitivity and therefore diagnose OIH.

For patients who have OIH, detoxification is possible using a single dose of buprenorphine/naloxone sublingually. Supportive care is important as opioid withdrawal may occur.

Are There Special Considerations with Regard to the Treatment of Pain in Patients with Congenital Heart Disease?

Children with congenital heart disease present a unique population for the management of acute postoperative pain. Unlike children with healthy cardiorespiratory status, the physiology of children with congenital heart disease can be impacted by common vital sign changes associated with acute pain.

This patient has uncontrolled postoperative pain from his initial operation. Nociceptive pain from tissue damage associated with the thoracotomy that is planned for him can lead to intensified, continued pain as reoperation is a risk factor for development of chronic postsurgical pain. Acute postoperative pain is associated with hypertension and tachycardia in addition to discomfort but is also life threatening given fresh suture lines. Additionally, inspiratory effort limited by pain increases the risk of developing atelectasis and eventually pulmonary infection especially if secretion clearance is poor.

Single ventricle physiology is another example of cardiorespiratory interdependence and one in which pain treatment can also impact physiology. Postoperative pain can result in increased pulmonary vascular resistance. Further, if splinting occurs, a paucity of negative intrathoracic pressure is generated with each breath and venous return to the lungs is compromised. Consequently, cardiac output can suffer. Treatment of pain with opioids may lead to hypoventilation, hypercarbia, elevated pulmonary vascular resistance, poor preload and, again, poor cardiac output.

What Is the Incidence of Persistent Pain After Surgery in Children?

Chronic postsurgical pain following surgery in childhood is approximately 16% after three months and 3% many years later. Specifically, persistent pain following thoracotomy is defined as pain that recurs or persists along a thoracotomy incision for at least two months.

Suggested Reading

Brislin RP, Rose JB. Pediatric acute pain management. *Anesthesiol Clin North America*. 2005;23(4):789–814.

Brooks MR, Golianu B. Perioperative management in children with chronic pain. *Paediatr Anaesth.* 2016 Aug;26(8):794–806. PMID: 27370517.

Ghai B, Makkar JK, Wig J. Postoperative pain assessment in preverbal children and children with cognitive impairment. *Paediatr Anaesth*. 2008;18(6):462–77. PMID: 18363630.

Greco C, Berde C. Pain management for the hospitalized pediatric patient. *Pediatr Clin North Am.* 2005;52(4):995–1027. PMID: 16009254.

Michelet D, Andreu-Gallien J, Bensalah T, et al. A meta-analysis of the use of nonsteroidal antiinflammatory drugs for pediatric postoperative pain. *Anesth Analg*. 2012;114 (2):393–406. PMID: 22104069.

Williams G, Howard RF, Liossi C. Persistent postsurgical pain in children and young people: prediction, prevention, and management. *Pain Rep*. 2017;2(5): e616. PMID: 29392231.

Chronic Pediatric Pain

Caro Monico

A 16-year-old girl arrives for follow-up after undergoing placement of a Nuss Bar via a minimally invasive approach. Her postoperative pain management course included: A T6 thoracic epidural placed intraoperatively with continuous ropivacaine infusion until postoperative day two (POD). On POD 2, she was transitioned to intravenous opioids and by POD 3, her pain was well-controlled with transition to PO pain medication. She was discharged on POD 5 and discharged with a two-week supply of oxycodone to be used PRN and instructed to take acetaminophen and ibuprofen PRN. On her two-week office visit, she was improving with pain well-controlled with PO medication. At her subsequent two-month appointment, she complained of some intermittent retrosternal pain that was enough to lead to some distress. Her mother is concerned about persistent pain after surgery. She has read that many patients have pain long after surgery and wants to know if her daughter is at risk. What will you tell her?

How Common Is Chronic Pain in Children?

Pediatric chronic pain, particularly when it develops after surgery, only recently entered the public consciousness as one of the factors contributing to the over-prescribing of opioids. The emerging understanding of the impact of pain on a young person's functional ability and quality of life reveals a physical, psychological, and social decline mirroring that of adult patients. The incidence of pediatric chronic pain is alarmingly high, with 20% of patients developing post-surgical chronic pain. As our appreciation of the multiplicity of pain presentations matures, we may reveal this to be an underestimation.

What Issue Should Be Considered Given the Preoperative Chronic Opioid Use?

Patients with chronic opioid dependence pose a unique perioperative challenge. Patients on chronic opioid therapy are at risk of suboptimal pain control due to increased opioid requirements, opioid tolerance, and iatrogenic under-dosing.

What Are the Implications of Poorly Controlled Postoperative Pain?

Patients with poorly controlled postoperative pain can have longer recovery times, increased risk of infection, unplanned readmissions, and development of chronic postsurgical pain. Additionally, poor pain control can leave a significant psychological footprint in the patient and family that can color future healthcare transactions. Whenever possible, effective treatment of these patients should include a combination of non-pharmacologic pain strategies (acupuncture, distraction, virtual reality, diaphragmatic breathing), neuraxial/regional anesthesia, multimodal analgesia, and maintenance and optimization of chronic opioid medication delivery during their hospital admission.

Would Your Discussion Be Different if You Learned that the Child Has Chronic Pain from Headaches or Abdominal Pain?

The underlying pathophysiology of pain can range from nociceptive pain or neuropathic pain to "functional pain" which is thought to be a result of an abnormal processing by both central and peripheral components of the nervous system. The International Association for the Study of Pain (IASP) defines pain as "an unpleasant sensory and emotional experience associated with actual or potential tissue damage, or described in terms of such damage," and can result from a combination of any of the aforementioned sources of pain. A primary pain disorder (often called "functional pain") is a term that is given to patient-reported pain which may or may not have an identifiable clear organic disease or to pain that is thought to have become its own separate disease or syndrome even when accompanied by a primary pathophysiology. Functional abdominal pain and chronic daily headaches are among the most commonly recognized of these pain disorders, and the perioperative clinician should pay special attention to these issues. Secondary pain disorders include pain states that clearly arise from and accompany an organic process. Examples of secondary pain disorders include polyneuropathy from type 2 diabetes mellitus and chemotherapy-induced neuropathy in blood cancers. The treatment of pediatric chronic pain disorders regardless of classification is anchored in the biopsychosocial model and necessitates an interdisciplinary or multidisciplinary care model that includes a medical, psychological, and functional evaluation. Parental education, cognitive behavioral therapy (CBT), behavior modification, improved coping, and avoidance of triggers have been shown to produce positive treatment responses in multiple pain conditions.

If the clinical environment allows for a preoperative visit and patients with known or suspected chronic pain can be identified, the clinician should obtain a pain consultation, and one preferably in conjunction with the chronic pain team. Given that chronic pain is a disease of the central nervous system which acts to alter and amplify pain messaging, especially in the context of stressful incidents, effective management of pain should also include cataloguing and addressing any mood disturbances, sleep disorders, functional state, family pain history, and stressors. Both pharmacologic and non-pharmacologic recommendations, including the importance of committing to physical therapy and biobehavioral treatment before and after surgery, should be candidly discussed with chronic pain patients and their families.

What Is Your Approach to a Chronic Pain History and Physical in the Perioperative Period?

Prompt recognition of chronic pain is the most important step in the management of chronic pain during the perioperative period. The clinician should begin this process by obtaining a focused history and physical examination that includes a detailed neurologic exam. Pain-related disturbances in sleep onset and maintenance, school functioning (school attendance, grades), physical activity (sports, physical education), mood disturbances (anxiety, depression), and social functioning should also be assessed. Additional high-yield questions are provided below:

1. Determine timing and goals of surgery
    - Is this a new or a repeat procedure?
    - Is the timing of the surgical procedure fixed or flexible?
    - Is the goal of surgery to decrease pain (important for preexisting pain)?
    - Is the goal of surgery to increase function?
    - What type of surgery is to occur?
        - Different types of surgeries result in varying levels of pain/chronic pain. Different anatomical approaches may impact the perioperative pain plan.
2. Inquire about pain. If pain is present, assess its location, radiation pattern, duration, character, intensity, exacerbation factors, and alleviating factors. If pain started as a result of an injury, it is important to learn about the mechanism of injury and any ongoing rehabilitation ("pre-hab") efforts.
3. Inquire about previous surgeries and in particular ask about any ongoing pain issues, previous regional anesthetics, and existing nerve damage.
4. Ask about previous and current pain therapies. This includes complementary and alternative medicine therapies (CAM) (e.g., acupuncture, massage), psychological support, pharmacologic therapies.
5. A complete past medical history should be collected to identify any comorbidities that may potentially contribute to pain. Some relevant

comorbidities include mood disorders, neurodevelopmental disorders, addiction, hepatic disease, renal disease, pulmonary disease, and gastrointestinal diagnoses.
6. A family history of chronic pain, mood disorders, psychiatric disorders, and addiction should be gathered.
7. Elicit family and patient goals of care for hospitalization. Set expectations for the surgical procedure and post-operative period.

What Is Chronic Postsurgical Pain?

Chronic postsurgical pain (CPSP) is an issue that has been gaining increasing recognition due to its impact on long-term disability. Patients undergoing surgery can have ongoing pain that does not improve within the usual time it takes to recover from surgery. The definition for CPSP as established by the International Association for the Study of Pain (IASP) is as follows:

- Pain must develop after surgical procedure
- Must be at least two months in duration
- Other causes must be excluded
- The possibility of pain from a preexisting condition is excluded

CPSP is a well-documented issue in adults with up to 40% of patients complaining about pain several months after surgery. Significantly, 5% of all patients undergoing surgery report severe debilitating pain after surgery. According to the IASP, one in every ten adult surgical patients experiences CPSP, and in one of every one hundred operations, this pain is intolerable. CPSP has known substantial economic effects (functional, days off, medical burden) in adult patients, but it has not been well studied in the pediatric population. Formerly, it was thought to be a much less prevalent issue in children; however, several studies have shown that the incidence of CPSP in the pediatric population may mirror that in the adult population, and a recent meta-analysis of 12 studies and 628 participants showed an incidence of 20% across all studies.

What Are the Risk Factors for CPSP in the Pediatric Population?

While studies looking at the risk factors associated with CPSP have been conducted in the adult population, little is known about which risk factors are significant within the pediatric population. The contributions of risk factors like gender, thoracotomy surgical subtype, breast surgery, and depression, which have been clearly delineated in the adult population, continue to be unknown in children. Recently, several studies have suggested that the presence of childhood anxiety, baseline level of pain before surgery, catastrophizing, and parental anxiety are significant risk factors for CPSP, over surgical type or pain cause. In adults, the type of surgery or the severity of a patient's disease process are thought to contribute to the severity and duration of pain after surgery. However, in the pediatric population, only the presence of preoperative pain has consistently been shown to be a risk factor for the development of CPSP.

While considering pediatric risk factors for CPSP, it is important to look at what risk factors have been identified in the adult population. Risk factors in the pre-, intra-, and postoperative phase have been more clearly identified in adults. Consistent with pediatric risk factors, the existence and severity of preoperative pain is a significant risk factor for the development of CPSP. In addition, the type of surgery tends to be important, with thoracotomy, amputation, hernia repair, and mastectomy resulting in the highest incidences of CPSP. Intraoperative factors such as longer and repeat surgeries tend to have higher rates of CPSP, and postoperative factors such as high levels of pain and adjuvant therapies such as chemoradiation lead to increased risk for CPSP. While psychosocial factors are thought to play a role in the development of CPSP, very few studies have been conducted looking at this effect in adults.

> The patient is a quiet and shy-appearing girl who frequently tracks the expressions of her mother and father. Her mother talks most during the conversation and appears very concerned about the procedure. When the anesthetic risks are discussed with the patient, the patient's mother bursts into tears and the patient also begins to cry.

What Is Pain Catastrophizing?

Pain catastrophizing is described as a maladaptive cognitive response to an actual or anticipated pain stimulus. The response itself is usually psychological or emotional in nature, and is often exaggerated in comparison to the usual response to the said pain stimulus. Pain catastrophizing is a significant issue due to the way it affects pain-related outcomes, and has been associated with increased pain sensitivity, pain severity, disability, and depression in both pain-free patients and patients with chronic pain. Significantly, pain catastrophizing has been shown to cause significant variance in patients during the postoperative period, often affecting pain severity, opioid usage, and willingness to undergo rehabilitation.

What Is Parental Catastrophizing?

While pain catastrophizing is an important issue in patient-related pain outcomes, parental catastrophizing may be a more significant contributor to pain outcomes in the pediatric population. Parental catastrophizing is, put simply, catastrophizing that is enacted by the parent in response to present or anticipated pain that the patient may experience. Catastrophizing is a maladaptive response, and can lead to potential worsening of the patient's pain. Firstly, children's thoughts and beliefs about pain are initially dictated by their interactions with parents. Different parents have differing perspectives about pain, how to react to pain, how to express pain, and how to alleviate pain, and such responses do not go unnoticed by children. High levels of parental anxiety in turn lead to high levels of child anxiety in the perioperative period. Pagé et al. showed that high levels of both parental and child anxiety lead to higher pain intensity, pain unpleasantness, and functional disability in the acute postsurgical phase. In addition, initial levels of parental catastrophizing correlated with the development of CPSP in children. Parental behavior is likely to reinforce the child's behavior and disposition towards pain.

What Is the Pediatric Fear-Avoidance Model?

The pediatric fear-avoidance model (p-FA model) for pain has become an increasingly salient explanatory model for how acute pain may transition to chronic pain. The FA model allows us to conceptualize how a patient could develop chronic pain as a result of pain-related fear. Take for example the patient who is experiencing acute back pain and diminishes that pain with a certain avoidant behavior (sitting, lying in bed); this avoidant behavior becomes positively enforced by a reduction in pain and anxiety. While this behavior may have initially been protective, as a way to prevent further damage to an injury or surgical site, after time the avoidant behavior becomes a maladaptive response that could potentially result in improper healing to the site of injury and decreased function even after the resolution of the acute pain.

Why Is the Psychosocial Model of Pain so Important?

The development of CPSP in the pediatric population has to be understood within the context of the biopsychosocial model. Historically, surgical pain was thought to be coupled with an identifiable and organic pathophysiology, where tissue injury or organic disease are prerequisite to the pain experience. However, we know that chronic pain is decoupled from tissue injury and can exist in the absence of nociceptive stimuli. It is easy to overlook this fundamental point when faced with a patient whose acute postoperative pain course appears to deviate from normal or when a patient's chronic pain state and attendant disability cannot be explained by a negative extensive medical workup. The most current definition of pain states that the pain experience is "an unpleasant sensory *and* emotional experience," and one that should never be purely segregated as medical vs. psychological or organic vs. non-organic or "supratentorial". Anxiety, depression, and catastrophizing are significant risk factors for CPSP in adults, though no definitive data on the incidence of CPSP in patients with anxiety or catastrophizing have been clearly delineated. Theunissen et al. showed that in a meta-analysis of 29 studies, there was a statistically significant association between anxiety or pain catastrophizing and CPSP in 67% of studies involving musculoskeletal surgery and 36% in all other types of surgery.

What Role Does Regional Anesthesia Play in CPSP?

Regional and neuraxial techniques have been implicated in improving pain in the immediate postoperative period and for some surgeries, can improve long-term surgical recovery. Both techniques involve the use of either local anesthetics or other adjunct analgesics perineurally to blunt the transmission, perception, and effects of pain (tachycardia, hypertension, nausea, infection, stress response, healing, etc.). Not only do patients report more comfort after both neuraxial and regional techniques, but several key benefits of these analgesic modalities have been well documented including antiinflammatory effects, faster recovery of bowel function, decreased systemic opioid use, and improved participation in physical therapy. The benefits of neuraxial analgesia are especially apparent in procedures that cause significant postoperative pain.

What Types of Chronic Medication Should the Patient Continue?

Pediatric patients may be on chronic opioid therapy (COT), antidepressants, or anticonvulsant medications. In terms of nonopioid adjunct medication such as NSAIDS or anticonvulsant medications like gabapentin, there are no formal pediatric guidelines on their use during the perioperative phase. However, because many of these drugs have been used in adult "multimodal analgesia" protocols, it is generally recommended that such medications are continued into the perioperative phase. Discontinuation or selective continuation of NSAIDS should be a mutual discussion with surgical colleagues given their impact on platelet function and potential threat to renal function.

Continuation of all chronic opioids is advised and higher perioperative opioid requirement in the perioperative phase should be anticipated. In a study conducted in 1995, Rapp et al. found that patients who were on chronic opioid therapy (with an average daily morphine equivalent of 13 mg IV morphine) required a three-fold greater dosage of opioids in the postoperative phase with worse pain scores than their nonchronic opioid counterparts.

There are several important considerations to optimize patients on chronic opioid therapy for the perioperative period. Management of opioids can be challenging because the patient's outpatient baseline chronic opioid requirement must be met on the inpatient setting on top of titrating opioids for acute and incident pain without increasing the baseline chronic, non-operative regimen. No data is currently available looking at the predicted postoperative opioid requirement based on preoperative daily opioid requirements, so the clinician must be vigilant about dosing during the perioperative period.

Which Adjuncts Should Be Considered Intraoperatively?

Intraoperative adjuncts such as ketamine, NSAIDs, α2-agonists, methadone, acetaminophen, ketorolac, and anticonvulsive agents have been used successfully to reduce opioid requirement both in the intraoperative and postoperative setting. The use of multimodal analgesia can allow the anesthesiologist to treat pain at receptors other than just opioid receptors, allowing for broader coverage of pain. In addition, regional anesthesia, neuraxial anesthesia, and even wound infiltration and lavage have been used to great effect in not only preventing the sensation of pain, but also the autonomic and inflammatory consequences of tissue damage, thereby preventing additional pain in the postoperative setting.

How to Prevent CPSP?

There is limited data on which modalities of anesthesia or chronic medication management prevent the development of CPSP. Overall, early and aggressive analgesic treatment after surgery has the potential to reduce the incidence of CPSP, but no specific pharmacologic agent or regional/neuraxial technique has yet been identified as a preventative therapy for the development of CPSP. Ketamine has shown some benefit in potentially preventing the development of CPSP, but no study has proven this effect. Gabapentin and pregabalin have been shown to be able to reduce the incidence of CPSP. A large systematic review showed that perioperative gabapentin decreased the incidence of chronic pain more than 2 months after surgery, and pregabalin similarly had a large decrease in the development of CPSP as well as a greater improvement in postsurgical patient function. Greater, more high-powered research will be required to properly determine how to best prevent the development of CPSP.

Suggested Reading

Clarke H, Bonin RP, Orser BA, et al. The prevention of chronic postsurgical pain using gabapentin and pregabalin: a combined systematic review and meta-analysis. *Anesth Analg.* 2012;115 (2):428–42. PMID: 22415535.

Liossi C, Howard RF. Pediatric chronic pain: Biopsychosocial assessment and formulation. *Pediatrics.* 2016;138(5). pii: e20160331. PMID: 27940762.

Pagé MG, Campbell F, Isaac L, et al. Parental risk factors for the development of pediatric acute and chronic postsurgical pain: a longitudinal study. *J Pain Res.* 2013;6:727–41. PMID: 24109194.

Rapp SE, Ready LB, Nessly ML. Acute pain management in patients with prior opioid consumption: a case-controlled retrospective review. *Pain.* 1995;61(2):195–201. PMID: 7659429.

Theunissen M, Peters ML, Bruce J, et al. Preoperative anxiety and catastrophizing: a systematic review and meta-analysis of the association with chronic postsurgical pain. *Clin J Pain.* 2012;28(9):819–41. PMID: 22760489.

Distraction Techniques for Pediatric Pain Management

Grace S. Kao and Emily R. Schwartz

A six-year-old female requires IV insertion. She appears tearful and anxious, clutching to and hiding behind her parents. Her parents, growing anxious, request guidance about strategies for nonpharmacologic pain management.

What Long-Term Issues Are Associated with Uncontrolled Pain?

Pain has come to be recognized as a substantial health problem, with pain treatment and relief noted as a human right by the World Health Organization and International Association for the Study of Pain. For children and adolescents, pain management is especially important, as untreated pain in infancy and childhood has been linked to lower pain thresholds as adolescents and adults. Therefore, it is imperative for healthcare providers to identify effective techniques and strategies to help alleviate pediatric pain. Non-pharmacological methods for pain management, including distraction techniques, have evidenced efficacy in contributing to pain relief, especially for acute medical procedures.

What Is Distraction?

Distraction is an effective pain management strategy and is defined (in the context of pain management) as a non-pharmacological cognitive or behavioral strategy that diverts attention from pain stimuli.

How Does Distraction Work to Reduce Pain?

Pain is modulated by various cognitive constructs, and distraction techniques make use of the brain's natural ability to differentiate attention in order to impact pain perception. Given the brain's restricted ability to process stimuli, engaging patients in distraction techniques limits their ability to experience painful stimuli. Distraction has been empirically shown to reduce pain perception, while increased attention to pain has been found to be associated with increased pain perception. Anesthesia providers are encouraged to implement the use of non-pharmacologic distraction activities as an effective and safe method, particularly for cases in which sedatives can pose substantial risks to the patient.

When and Where Can Distraction Techniques Be Used for Pain Management?

Distraction techniques have been deemed effective in multiple settings, including laboratory settings, during acute medical procedures, with burn patients, and in the context of chronic pain. Techniques provide pediatric patients and their parents tools for self-managing pain. Further, they help to alleviate not only self-reported pain, but also distress and anxiety, which are often potent contributors to pain exacerbation.

Distraction activities can aid the anesthesiologist when patient cooperation proves challenging and can be used to alleviate procedural distress in pediatric patients, which has been linked to lasting behavioral and emotional maladaptation in children. A systematic review and meta-analysis recently demonstrated that children's self-reported pain and behavioral indicators of distress significantly decreased with the use of distraction techniques during painful procedures.

What Is the Role of a Child Life Specialist When Considering Distraction?

Child life specialists are trained to use age-appropriate and specifically tailored preparation methods based on the child's chronological and developmental age, anxiety levels, and prior hospital experiences. Their involvement can benefit pediatric patients who typically respond well to instructional coaching through painful experiences.

Pain-related anxiety prior to surgery often predicts poor recovery outcomes and/or development of chronic post-surgical pain. Preoperative distraction techniques to allay anxiety range from humor to breathing to use of video games. Humorous environmental distractions and video glasses have been found to have a similar anxiolytic effect as oral midazolam, underscoring the benefit and cost-effectiveness of distraction technique teaching in the preoperative setting.

In chronic pain management, psychologists work with patients and parents to learn how to apply pain distraction techniques in daily life for purposes of restoring function.

How Do Distraction Techniques Work?

Multiple theories contribute to the understanding of how distraction techniques may affect undesired sensations and perceptions (such as pain). The gate control theory of pain, developed by Melzack and Wall in 1956, postulates that pain travels through various physiological "gates" that modulate pain signal intensity. Pain signals may be modulated as an ascending signal through the spinal cord or as a descending signal via interpretation by the brain. It is thought that when distraction is used for pain management, pain-inhibitory processes are triggered that affect nociceptive transmissions, helping to "close the gate" on pain signaling.

From a cognitive processing standpoint, distraction is thought to be effective because it steers cognitive resources away from painful stimuli. The role of attention in pain perception is key, and several models have been proposed to explain how distraction affects the pain experience. First, the capacity model of attention, proposed by McCaul and Malott (1985), suggests that one must actively attend to a painful stimulus in order for it to incur distress, as attention capacity is limited. Thus, if a distraction activity is able to use enough attention processing resources to lessen focus on the pain stimulus, distress will in turn be lessened. Cognitive-affective and neurocognitive models of attention and pain postulate that pain is "evolutionarily disposed to interrupt attention" and thus, distraction activities must be intentional, goal-directed tasks that engage "top-down" attentional control in order to be effective. A top-down approach entails a goal-directed process that engages working memory, as opposed to a bottom up approach, which is an unintentional capture of attention by stimuli.

What Are Common Distraction Techniques for Children and Adolescents?

A multitude of techniques and technologies may be used for distraction from pain including:

- Controlled breathing
- Imagery
- Counting backwards
- Coping statements
- Solving problems
- Distraction stimuli
  - Movies and/or television
  - Interactive toys
  - Virtual reality technology
  - Music
- Bubble-blowing
- Short stories

How Are the Different Distraction Techniques Distinguished?

Distraction techniques may be distinguished by level of interaction required and are often categorized as interactive/active versus passive distraction. Generally, active distraction involves a patient's participation and involvement in an activity, whereas passive distraction consists of the patient's observance of a stimulus. Both forms of distraction have been found to be effective for pain management, though several studies have concluded that engagement in active distraction resulted in higher pain thresholds and greater pain tolerance, as compared to passive, especially for younger children.

Active distraction techniques increase tolerability and decrease pain scores and distress for pediatric and adult populations. Audiovisual distractions (tablet devices/movies) are particularly successful in reducing procedural distress in children. In accordance with the cognitive-affective and neurocognitive models of attention and pain models mentioned above, activities that engage central cognitive processing (e.g., virtual reality video games) improve pain tolerance over and above passive distraction.

Distraction types may also be categorized as cognitive versus behavioral. Cognitive strategies include mind-based strategies to refocus attention such as listening to music, counting, and conversation. Behavioral strategies utilize activities-based techniques, such as focused breathing, interactive toys and games, and virtual reality technology.

How Will You Select the Most Appropriate Distraction Technique?

Selection of distraction techniques should include consideration of developmental level and individual patient preferences and temperament. For example, an interactive video game distraction is more effective if the game has capability to shift toward the ability level of the child. Young children typically respond well to distraction activities that are task-oriented, whereas older children respond better to techniques like controlled breathing and reimagination. A patient's ability to self-select their strategy of choice may also, in and of itself, provide a sense of empowerment and control in the pain management process. Distraction methods should be chosen based on the patient's developmental stage, cognitive capacity, and personal preferences in addition to practicality based on the setting of the procedure.

The use of passive or active music therapy as a distraction technique is one of many nonpharmacological interventions which is highly successful in relieving procedural pain in patients of all ages. In both pediatric and adult populations, the activity of listening to music has been shown to decrease pain and anxiety. In that process, patients gain the ability to cope better with their circumstance and gain a sense of autonomy because the distraction aids them in altering the underlying meaning that they associate with the pain and distress that they are experiencing. Music interventions help children gain a sense of control by providing them comfort and familiarity in an otherwise unfamiliar environment.

What Is the Recommended Implementation of Distraction Techniques for Pain Management for Children and Adolescents?

Before the procedure begins, the distraction method deemed most appropriate for the patient should be thoroughly discussed with the child, preferably while the parents are present. The medical team should provide age-appropriate information regarding the nature of the procedure, what the child can expect to experience, as well as details regarding type of distraction strategy that will be used for the patient's comfort. Within the medical team itself, extensive communication and preparation is vital for a successful outcome. When applicable, the use of topical local anesthetic should be used for the patient's maximal comfort. The medical team should provide constant reassurance and praise of the patient throughout the procedure, preferably led by child life or behavioral health professionals. Should the non-pharmacologic distraction approach not suffice, backup plans should be discussed and prepared by the medical team.

What Barriers Should Be Considered in Implementation of Distraction Techniques for Pain Management?

Other cognitive factors may impact the analgesic effects of distraction. For example, catastrophizing – a set of negative emotional/cognitive processes such as magnification, rumination, and pessimism about pain sensations and feelings of helplessness when in pain – has been found to predict delay in distraction-induced pain relief. In adults, attentional bias towards pain -related information has also been found to dampen analgesic effects of distraction. Similarly, chronic pain history, which has been significantly linked to attentional bias toward painful stimuli and higher pain sensitivity and catastrophizing, may also serve as a barrier for optimal use of distraction techniques. Finally, researchers suggest the affective experience of pain also affects effectiveness of distraction and that activities which generate positive affect may impede pain more effectively than those which produce neutral affect.

Suggested Reading

Adler AC, Schwartz E, Waters JM, Stricker PA. Anesthetizing a child for a large compressive mediastinal mass with distraction techniques and music therapies as the sole agents. *J Clin Anesth.* 2016;35:392–7.

Kennedy RM, Luhmann J, Zempsky WT. Clinical implications of unmanaged needle-insertion pain and distress in children. *Pediatrics.* 2008;122:S130–S133.

Kerimoglu B, Neuman A, Paul J, Stefanov DG, Twersky R. Anesthesia induction using video glasses as a distraction tool for the management of preoperative anxiety in children: anesth. *Analg.* 2013;117:1373–9.

Koller D, Goldman RD. Distraction techniques for children undergoing procedures: a critical review of pediatric research. *J Pediatr Nurs.* 2012;27:652.

Litman RS. Allaying anxiety in children: when a funny thing happens on the way to the operating room. *Anesthesiology.* 2011;115:4–5.

McCaul KD, Malott JM. Distraction and coping with pain. *Pain.* 1985;23 (3):315.

Ruda MA, Ling QD, Hohmann AG, Peng YB, Tachibana T. Altered nociceptive neuronal circuits after neonatal peripheral inflammation. *Science.* 2000;289:628–31.

Schreiber, KL, et al. Distraction analgesia in chronic pain patients: the impact of catastrophizing. *Anesthesiology.* 2014;121:1292–301.

Chapter 58

Transitional Circulation

Eric L. Vu and Zoel A. Quiñónez

A 38-week-old, 3.67 kg boy born to a G15P4 mother had the prenatal diagnosis of a large vein of Galen malformation. The child was found to have high output cardiac failure on a fetal echocardiogram (hydrops faetalis), which required maternal digoxin therapy during pregnancy. Due to significant hydrocephalus, the child was delivered via cesarean section, with Apgar scores of 2 and 7.

The neonatologist intubated the child at birth due to poor respiratory effort, and placed arterial and venous umbilical catheters. The child now requires assisted ventilation with an FiO_2 of 0.50. The chest X-ray reveals cardiomegaly and poorly aerated lungs. The transthoracic echocardiogram reveals a large patent ductus arteriosus and a patent foramen ovale, both with right to left shunting, as well as moderate tricuspid regurgitation with estimated suprasystemic right ventricular systolic pressures, moderately depressed right ventricular function, and normal left ventricular systolic function.

Vital signs include: UAC: 69/30, HR 120, SpO_2 92% (FiO_2: 0.50)

Describe the Pathway of Normal Fetal Circulation

Oxygenated blood leaves the placenta from one umbilical vein. Most of the oxygenated blood bypasses the hepatic circulation via the ductus venosus and enters the inferior vena cava (IVC). At this juncture, oxygenated blood from the ductus venosus mixes with deoxygenated blood from the lower extremities. Blood from the IVC enters the right atrium, a majority of which is directed by the Eustachian valve across the foramen ovale, through the left atrium and into the left ventricle. Here, the left ventricle pumps blood across the aortic valve to supply the coronary vessels and aortic arch, supplying blood to the upper and lower body.

The superior vena cava (SVC) directs deoxygenated blood from the upper body to the right atrium. As opposed to IVC blood, the majority of SVC blood crosses the tricuspid valve and enters the right ventricle. From the right ventricle, the blood enters the pulmonary arteries, and, due to high pulmonary vascular resistance (PVR), the blood crosses the ductus arteriosus to the distal aortic arch. At this point, this blood mixes with blood from the left ventricle as it travels down the descending thoracic aorta towards the internal iliac arteries and back to the placenta. An umbilical artery originates from each of the internal iliac arteries to deliver fetal blood to, and oxygenate, the placenta (Figure 58.1).

What Are the Important Physiological Differences between Fetal and Adult Circulations?

Fetal circulation is characterized by a high PVR state due to fluid filled lungs and a hypoxic environment. In addition, systemic vascular resistance (SVR) is low due to the large surface area and low resistance of the utero-placental interface. There is shunting across the:

- Liver via the ductus venosus (oxygenated blood)
- Right heart across the foramen ovale (oxygenated blood)
- Lungs and upper body across the ductus arteriosus (deoxygenated blood)

The physiologic shunts allow for the more oxygenated blood from the umbilical vein to preferentially perfuse the brain and heart and the less oxygenated blood from the SVC to perfuse the lower body. Taken as a whole, the placenta, rather than the lungs, provides oxygenated blood for systemic oxygen delivery, and as such pulmonary blood flow is diminutive (8–10 fold) compared to that of postnatal life. Shunts carry fully oxygenated blood (ductus venosus) to the heart and blood with mixed oxygenation (foramen ovale and

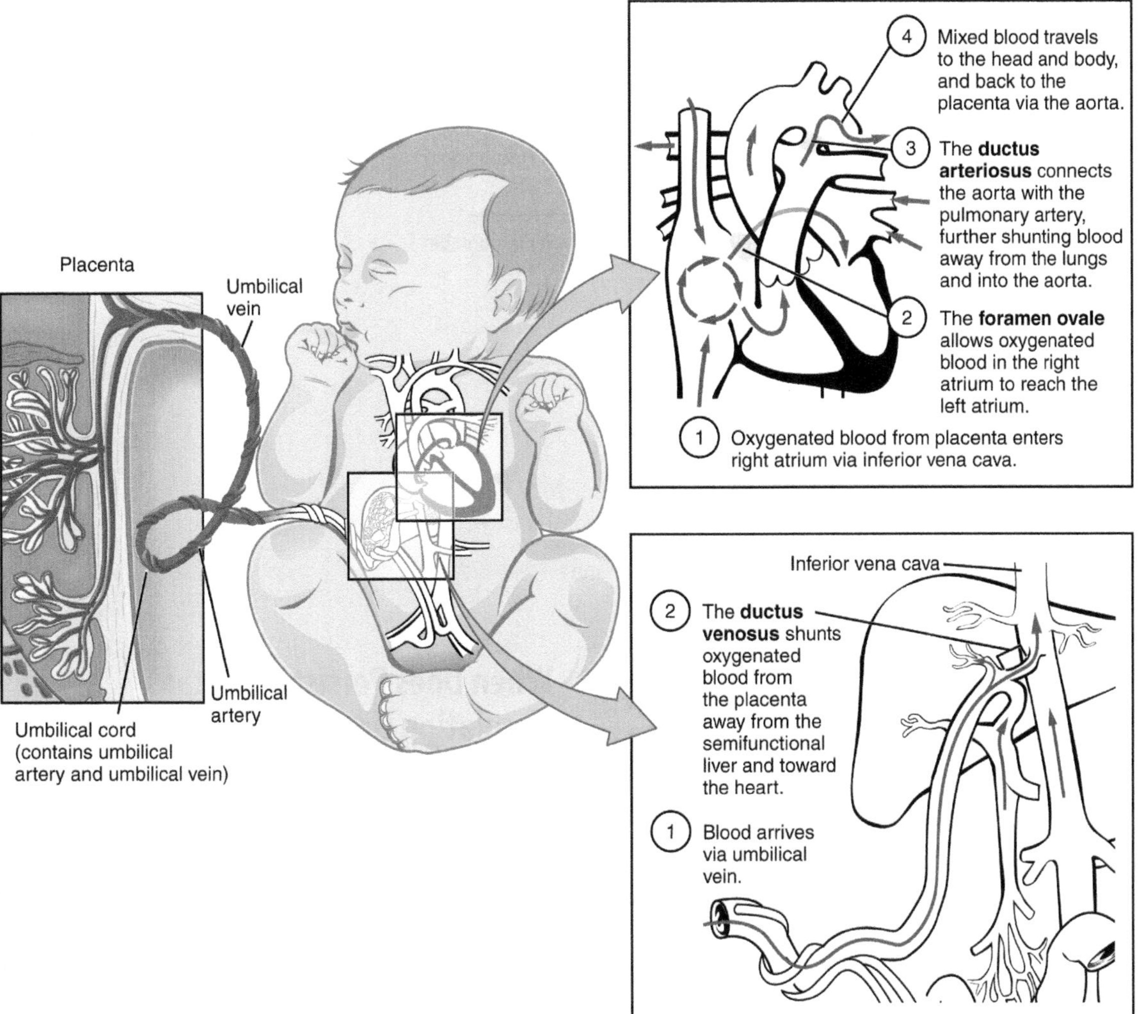

Figure 58.1 Schematic representation of fetal circulation. Image by OpenStax College, reproduced here under CC BY https://upload.wikimedia.org/wikipedia/commons/b/be/2916_Fetal_Circulatory_System-02.jpg

ductus arteriosus) to the body and ultimately back to the placenta via the iliac vessels for oxygenation.

How Is the Fetal Oxygen Carrying Capacity Regulated?

For oxygen transport to occur in the fetal hypoxic environment (normal umbilical vein PaO_2 is 30–35 mmHg), the majority (80%) of hemoglobin (Hgb) is Hgb F, whereas Hgb A accounts for 90% of adult hemoglobin. The different protein structure of fetal hemoglobin confers its greater affinity for oxygen, represented as the PaO_2 at which the hemoglobin molecules are 50% saturated, or the P50 value. Hgb F has a P50 of approximately 19 mmHg whereas Hgb A has a P50 of approximately 26 mmHg (Figure 58.2). This improves fetal oxygen uptake at the placenta. In addition, normal fetal pH (7.25–7.35) is lower compared to adults (7.35–7.45). This acidosis also shifts the oxygen-hemoglobin dissociation curve to the right, facilitating the unloading of oxygen at the fetal tissue level (Figure 58.2).

What Is Transitional Circulation?

Transitional circulation refers to the period of time when the fetal circulation transitions to adult circulation. This period begins immediately after delivery; the

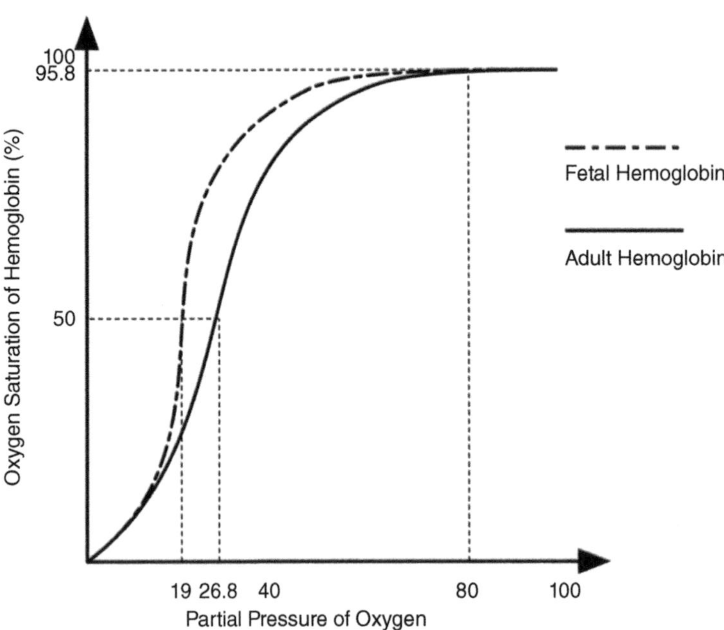

Figure 58.2 Oxyhemoglobin dissociation curve for fetal and adult hemoglobin. Courtesy of Adam C. Adler, MD

umbilical cord is clamped, and the lungs inflate with initial breaths. Umbilical cord clamping increases SVR, and increased PaO_2 reduces PVR. The reduction of PVR increases blood flow to the lungs and left atrium. The increased left atrial pressures functionally close the foramen ovale, eliminating the shunting across the atrial septum. Over the next six to twelve months, the foramen ovale is closed and becomes the fossa ovalis. In approximately 25–35% of adults, closure does not occur, and a probe-patent foramen ovale exists.

While in utero, the ductus arteriosus remains open due to hypoxia, acidosis, and placental prostaglandins. Postnatally, the ductus arteriosus begins to close over the first one to four days of life in the majority of neonates. Functional closure initially occurs as the left atrial and aortic root pressures become greater than the right atrial and pulmonary arterial pressures, and the concomitant increase of PaO_2 and loss of prostaglandin E_2 leads to muscular wall contraction. Over the next one to three months, anatomic closure occurs as proliferation of fibrous tissue occludes the ductus arteriosus lumen. The ductal remnant becomes the ligamentum arteriosum. Indomethacin, a nonsteroidal anti-inflammatory agent, can be used to facilitate closure of a patent ductus arteriosus though inhibition of prostaglandin synthesis. Alternatively, when medical management is unsuccessful, surgical ligation may be required for a patent ductus arteriosus.

When Does Persistent Fetal Circulation Occur?

Persistent fetal circulation (failure in the conversion of fetal to adult circulation) can occur in any condition with severe physiological derangement where there is hypoxia and acidosis. In the vein of Galen malformation (VOGM), one or more branches of arteries of the carotid or vertebral system bypass the cerebral capillary system to feed directly into the Median Prosencephalic Vein of Markowski, an embryologic remnant, creating a left-to-right shunt. In neonates with VOGM, cerebral blood flow may account for up to 80% of cardiac output. Consequently, this lesion can result in high output congestive heart failure, hydrocephalus, and seizures. This high output congestive heart failure due to VOGM may quickly progress to cardiogenic shock during the neonatal period. A persistent transitional circulation, represented here by the presence of a patent ductus arteriosus, patent foramen ovale, and severe pulmonary hypertension, may further complicate the disease process. The increased systolic and diastolic wall stress worsens the cardiogenic shock, which maintains the transitional circulation.

Any condition with pulmonary hypertension (persistent pulmonary hypertension of the newborn) may cause a persistent fetal circulation. The increase in right ventricular afterload leads to right-to-left shunting through a patent foramen ovale and/or patent ductus arteriosus, as well as right ventricular dysfunction. Underdevelopment, maldevelopment or maladaptation of the pulmonary vasculature due, for instance, to pulmonary hypoplasia, meconium aspiration, severe respiratory distress syndrome, pneumonia, or episodes of hypoxia can also lead to persistent pulmonary hypertension of the newborn (PPHN).

In congenital heart disease, there are lesions incompatible with postnatal circulation. These could include ductal dependent lesions (such as pulmonary atresia or hypoplastic left heart syndrome) or parallel systemic and pulmonary circulations (such as transposition of the great arteries). In these cases, prostaglandin E_1 is often used to maintain a patent ductus arteriosus until an intervention can occur. Infants receiving prostaglandin E_1 are at risk for apnea, fevers, and generalized edema.

What Are the Anesthetic Considerations in Caring for a Child with a Persistent Transitional Circulation?

A thorough understanding of the disease pathophysiology guides management. For the VOGM, endovascular treatment is often attempted to reduce or eliminate the degree of arteriovenous shunting. Oftentimes, this requires multiple interventional radiology sessions.

Assessment of end-organ function is paramount to the preoperative assessment, not only to tailor anesthetic care, but also to determine whether a patient is a candidate for intervention. Given a wide spectrum of disease, providers must determine the likely long-term outcomes for each patient. A trans-fontanelle ultrasound, brain MRI, head CT, EEG, postnatal TTE, renal and hepatic studies, and a thorough clinical exam can augment decision-making with regard to intervention and anesthetic management. The prenatal ultrasound can help determine the degree of intracranial shunt, as well as the degree of cardiac dysfunction. While conventional angiography is the gold standard for imaging of VOGM, this exam is usually only undertaken if an intervention is planned.

Preoperatively, neonates may require respiratory support with high-flow nasal cannula or endotracheal intubation. Heart failure is managed with diuretics (e.g., furosemide) and inotropic support (e.g., epinephrine, dopamine, milrinone). The patient is closely monitored for multi-organ failure while awaiting endovascular treatment. With very severe heart failure and pulmonary hypertension, inhaled nitric oxide (iNO) may be necessary to reduce pulmonary vascular resistance to maintain oxygenation.

Intraoperative management necessitates balancing competing physiologic goals and mitigating the effects of a persistent transitional circulation. Avoiding intermittent increases in pulmonary arterial pressures (pulmonary hypertensive crises) requires adequate oxygenation, ventilation, analgesia, and iNO as needed. Treatment with sodium bicarbonate of the severe acidosis due to hypoxia and a low cardiac output state may also be necessary.

Ensuring adequate coronary perfusion pressures requires close monitoring for ECG changes indicative of ischemia. Diastolic runoff that compromises coronary perfusion may occur with a patent ductus arteriosus. In this case, blood pressure may need to be augmented or additional oxygen carrying capacity may be required with a transfusion of red blood cells. Excessive reduction in PVR may lead to increased diastolic runoff, which stands in opposition to minimizing the PPHN seen with a persistent transitional circulation. Clinical signs and symptoms (delayed capillary refill, low diastolic blood pressure, worsening end-organ damage) may prompt scaling back of interventions that decrease PVR to reduce diastolic runoff.

In addition to standard ASA monitors, recommended access and monitors include:

- Adequate intravenous access for blood transfusion.
- Arterial line for close hemodynamic monitoring and arterial blood gases.
- Central line for infusion of inotropes.

With regard to patients with VOGM, a large amount of saline may be infused by the interventionalist during the endovascular procedure. It is imperative to monitor for volume overload and consider diuretic administration during the procedure. In addition, consequences of volume overload should be anticipated including: dilutional anemia, dilutional coagulopathy, and electrolyte imbalances.

After the procedure, the patient is left intubated and transported to an intensive care unit for continued critical care and monitoring.

Suggested Reading

Fuloria M, Aschner JL. Persistent pulmonary hypertension of the newborn. *Semin Fetal Neonatal Med.* 2017;22(4):220–6. PMID: 28342684.

Jain A, McNamara PJ. Persistent pulmonary hypertension of the newborn: Advances in diagnosis and treatment. *Semin Fetal Neonatal Med.* 2015;20(4):262–71. PMID: 25843770.

Lakshminrusimha S, Mathew B, Leach CL. Pharmacologic strategies in neonatal pulmonary hypertension other than nitric oxide. *Semin Perinatol.* 2016;40(3):160–73. PMID: 26778236.

Puthiyachirakkal M, Mhanna MJ. Pathophysiology, management, and outcome of persistent pulmonary hypertension of the newborn: a clinical review. *Front Pediatr.* 2013;1:23. PMID: 24400269.

Stayer SA, Liu Y. Pulmonary hypertension of the newborn. *Best Pract Res Clin Anaesthesiol.* 2010;24 (3):375–86. PMID: 21033014.

Wu TW, Azhibekov T, Seri I. Transitional hemodynamics in preterm neonates: clinical relevance. *Pediatr Neonatol.* 2016;57(1):7–18. PMID: 26482579.

Chapter

59

Patent Ductus Arteriosus

Adam C. Adler

A 12-week-old female, born at 32 weeks' gestation, is being evaluated for poor weight gain and "fussiness" with feeds. BP: 60/17 mmHg; HR: 146/min; RR: 45/min increasing to 60/min with feeds; SpO_2: 100% on room air. Weight: 2.6 kg. CXR: prominent pulmonary vascular markings.

What Is the Function of the Ductus Arteriosus?

The ductus arteriosus (DA) is a vascular connection between the aorta and the pulmonary arterial circulation. During fetal life, prior to lung expansion, high pulmonary venous resistance (PVR) forces blood to bypass the lungs via the ductus arteriosus. It is usually located proximal to the take-off of the left subclavian artery; however, this location may vary in a small percentage of the population.

How Is a PDA Diagnosed?

The history of prematurity, feeding intolerance, and wide pulse pressure all point in the direction of a patent ductus arteriosus (PDA). PDAs may be identified as a murmur in an asymptomatic patient or may present as heart failure. Most commonly, echocardiography is performed to visualize the PDA and exclude other structural heart disease lesions.

What Are the Important Diagnoses to Consider?

Other forms of structural heart disease that should be excluded include atrial septal defect (ASD), aortopulmonary window, and aortic insufficiency.

What Are the Signs/Symptoms of a PDA?

Patients often present with a murmur that can be heard across the entire precordium although best auscultated in the upper left sternal border and infra-clavicular regions. As pulmonary pressures fall in the first few days to weeks of life, aortic pressure exceeds pulmonary pressures in both systole and diastole, producing a continuous flow murmur, often referred to as a "machine-like" murmur.

Patients may also have widened pulse pressure due to diastolic run-off, bounding pulses, tachypnea, pulmonary edema, and/or a history of poor feeding.

Findings associated with other diseases of prematurity, i.e., necrotizing enterocolitis (NEC), intraventricular haemorrhage (IVH), bronchopulmonary dysplasia (BPD), should be considered.

What Is the Incidence of PDA?

The incidence of an isolated PDA is approximately 1 in 2,500–5,000 cases and is more common in females than males. The incidence of PDA is highest in premature infants.

What Is the Most Likely Age for Presentation?

The age at presentation is variable. Symptoms usually appear as the PVR decreases in the first weeks of life.

Describe the Anatomic Location of the Ductus Arteriosus

The DA most often originates from the aorta, immediately distal to the left subclavian artery take-off, and attaches to the left pulmonary artery. The location of the ductus arteriosus may vary, complicating surgical identification at times.

What Is the Pathophysiology of a PDA?

Most often, a PDA results in a left-to-right cardiac shunt. As the PVR decreases in the first few days to months of life, the volume shunted from left to right may increase significantly. The volume of blood shunted is generally proportional to the length and diameter of the PDA as well as the balance of systemic vascular resistance (SVR) and PVR.

What Are the Major Hemodynamic Consequences of a PDA?

Large PDAs result in large left-to-right cardiac shunts and pulmonary overcirculation. These children can have dyspnea with feedings, poor weight gain, and pulmonary vascular enlargement from increased flow. Additionally, diastolic run-off (L→R flow through the PDA in diastole) reduces the coronary perfusion pressure which can result in myocardial ischemia, especially in the presence of anemia or reduced SVR. Reduced systemic blood flow as a result of pulmonary overcirculation may result in decreased renal and splanchnic perfusion with resulting necrotizing enterocolitis.

What Factors Contribute to Spontaneous Closure of the DA?

Postnatally, drop in PVR with lung aeration and expansion, reduction in placental prostaglandins, rising arterial PaO_2, and release of vasoactive substrates (thromboxane, bradykinin, etc.) all promote closure of the DA.

Review the Available Medical Therapies for PDA Closure

The most commonly used medical therapies include indomethacin and other NSAID medications. Infants born preterm are more likely to have PDA lesions that require surgical closure after failure of medical therapy when compared to full term infants.

What Is the Treatment to Maintain the DA in Patients with Ductal Dependent Lesions?

These patients are maintained on intravenous prostaglandins to promote ductal patency until the primary lesions may be surgically corrected or a more stable form of pulmonary blood flow established in the form of a conduit (BT shunt).

What Are the Major Risks of IV Prostaglandins?

Intravenous prostaglandins should be started and maintained as a slow continuous infusion. Care must be taken to avoid bolus doses, which may result in hypotension or seizure activity. Due to the long half-life of prostaglandin, the infusion is often stopped before transport to the operating room for definitive treatment to avoid accidental bolus dosing.

What Are the Main Indications for Closure of a PDA?

Patients with moderate or large PDAs associated with symptoms of L→R shunting, left-sided volume overload and those with mild to moderate pulmonary hypertension should be considered for elective closure. Patients with a previous history of infective endocarditis should also be considered for elective closure.

What Are the Main Reasons to Avoid Closing the Ductus?

Patients with mild signs (small audible murmur) or those with incidentally found PDA ("silent PDA") are often managed by observation alone.

Patients with severe and irreversible pulmonary hypertension should also not undergo closure as the ductus is often required to allow right to left shunting during episodes of elevated pulmonary vascular resistance.

Describe the Three Main Invasive Approaches for Closure of PDAs

Common approaches for closure of PDAs include surgical closure or occlusion via catheter-based interventions.

Endovascularly, a catheter can be placed in the femoral or umbilical vessels and directed toward the DA. Endovascular coils can be deployed in the DA causing thrombosis and closure (Figure 59.1). Risks of the procedure include size limitation based on the catheter size and venous vessel size and large ducts >4 mm. Additionally, coils have been reported to

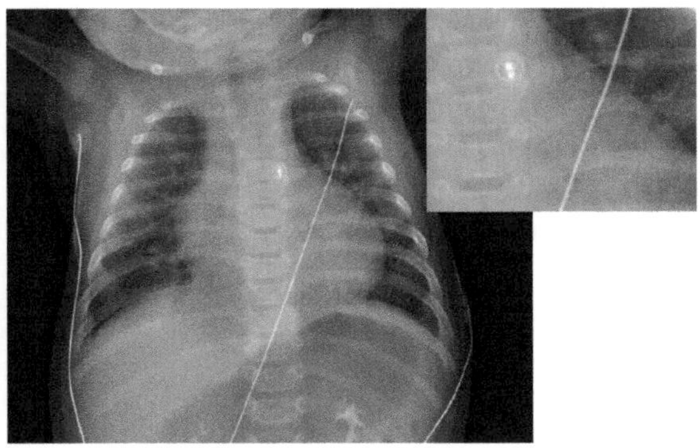

Figure 59.1 Portable chest X-ray of a four-month-old male after PDA Amplatzer device closure.

embolize or project out of the DA, causing occlusion of surrounding structures such as the left pulmonary artery. Antibiotic prophylaxis should be administered in these cases prior to device deployment.

Surgical techniques include open division and ligation of the duct or video assisted thoracoscopic (VATS) PDA ligation.

For either surgical technique, the patient assumes the right lateral decubitus position. The duct is visualized by open surgical technique or by video assist.

Compare the Advantages/Disadvantages to Open Surgical Technique vs. VATS

Open surgical technique may be performed at the bedside which may be beneficial in neonates who are hemodynamically unstable, of extremely low birth weight, or require nonconventional methods of ventilation. Open techniques allow for direct visualization and division and ligation of the duct which reduces risk of ductal recanalization. Open techniques may be beneficial for patients with aberrant anatomy and/or esophageal disorders which may require more extensive dissection of the PDA from surrounding esophageal and aortic structures.

The ability for immediate hemorrhage control using the open technique is obviously present when compared to the VATS technique.

VATS technique allows for a less invasive chest wall incision and potentially reduced pain postoperatively. In this technique, the surgeon places a vascular clip on the duct causing occlusion. However, it may be possible to only partially clip the DA resulting in an incomplete closure.

What Are the Major Anesthetic Considerations for Surgical PDA Ligation Procedures?

Aside from the general anesthetic considerations in premature infants and patients requiring remote site anesthesia, there are a few specific considerations for PDA closures.

With the proximity to the great vessels and potential for brisk bleeds, cross-matched blood should be at the bedside, cross-checked with a warmer immediately available for transfusion.

Arterial access, while beneficial for monitoring and sampling, is not necessarily required for this procedure and is largely institution dependent.

Ideally, a monitoring device should be applied to each extremity in the form of a non-invasive blood pressure (NIBP) cuff, arterial line, or pulse oximeter. As highlighted below, a major risk during PDA ligation is accidental ligation or damage to surrounding vessels including the aorta and branch pulmonary arteries. After ligation, loss of blood pressure or saturation on the lower extremity may signify aortic rather than DA occlusion. The surgeon will often apply a temporary clip or ligature to the DA while monitoring the lower extremity pressure or oximeter to identify changes prior to definitive ligation. Additionally, new gradients between upper and lower extremity measured pressures may indicate the formation of an aortic coarctation and should be addressed.

After the ligation of the DA, the diastolic blood pressure should be compared to the preligation value to assess for diastolic pressure increase as well as reduction in pulse pressure, a sign of successful PDA closure.

Is Endocarditis Prophylaxis Required for Patients with PDAs Or Those with Device Closure History?

Isolated PDAs are not an indication for endocarditis prophylaxis. However, antibiotics should be considered in the first six months following device closure.

What Becomes of the Ductus Arteriosus in Postnatal Life?

Shortly after birth (usually within 10–15 hours), due to the combination of decreased PVR, higher pO_2, and cessation of circulating maternal prostaglandins, the smooth muscle within the ductus arteriosus begins to contract, which causes its *functional* (reversible) closure. It achieves *anatomic* (irreversible) closure by two to three weeks of life. The ductus arteriosus then becomes the ligamentum arteriosum, the fibrous connection between the aorta and pulmonary artery.

POSTOPERATIVE CONSIDERATIONS

What Are the Most Common Complications Associated with Surgical PDA Closure?

- Major bleeding can complicate this delicate surgery.
- Esophageal damage or accidental ligation.
- Injury or ligation of the recurrent laryngeal nerve.
- Accidental ligation of other vessels including the aorta or branch pulmonary artery.
- Chylothorax from damage to lymphatic networks crossing the pleural of peri-aortic regions.
- Residual ductal patency.
- Pneumothorax.

Suggested Reading

Francis E, Singhi AK, Lakshmivenkateshaiah S, et al. Transcatheter occlusion of patent ductus arteriosus in pre-term infants. *JACC Cardiovasc Interv.* 2010;3(5):550–5. PMID: 20488412.

Jain A, Shah PS. Diagnosis, evaluation, and management of patent ductus arteriosus in preterm neonates. *JAMA Pediatr.* 2015;169(9):863–72. PMID: 26168357.

Schneider DJ, Moore JW. Patent ductus arteriosus. *Circulation.* 2006;114(17):1873–82. PMID: 17060397.

Chapter 60

Coarctation of the Aorta

Adam C. Adler

A 16-day-old female presents for a sedated echocardiogram. She was at the pediatrician for a well-child visit when the physician noted weaker femoral pulses compared with her radial pulses. Vital signs are: BPs: RUE: 98/60 LUE: 62/31 RLE: 66/32 LLE: 66/30; HR 126/min; RR 25/min; SpO_2 100% on room air. Weight 4.2 kg. Physical examination was notable for excessive tissue over the posterior neck. Chest X-ray reveals prominent pulmonary vascular markings.

What Is Coarctation of the Aorta?

Coarctation is simply a narrowing of the aorta. Most commonly, the narrowing is present at the site of the ductus arteriosus attachment (or former attachment; Figure 60.1). Less commonly, the coarctation appears in the ascending aorta and is also known as a preductal coarctation. Coarctation may present in the neonatal period (first 30 days of life) or at any time following. Sometimes it is undiagnosed until later in life. Coarctation may be associated with other congenital heart defects, such as hypoplastic left ventricle (LV), ventricular septal defect (VSD), or atrial septal defect (ASD). Up to 30% of children with Turner syndrome have coarctation.

What Are the Clinical Manifestations of Turner Syndrome?

Turner syndrome is a genetic mosaicism in which part or all of an X chromosome is lost. These patients can be monosomy X or contain a chromosomal mosaicism (e.g., 45,X/46,XX). Common clinical signs are:

- Wide-spaced nipples
- Short stature
- Congenital lymphedema of hands and feet
- Webbed neck
- Low hairline
- Hearing loss
- Ovarian insufficiency
- Hypertension
- Prolonged QT interval
- Renal anomalies
- Cardiovascular anomalies
- Metabolic syndrome

What Are the Common Cardiac Issues Affecting Patients with Turner Syndrome?

Cardiovascular anomalies are exceedingly common in patients with Turner syndrome. In addition to coarctation, aortic valve anomalies, especially bicuspid aortic valves, are present in as many as 30%. These patients are also at a higher risk for progressive aortic dilation and aortic dissection.

What Are the Major Hemodynamic Consequences of a Preductal Coarctation?

Coarctation of the aorta essentially functions as an LV outflow tract obstruction. Severe coarctation may result in LV failure and poor distal perfusion.

Critical coarctation in infancy generally requires early intervention. The patient is stabilized with prostaglandin to promote ductal patency which allows for perfusion to the lower extremities. Inotropic agents are administered when needed to improve myocardial contractility, especially in the setting of heart failure.

What Is Differential Cyanosis?

In the absence of an intracardiac mixing lesion (e.g., VSD), the upper body is oxygenating via the LV and ascending aorta while the lower body is perfused with deoxygenated blood from the RV via the PDA. This

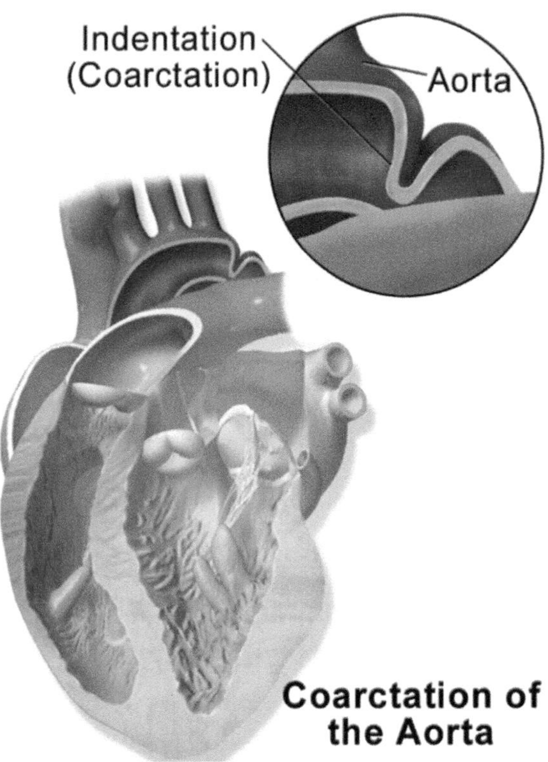

Figure 60.1 Pictorial illustration of aortic coarctation which can occur as illustrated or as a circumferential narrowing of the aortic lumen. Image reproduce from Blausen.com staff (2014). "Medical gallery of Blausen Medical 2014". *WikiJournal of Medicine* 1 (2) under CC BY 3.0 license https://creativecommons.org/licenses/by/3.0/

results in a differential cyanosis between the lower and upper extremities.

How Is the Diagnosis of Coarctation Made?

Coarctation is diagnosed prenatally by ultrasound or suspected postnatally based on physical examination findings such as radial-femoral pulse delay or discrepant blood pressures particularly between the right upper extremity and lower extremities. Transthoracic echocardiography can often identify the region of coarctation, especially in the neonate as well as resultant LV hypertrophy. Gradients across the narrowing are estimated by Doppler to assess the severity of the narrowing. In the setting of LV failure, the estimated gradient may be artificially low. In larger children, CT angiography or cardiac MRI may be done to assess the location and extent of the coarctation and resultant collateral vessels. Cardiac catheterization allows for direct measurement of pressures pre- and post-narrowing and calculation of the true gradient.

Describe the Setting in Which Administration of Prostaglandin E1 (PGE1) Is Indicated in Children with a Coarctation

In cases of preductal coarctation (often with a co-existing hypoplastic aortic arch) identified at birth, flow to the descending aorta may be dependent on blood flow through a PDA. If the PDA closes in the first days of life, blood flow past the coarctation may be restricted and the child may suffer a shock-like condition of poor tissue perfusion. Administration of PGE1 as a continuous infusion will maintain patency of the PDA and enable distal tissue perfusion until the coarctation can be surgically dilated.

Initiation of PGE1 causes central apnea in 15–20% of neonates and thus requires close monitoring. Boluses of PGE1 may result in hypotension or seizure activity. Due to the long half-life of prostaglandin, the infusion is often stopped before transport to the operating room for definitive treatment to avoid accidental bolus dosing.

Continued dilatation of the PDA will also allow for decompression of the pulmonary circulation and RV. When the ductus remains patent, a pressure gradient between the upper and lower extremities may exist (Figure 60.2).

What Are the Surgical Approaches to Repair an Aortic Coarctation?

The main surgical approach is an end-to-end anastomosis. This approach allows the surgeon to avoid graft material (which does not grow with the child) and it avoids division of the subclavian artery (an older technique). The end-to-end anastomosis technique allows for the resection of any remaining ductal tissue that may serve to be a lead point for a future restenosis. The disadvantage of the end-to-end anastomosis is a 10–15% rate of restenosis. Balloon dilation can be used to dilate areas of restenosis, however there is an increased risk of subsequent aortic aneurysmal formation.

The other method of repair is placement of an interposition graft. This technique utilizes a graft that closes the gap after the narrowed section of the aorta

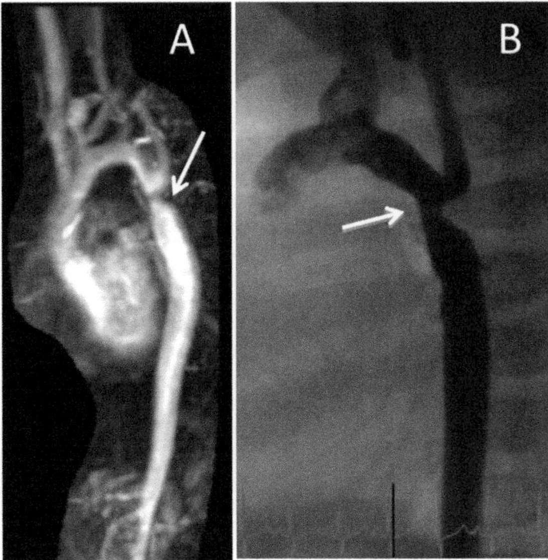

Figure 60.2 (A) Computed tomographic angiography demonstrating a distinct area of coarctation in the "juxta-ductal" region of the aorta distal to the left subclavian artery (arrow). (B) Cardiac catheterization with area of narrowing in the proximal segment of the descending aorta (arrow)

is resected. This may be necessary in older children in whom a larger segment of the aorta is narrowed, resulting in an area too long for end-to-end anastomosis without tension on the sutures. This technique is generally reserved for patients large enough to get a full size (diameter) aortic tube graft.

The main surgical approach is via a left chest thoracotomy. One-lung ventilation is generally unnecessary, as the surgeon will usually retract the left lung for visibility. Alternatively, the approach may be via sternotomy and utilization of cardiopulmonary bypass (CPB). This may be required due to the location of the coarctation or the need for work on the aortic arch or other cardiac defects.

What Are the Major Anesthetic Considerations for Coarctation Procedures?

With the proximity to the great vessels and potential for brisk bleeding, cross-matched blood should be at the bedside, with a warmer immediately available for transfusion. Arterial access, while beneficial for monitoring and sampling, is not necessarily required for this procedure and is largely institution dependent. Ideally, a monitoring device should be applied to each extremity in the form of a NIBP cuff or pulse oximeter to assess for residual gradients postoperatively. Heparin is generally given during cross-clamping with the dose being institution dependent. A cooling blanket can be employed to avoid hyperthermia during aortic cross-clamp.

Older patients develop collaterals to bypass the area of coarctation. These collaterals increase spinal cord and distal perfusion during aortic cross-clamping and reduce the incidence of hemodynamic changes generally associated with cross-clamping. However, large collaterals can pose an increased bleeding risk during thoracotomy.

Postoperative pain after thoracotomy may be severe. PCA should be used for older developmentally appropriate patients. Some centers prefer regional anesthesia in the form of paravertebral single-shot injection or placement of a catheter.

What Are the Most Common Side Effects or Complications Associated with Coarctation Repair?

- The most catastrophic complication of coarctation repair is paraplegia resulting from ischemia of the distal aorta and spinal cord blood supply. The risk is greater in the absence of collaterals and with prolonged cord clamp time (>20–30 minutes);
- Hyperthermia during aortic cross-clamp is associated with poor neurologic outcome. Postoperative hypertension may occur and is treated with nicardipine or nitroprusside (institution dependent);
- Postoperative abdominal pain from mesenteric reperfusion;
- Esophageal damage or accidental ligation;
- Injury or ligation of the recurrent laryngeal nerve;
- Accidental ligation of other vessels;
- Chylothorax from damage to lymphatic networks crossing the pleura of peri-aortic regions;
- Residual aortic coarctation (residual gradient of > 20 mmHg).

What Is Re-coarctation?

The incidence of recurrent coarctation is approximately 5–20%. Intervention is often reserved for re-coarctation with residual gradients of >20 mmHg by cardiac catheterization or 35 mmHg by echocardiography. Initial intervention for re-coarctation is generally via balloon dilatation.

Suggested Reading

Milbrandt T. Thomas E. Turner syndrome. *Pediatr Rev.* 2013;34 (9):420–1. PMID: 24000347.

Sybert VP, McCauley E. Turner syndrome. *NEJM.* 2004;351:1227–38. PMID: 15371580.

Torok RD, Campbell MJ, Fleming GA, et al. Coarctation of the aorta: management from infancy to adulthood. *World J Cardiol.* 2015;7 (11):765–75. PMID: 26635924.

Chapter 61

Atrial Septal Defects

Adam C. Adler

A six-year-old female presents for annual physical examination.

Her current vital signs are: blood pressure 98/62 mmHg; heart rate 97/min; respiratory rate 15/min; SpO_2 100% on room air. On auscultation, there is a systolic murmur with a split S2. Upon further questioning, the mother reports that she does have some shortness of breath with strenuous activity.

Chest X-ray reveals prominent pulmonary vascular markings and mild enlargement of the right-sided cardiac silhouette. An EKG is performed showing right axis deviation and right ventricular hypertrophy. The patient is sent for transthoracic echocardiography revealing a 7 mm secundum type atrial septal defect.

What Is the Incidence of Atrial Septal Defects (ASDs)?

The incidence of atrial septal defects (ASDs) is approximately 50–100 per 100,000 live births. ASDs are the third most common congenital heart defect and have a female predominance. While most cases are sporadic, a familial inheritance appears in affected families. While most ASDs occur in isolation, they may occur in association with many genetic syndromes, e.g., Down, Holt–Oram, Noonan among others, or as part of more complex congenital heart disease (CHD).

What Is the Most Likely Age for Presentation?

ASDs may occur as isolated defects or as part of a larger continuum of congenital structural defects. It may take decades before an unrepaired ASD causes symptoms that necessitate cardiac evaluation. ASDs can often be diagnosed early in life by an astute clinician auscultating a murmur prompting further evaluation. ASDs associated with larger congenital heart defects, e.g., complete AV canal defects, are often diagnosed in the early neonatal period or prenatally.

Identify the Four Main Types of Atrial Septal Defects

ASDs are classified based on the anatomic location of the defect (Figure 61.1). The main types of atrial septal defects are:

- Primum
- Secundum
- Sinus Venosus (SV)
- Coronary Sinus

Describe the Formation of the Atrial Septum

The atrial septum primum begins to develop at around day 28 of gestation. It grows from the superior portion of the common atrium toward the central endocardial cushions. Septum secundum develops as an atrial infolding to the right of the septum primum. The inferior segment of the atrial septum is an upward extension of the endocardial cushions. The foramen ovale, a normally occurring atrial septal defect in fetal development, is a small opening in the septum primum.

Describe the Defect Associated with a Secundum Type ASD

A secundum ASD is really a defect in the septum primum. There are often one or more small holes in the septum primum in the center of the fossa ovalis. Secundum ASDs are the most common atrial septal defect (Figure 61.2).

Ostium Primum/
Secundum ASD
Primum ASD
Tricuspid
Valve
Sinus
Venosus
Coronary
Sinus

Figure 61.1 Drawing highlighting the types and locations of the four types of atrial septal defects. © Adam C. Adler, MD, drawn by J. Daynes

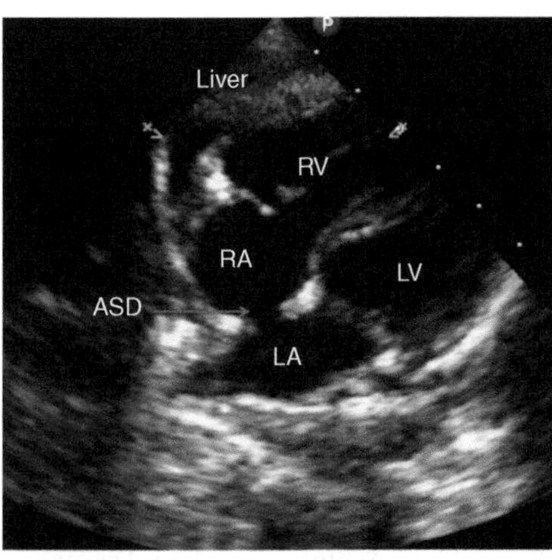

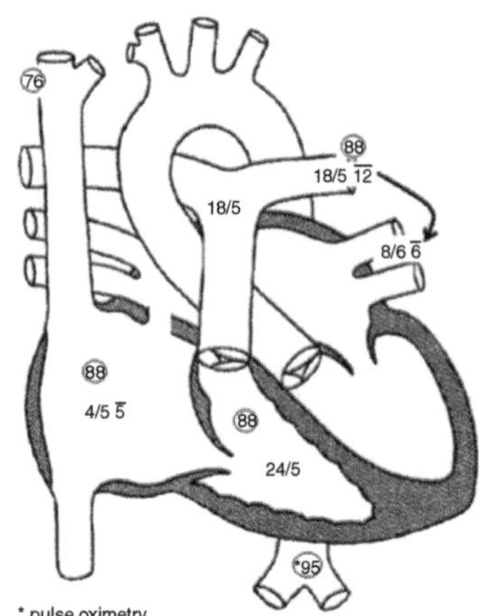

Figure 61.2 Left: Subcostal transthoracic echocardiography demonstrating a secundum type ASD. Right: Cardiac catheterization pictorial of a patient with a moderate ASD. There is a "step up" in saturation from the superior vena cava (76%) to the right atrium (88%).

Describe the Defect Associated with a Primum ASD

A primum ASD, because of its association with the endocardial cushions, may involve a cleft within the anterior leaflet of the mitral valve. If severe, this defect may be addressed during surgical intervention (Figure 61.3).

Describe the Defect Associated with a Sinus Venosus ASD

This defect does not actually involve the atrial septal tissue. Sinus venosus ASDs are actually a connection between the right-sided pulmonary veins and the superior vena cava (SVC) or right atrium. Sinus venosus ASDs account for <10% of ASDs. The most common defect involves connection between the right upper pulmonary vein and the SVC. This defect is a left-to-right shunt at the atrial level as oxygenated blood returning from the lungs is directed to the right atrium instead of the left.

Describe the Defect Associated with a Coronary Sinus ASD

Similar to a SV ASD, a coronary sinus ASD is not a defect in the atrial septal tissue. Rather, the coronary

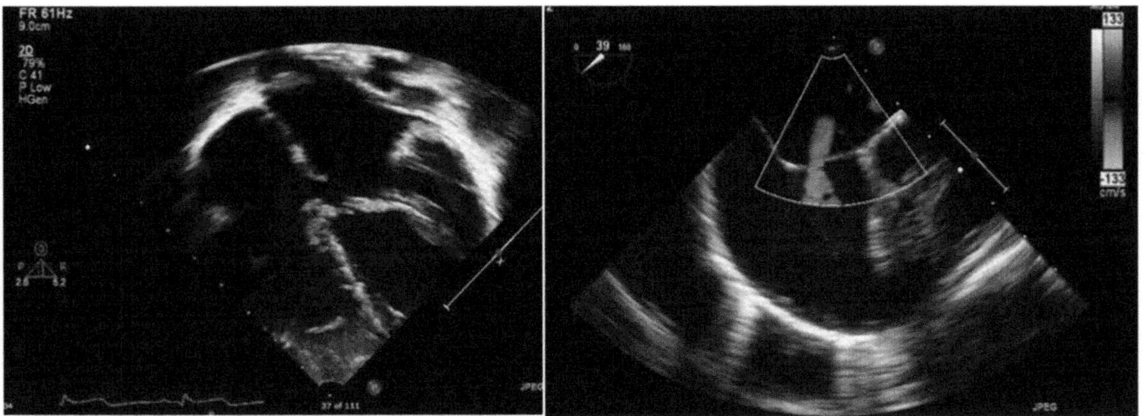

Figure 61.3 Transthoracic echocardiogram demonstrating a primum ASD (left) with large left to right shunting across the defect (right)

sinus is unroofed to drain into the left atrium. Normally, the coronary sinus directs the venous return from the heart into the right atrium. In coronary sinus ASDs, the coronary sinus is opened to the left and right atria allowing the two atria to communicate through this structure. This generates left-to-right shunting at the atrial level.

When a Coronary Sinus ASD Is Identified, What Other Anomaly Must Be Excluded?

Coronary sinus ASDs are associated with a persistent left superior vena cava (LSVC). An LSVC, is a normal structure during fetal life generally in involutes during fetal development. When present, it often communicates with the coronary sinus and/or left atrium. If the coronary sinus communicates directly with the left atrium, a right-to-left shunt exists. Often, a bridging vein between the right and left SVC exists. Identification of a persistent LSVC is important when planning the strategy for cardiopulmonary bypass as the LSVC can provide unwanted venous return and obscure the surgeon's view. Typically, the surgeon will choose to snare the LSVC, especially in the presence of a bridging vein, and direct the flow toward the SVC cannula.

What Is the Pathophysiology of an ASD?

An ASD serves as a left-to-right shunt. The degree of shunting is determined by the size of the defect, relative diastolic compliance of the ventricles, presence of pulmonary valve stenosis, and pulmonary vascular resistance.

What Are the Major Hemodynamic Consequences of an Unrepaired ASD?

With an ASD, both atria and the right ventricle are subjected to chronic volume overload. This results in atrial and ventricular dilation resulting in right ventricle (RV) dysfunction and atrial arrhythmia. The pulmonary vasculature also undergoes changes from the chronic volume overload resulting in muscularization of the pulmonary vascular bed and elevated pulmonary vascular resistance. Over time, elevated pulmonary vascular resistance results in RV pressure elevations and hypertrophy. In severe cases, this can result in reversal of flow (right-to-left shunting) across the ASD, a condition known as Eisenmenger syndrome.

Describe the Appearance of a Chest X-Ray in a Patient with a Large and Unrepaired ASD

Generally, these patients will have right ventricular hypertrophy and enlargement of the cardiac silhouette, especially of right-sided structures. There may be prominence of pulmonary vasculature due to pulmonary overcirculation.

What Is the Characteristic Murmur in Patients with an ASD?

The most characteristic murmur in patients with an ASD is the fixed split S2. The S2 sound (closure of the semilunar valves) is physiologically split during inspiration. During inspiration, the increase in venous return

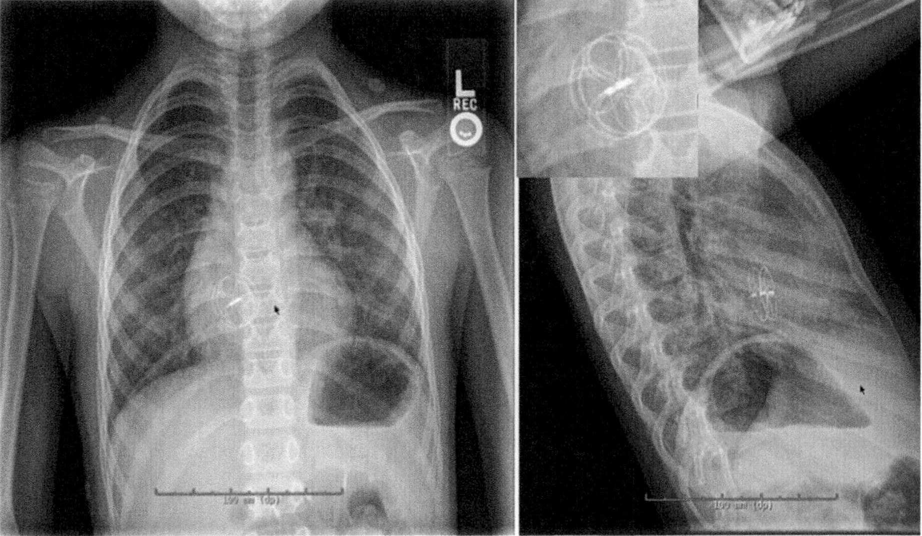

Figure 61.4 Chest X-ray demonstrating an Amplatzer device in situ

overloads the right ventricle and delays the closure of the pulmonary valve. In patients with an ASD, the RV is continuously overloaded from left-to-right shunting, producing a widely split S2.

What Is the Natural History of Unrepaired ASDs?

Secundum ASDs <5 mm may close spontaneously. Primum, large secundum, sinus venosus, and coronary sinus defects generally do not close and usually require intervention.

Describe the Two Main Invasive Approaches for Closure of ASDs

Common approaches for closure of ASDs include surgical closure or catheter-based device closure.

Secundum type ASDs are generally the only type that are amenable to catheter-based device closure at present, most commonly using an Amplatzer device (bilobed disk) (Figure 61.4). A preintervention echocardiogram is performed which is often a transesophageal echocardiography (TEE) to evaluate the rims on either side of the defect. Intraoperatively, a TEE is used throughout the procedure to: evaluate the regions surrounding the defect, guide device positioning, evaluate the atrial septum for evidence of residual shunting, and assure surrounding structures, e.g., AV valves, are intact.

Surgical intervention is done using cardiopulmonary bypass most commonly with bicaval cannulation to optimize visualization. The ASD is approached by right atriotomy and closed using an autologous pericardial patch.

Repair of a sinus venosus defect requires the surgeon to baffle the anomalous venous drainage across the ASD to the left atrium. This baffle is generally accomplished using either autologous pericardium or the atrial tissue itself to create a baffle shunting this blood across the area of the ASD without suturing the pulmonary vein itself. The ASD is closed to the right of the baffle, reestablishing atrial isolation.

A coronary sinus defect (unroofed coronary sinus) is closed by a "roofing" procedure. The coronary sinus is exposed through the right atrium and generally requires excision of the atrial septum. The coronary sinus, which is freely open to both the right and left atria, is closed or "roofed" on the left atrial side using pericardium. The atrial septum is closed leaving the coronary sinus draining solely to the right atrium as intended.

What Are the Major Anesthetic Considerations for Catheter-Based Repair of ASDs?

Aside from the routine risk associated with any catheter-based intervention, the primary risks include damage to the atrial septum (and creation of a larger ASD), device migration/embolization, and damage to the aortic valve. Prior to placing a transcatheter ASD device, an echocardiogram is performed to evaluate the retro-aortic rims. Insufficient rims are associated with long-term erosion into the aortic valve. Long-term issues following transcatheter device closure include: local tissue erosion, arrhythmias, endocarditis, and in situ device thrombosis.

What Are the Major Anesthetic Considerations for Surgical Repair of ASDs?

Generally, patients with ASDs are asymptomatic and do not have pulmonary hypertension. These patients may be managed with diuretics if significant pulmonary congestion is present. Mask induction is usually performed with premedication as needed. Presence of an LSVC should be noted as it may interfere with cannulation. If the surgeon snares the LSVC, careful and continued examination of the head for signs of venous congestion should be monitored and communicated with the surgeon.

In general, the repair of routine ASD is uneventful. The patient should be prepared for extubation either in the operating room or shortly afterwards in the intensive care unit. Repair of coronary sinus ASDs may result in damage to the conduction system.

Suggested Reading

Deen JF, Jones TK. Shunt lesions. *Cardiol Clin.* 2015;33(4):513–20. PMID: 26471816.

O'Byrne ML, Glatz AC, Sunderji S, et al. Prevalence of deficient retro-aortic rim and its effects on outcomes in device closure of atrial septal defects. *Pediatr Cardiol.* 2014;35(7):1181–90. PMID: 24823883.

Ventricular Septal Defects

Adam C. Adler

A 23-month-old female presents for annual physical examination. Her current vital signs are: blood pressure 78/22 mmHg; heart rate 97/min; respiratory rate 26/min; SpO_2 100% on room air. On auscultation, there is a holosystolic murmur at the left sternal border with a split S2. Upon further questioning, the mother reports that she has "fast breathing" when eating with occasional sweating at meal times.

Chest X-ray reveals prominent pulmonary vascular markings and mild enlargement of the right-sided cardiac silhouette. The patient is sent for transthoracic echocardiography revealing a large conoventricular type ventricular septal defect.

DIAGNOSIS

What Is the Incidence for VSDs?

The incidence of ventricular septal defects (VSDs) is approximately one to two per 1,000 live births making it one of the most common congenital heart defects. Isolated VSDs account for nearly 20–30% of all congenital heart defects. VSDs are also present in a wide range of other cardiac defects, e.g., atrioventricular (AV) canal defects and pulmonary atresia with VSD. Approximately 25% of isolated VSDs are in association with another anomaly either genetic or morphologic (trisomy 21, VATER syndrome, VACTERL).

What Is the Most Likely Age for Presentation in Patients with VSDs?

As opposed to atrial septal defects, VSDs can relay symptoms more readily in the neonatal period. VSDs may occur as isolated defects or as part of a larger continuum of congenital structural defects. Smaller VSDs can often be diagnosed early in life by an astute clinician auscultating a murmur prompting further evaluation. VSDs in associated with larger congenital heart defects, e.g., complete AV canal defects, are often diagnosed in the early neonatal period.

Identify the Four Main Types of VSDs

VSDs are classified based on the anatomic location of the defect (Figure 62.1). There are two main types of basic nomenclature for VSDs, and this is somewhat institution dependent. The main types will be listed here with the lesser-used classification in parentheses. The main types of ventricular septal defects are: conventricular (perimembranous), conotruncal (outlet), inlet (AV canal type), and muscular (trabecular).

Briefly Describe the Three Main Segments of the Ventricular Septum

The ventricular septum has three primary components:

- The ***inlet portion*** of the septum extends from beneath the septal leaflet of the tricuspid valve to the tricuspid valves, papillary muscle attachment.
- The ***trabecular or muscular portion*** extends from the chordal attachment of the tricuspid valve to the apex of the ventricles and cephalad toward the conal septum.
- The ***outlet portion*** is the infundibular septum extending to the pulmonary and aortic annuli.

What Is the Natural History of Untreated VSDs in the Neonatal Period?

Approximately 50–70% of VSDs identified in the neonatal period will close spontaneously or regress in size by 6–12 months, specifically the conventricular and muscular type VSDs.

VSDs of the conotruncal (outlet) and inlet (AV canal type) generally do not close spontaneously and require intervention.

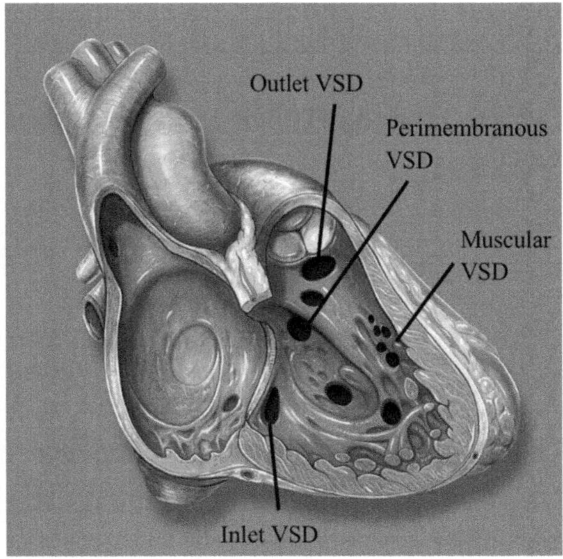

Figure 62.1 Types of ventricular septal defects. Image credit: Patrick J. Lynch, medical illustrator, and C. Carl Jaffe, MD, cardiologist. Reproduced here under CC BY 2.5 license https://creativecommons.org/licenses/by/2.5/

Describe the Typical Presentation of Children with Large Unrepaired VSDs

With a large and unrestrictive VSD, there is often significant left-to-right shunting. As the pulmonary vascular resistance (PVR) falls in the first days to weeks of life, left-to-right shunting increases. If the VSD is moderate and the PVR is high, it can be missed during early auscultation. The shunt results in excessive pulmonary blood flow (overcirculation) and these neonates can present with tachypnea and dyspnea especially with feeding.

Often, these children have sweating during feeding and are generally small for their age due to excessive work of breathing. The excessive overcirculation results in congestive heart failure that can be severe. For small patients, medical management with diuretics and feeding through an indwelling nasogastric tube to reduce the work of breathing can allow for the child to grow, making the surgical repair technically easier to perform.

What Is the Meaning of the Qp:Qs Ratio in Patients with VSDs?

The Qp:Qs ratio is the ratio of the pulmonary blood flow to systemic blood flow (Figure 62.2). Normally this ratio equals one with the entire preload to the right ventricle (RV) eventually becoming the preload to the left ventricle (LV). With large mixing lesions, it is important to determine the % of blood that is recirculating.

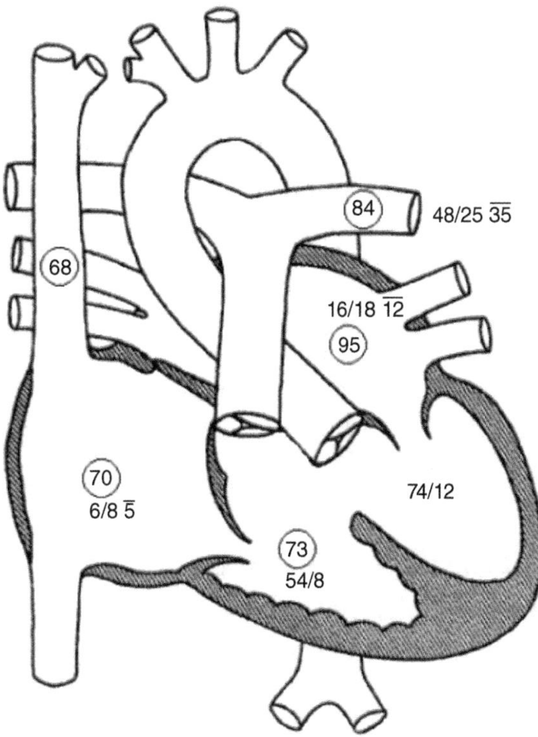

Figure 62.2 Diagram of cardiac catheterization findings for a patient with perimembranous VSD

A simplified formula for determining the Qp:Qs can calculated using only oxygen saturations.

$$\text{Qp} : \text{Qs} = (\text{Aortic sat\%} - \text{Right atrial sat\%}) / (\text{Pulmonary venous sat\%} - \text{Pulmonary artery sat\%}).$$

Small VSDs will have a Qp:Qs ratio of <1.5:1

Medium VSDs have a large Qp:Qs of 2–3:1

Large VSDs can have Qp:Qs ratios exceeding 3:1 or greater.

For Figure 62.2, What Is the Calculated Qp:Qs Ratio When the Saturation in the Aorta Is 100%?

From the formula,

$$\text{Qp} : \text{Qs} = (\text{Aortic sat\%} - \text{Right atrial sat\%}) / (\text{Pulmonary venous sat\%} - \text{Pulmonary artery sat\%})$$

In this case, the formula becomes Qp:Qs = (100–70)/(95–84) giving a Qp/Qs of 2.7.

Notice that from the right atrium to the RV, the saturation increases from 70 to 73. This is known as a step-up. Normally, the saturation from the right atrium to ventricle should be identical. The fact that there is an increase, or step-up, signifies the presence of a mixing lesion.

What Is the Consequence of Leaving a Large VSD Unrepaired?

Aside from the issues with feeding and poor weight gain, significant overcirculation leads to pulmonary vascular occlusive disease. The muscularization of the pulmonary vasculature develops over time from persistent elevations in blood volume and pressure within this normally low-pressure system. Over time, this leads to pulmonary hypertension, right ventricular hypertrophy and even flow reversal across the VSD in severe cases (right-to-left shunting).

List the Indications for Closing a VSD in the Neonatal Period

- Large VSDs
- Symptomatic VSDs
- VSDs with associated aortic insufficiency
- Medium-sized VSDs with failure to thrive
- Conotruncal (outlet), inlet (AV canal type)
- Residual VSDs >3 mm and those with associated Pulmonary artery pressure elevation
- Smaller VSDs when the patient is already undergoing cardiac surgery

Smaller lesions that are less symptomatic may be managed by diuretics while allowing the child to grow with the hopes of spontaneous closure. Delay until the child is two to three years of age provides a larger patient that is surgically more appealing and avoids cardiopulmonary bypass in the neonatal period.

My Patient Is Three Years Old at the Time of Diagnosis. Why Are They Doing a Cardiac Catheterization?

For patients older than one to two years when a large VSD is discovered, a cardiac catheterization is recommended to evaluate if the lesion is amenable to closure. Patients with high pulmonary vascular resistance and those with desaturation during physical activity should not have their VSD closed immediately. If the patient's PVR is elevated from prolonged overcirculation, the Qp:Qs may be decreased indicating that right-sided (RV) pressure is elevated. Desaturation during activity signifies reversal of flow across the VSD (right heart pop-off) and closure of the VSD can result in right heart failure.

List the Types of VSDs from Most to Least Frequent

- Conventricular (perimembranous) approximately 70–80% of VSDs.
- Muscular (trabecular) approximately 10–20% of VSDs.
- Conotruncal (outlet) approximately 5% of VSDs.
- Inlet (AV canal type) approximately 5% of VSDs.

Describe the Defect Associated with a Conventricular (Perimembranous) VSD

These VSDs are defects between the conal portion of the septum and extend toward the tricuspid valve annulus. The aortic valve can be visualized through the defect and occasionally, the noncoronary leaflet of the aortic valve may prolapse through the defect leading to aortic insufficiency.

Describe the Defect Associated with a Conotruncal (Outlet) VSD

These VSDs are in the conotruncal region of the septum immediately beneath the pulmonary valve. Occasionally, these VSDs are referred to as subpulmonary or infundibular VSDs due to their location. In this defect, the tissue separating the aortic and pulmonary valves is deficient and can lead to aortic insufficiency due to prolapse of the aortic valve leaflet into the defect.

Describe the Defect Associated with an Inlet (AV Canal Type) VSD

These VSDs are situated at the level of the tricuspid valve with the septal leaflets and annulus forming their border. The conduction tissue is located near the posterior border of the defect at the point of division into the right bundle branch. Occasionally, there may be an associated cleft of the anterior mitral valve leaflet.

Describe the Defect Associated with a Muscular VSD

These defects are located at any place within the muscular septum. They can be a single defect or multiple defects. These defects can have numerous openings on the RV side of the septum but usually one opening on the LV side of the septum. Generally, muscular VSDs are not notable for their proximity to the conduction system unless there is an associated conventricular VSD or the muscular VSD is located near the tricuspid valve.

What Is the Pathophysiology of a VSD?

A VSD serves as a left-to-right shunt. The degree of shunting is determined by the size of the defect, relative diastolic compliance of the ventricles, presence of pulmonary valve stenosis and pulmonary vascular resistance.

What Are the Major Hemodynamic Consequences of an Uncorrected VSD?

With a VSD, the right ventricle is subjected to chronic volume overload. This results in ventricular hypertrophy and dilation resulting in RV dysfunction and atrial arrhythmia. The pulmonary vasculature also undergoes changes from the chronic volume overload resulting in muscularization of the pulmonary vascular bed and elevated pulmonary vascular resistance. Over time, elevated pulmonary vascular resistance results in RV pressure elevations and hypertrophy. In severe cases, this can result in reversal of flow (right-to-left shunting) across the VSD, a condition known as Eisenmenger syndrome.

Describe the Appearance of a Chest X-Ray in a Patient with a Large VSD

Generally, these patients will have right ventricular hypertrophy and enlargement of the cardiac silhouette. There may be prominence of pulmonary vasculature due to pulmonary overcirculation.

What Is the Characteristic Murmur in Patients with a VSD?

With the increase in left-to-right flow, the right ventricle experiences an excessive volume overload and takes longer to eject its stroke volume. This leads to delayed closure of Pulmonary valve and thus a split S2 may result. A holosystolic systolic murmur best heard at the left sternal border may be observed.

Describe the Two Main Invasive Approaches to Closure of VSDs

Common approaches for closure of VSDs include surgical closure or catheter-based device closure.

Some muscular type VSDs may be amenable to a catheter-based closure using a device similar to ones used for secundum ASDs. More commonly, surgical intervention is done using cardiopulmonary bypass most commonly with bicaval cannulation to optimize visualization. The VSD is approached by right atriotomy and generally through the tricuspid valve. These defects are closed with a Dacron patch, homograft patch, occasionally with a PTFE-based Gore-Tex patch or simply sutured closed with or without a pledget.

What Are the Major Anesthetic Considerations for Surgical Repair of VSDs?

Generally, patients with VSDs have pulmonary overcirculation. These patients may be managed with diuretics if significant pulmonary congestion is present. Mask induction is usually performed with a premedicant if needed.

Most often, the repair of a routine VSD is uneventful. The patient should be prepared for extubation either in the operating room or shortly afterwards in the intensive care unit. Repair of conotruncal and conventricular VSDs can affect the aortic valve due to its close proximity to the sutures required for the repair. Repair of inlet VSDs can affect the conduction system and means of artificial pacing should be readily available. A transesophageal echocardiograph (TEE) is often performed at the termination of cardiopulmonary bypass and should specifically evaluate for residual VSDs and damage to the anterior mitral valve leaflet, aortic non and right coronary leaflets and the septal leaflet, of the tricuspid valve.

Suggested Reading

Minette MS, Sahn DJ. Ventricular septal defects. *Circulation*. 2006;114:2190–7. PMID: 17101870.

Spicer DE, Hsu HH, Co-Vu J, et al. Ventricular septal defect. *Orphanet J Rare Dis*. 2014;9:144. PMID: 25523232.

Chapter 63

Anesthesia for Cardiac Catheterization

Jamie W. Sinton

A 17-day-old, full-term male with Trisomy 21, transitional atrioventricular canal defect (TAVC), secundum atrial septal defect (ASD), and aortic arch hypoplasia presents for hemodynamic cardiac catheterization. This infant is currently in the neonatal intensive care unit, tachypneic and saturating 92% on room air. His echocardiogram is suggestive of pulmonary hypertension. His Hgb is 10.7 g/dl and his assumed oxygen consumption is 170 mL/min/m^2. His catheterization diagram is shown in Figure 63.1.

What Is a Transitional Atrioventricular Canal Defect?

An atrioventricular canal (AVC) defect, also known as an atrioventricular septal defect, is a defect involving the endocardial cushions. These defects are categorized into partial, transitional, and complete AVC defects (Table 63.1).

What Are the Rastelli Classifications for Complete Atrioventricular Canal Defects?

The normal AV valves (mitral and tricuspid) form one valve referred to as the common AV valve. This valve straddles the ventricular septal defect with varying choral attachments. The leaflets that overlie the septate are referred to as "bridging leaflets." The variations of the attachments determine the Rastelli classification which is helpful in surgical planning.

What Is the Natural History of AVC Defect Physiology?

Atrioventricular canal defects begin as a left-to-right shunt at the atrial (ASD) and ventricular (VSD) levels. In this patient, only an inlet (type III) VSD is present. With the normal age-related decline in pulmonary vascular resistance, nadir around two months of age, the left-to-right shunt increases and pulmonary over-circulation develops. Infants develop congestive heart failure and failure to thrive. Surgical correction is undertaken in infancy, often around four months of age. If surgical correction is deferred, longstanding pulmonary over-circulation can lead to pulmonary hypertension, Eisenmenger's syndrome, and arterial oxygen desaturation.

Is This Patient's Presentation Consistent with the Natural History of AVC?

No. This patient has a left-to-right shunting lesion. He should not have arterial oxygen desaturation nor echocardiographic evidence of pulmonary hypertension at age 17 days.

What Echocardiographic Findings May Suggest Pulmonary Hypertension?

Pulmonary arterial hemodynamics cannot be directly measured using echocardiography. However, several echo findings are suggestive of pulmonary hypertension. Flattening of the interventricular septum during systole, tricuspid regurgitation, and right ventricular hypertrophy may all indicate a hypertensive right ventricle and could suggest pulmonary hypertension depending on the rest of the clinical and echo features.

Is Cardiac Catheterization Routinely Performed Prior to Surgical Repair of AVC?

No. This patient has echo findings of pulmonary hypertension which is unexpected, therefore catheterization is indicated to clarify hemodynamics and assess for suitability of complete repair (or medical optimization prior to complete repair). Angiograms are also taken to determine anatomic relationships and morphology as needed.

Table 63.1 Description of the types of AV canal type defects.

Canal defect type	Defect location	Associated issues
Partial canal	Primum ASD Cleft anterior mitral valve leaflet	tricuspid valve (TV) often abnormal Mitral regurgitation due to cleft leaflet
Transitional canal	Primum ASD AV valve anomaly VSD (restrictive) Cleft anterior mitral valve leaflet	Mitral regurgitation due to cleft leaflet
Complete canal	Primum ASD Common AV valve VSD (non-restrictive)	Mitral regurgitation due to cleft leaflet Classified according to Rastelli types A,B,C

What Measurements Are Taken during a Hemodynamic Catheterization? What Ventilation Strategy Is Helpful to Ensure Accuracy of Catheterization Measurements?

Oxygen saturations and pressure measurements are obtained in sequence from the superior vena cava (SVC), right atrium (RA), right ventricle (RV), pulmonary artery (PA), and pulmonary capillary wedge (PCW) during a right heart cath eterization. This is followed by a left heart catheterization in which measurements are taken from the descending, transverse and ascending aorta, left ventricle (LV), and left atrium (LA).

Ventilation with room air and measurements taken at end expiration help to ensure consistency and accuracy of hemodynamic catheterization data. Ideally, positive pressure ventilation is minimized or

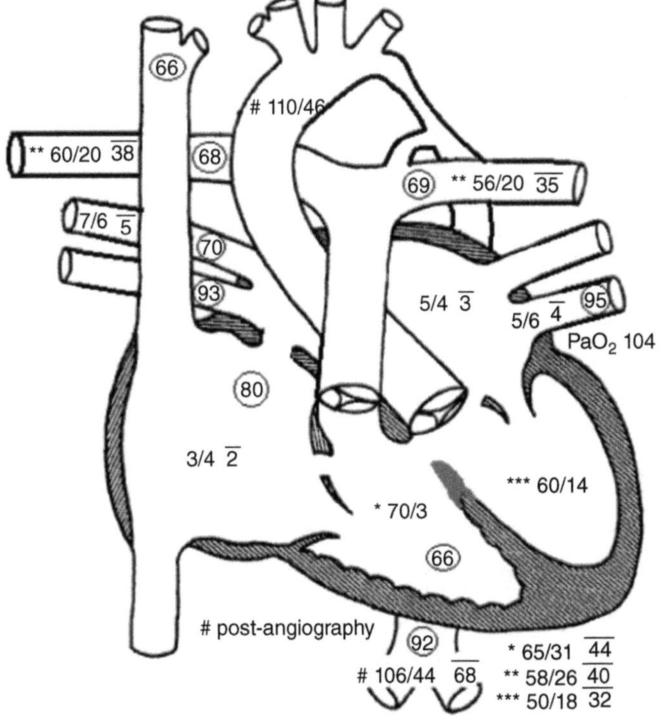

Figure 63.1 Cardiac catheterization diagram. Encircled values represent oxygen saturation, pressures are denoted as systolic / diastolic, mean pressures are overlined. Courtesy of Adam C. Adler, MD.

avoided completely as is excess positive end-expiratory pressure (PEEP). Similarly, obstruction during spontaneous ventilation may result in abnormally high intracardiac pressure measurements.

What Calculations Are Made from the Hemodynamic Data?

Oxygen saturations are used to calculate oxygen carrying capacity, oxygen content, and cardiac output. In patients with shunt lesions such as this patient, the ratio of pulmonary to systemic blood flow, Qp:Qs, can be calculated. Pressure measurements are used to calculate pulmonary and systemic vascular resistances, transpulmonary gradient, and peak-to-peak gradient.

Oxygen Saturation in the SVC Is 66%, in the RA Is 80%, and in the RV Is 66%. Would These Values Be Expected in a Patient with a Structurally Normal Heart?

No. Oxygen saturations on the systemic venous (right) side of the heart should decline slightly as blood progresses toward the pulmonary artery. In this case, the saturation in the right atrium exceeds the SVC. This implies the existence of a left-to-right shunt at the atrial level. This is consistent with the patient's known ASD.

The RV saturation of 66% is much less than the RA saturation of 80%. This is inconsistent with left-to-right shunting through his VSD. This is concerning for flow reversal through the VSD, e.g., bidirectional or right-to-left at some point in the cardiac cycle. Ventricular pressure measurements and/or ventriculograms are helpful to clarify this.

What Can Be Concluded from the Right Upper Pulmonary Vein Saturation of 70%?

Normally, pulmonary vein saturation should approach 100%. Pulmonary vein desaturation indicates pulmonary pathology at least in a segmental lung section.

What Is the Expected Qp/Qs in a Patient with a Left-to-Right Shunt (Such as Most Patients with TAVC)? <1, =1, or >1?

Left-to-right shunt physiology produces excessive pulmonary blood flow. When pulmonary blood flow exceeds systemic blood flow, Qp/Qs is > 1.

What Is the Qp:Qs Ratio?

The Qp:Qs is a ratio of pulmonary (Qp) to systemic (Qs) blood flow (or cardiac output).

How Is Qp:Qs Calculated?

To calculate the pulmonary or systemic blood flow, oxygen consumption is divided by the absolute value of the difference in oxygen content between arterial and venous blood. In general, flow = oxygen consumption / (difference in arterial and venous oxygen content).

Pulmonary flow (Qp):

$$\begin{aligned} Qp &= VO_2/[Hb \times 1.34 \times 10 \times (SpvO_2 - SpaO_2)] \\ &= 4.6\ L/\min/m^2 \end{aligned}$$

Systemic flow (Qs):

$$\begin{aligned} Qs &= VO_2/[Hb \times 1.34 \times 10 \times (SaO_2 - SvO_2)] \\ &= 4.6\ L/\min/m^2 \end{aligned}$$

Because the right and left sides of the heart each have the same hemoglobin and oxygen consumption, a rearrangement and simplification of this calculation can be made:

$$Qp : Qs = (SaO_2 - SvO_2)/(SpvO_2 - SpaO_2)$$

In our patient, the oxygen saturations are SaO_2 = 92%, SvO_2 is usually taken from the SVC and = 66%, $SpvO_2$ = 93–95%; use 95% for calculations, $SpaO_2$ = 69%.

Using the above formula, Qp:Qs = 1.

This patient is ventilated with room air, so any contribution of dissolved oxygen to oxygen content is negligible.

Is a Qp:Qs of 1 to Be Expected in This Patient? What Can Be Concluded from This Value?

Patients with AVC defects are expected to have left-to-right shunts with Qp:Qs >1. Our patient's Qp:Qs equals 1. This finding, along with a desaturated right ventricle (compared to the right atrium), and suprasystemic right ventricular pressure suggests some pulmonary obstruction such as pulmonary hypertension.

How Can Pulmonary Obstruction Due to Pulmonary Valve Pathology Be Differentiated from Pulmonary Hypertension by Catheterization?

Certainly, echo images of the pulmonic valve may adequately rule out pulmonary valvular obstruction or stenosis. Without echo findings of pulmonary stenosis, pulmonary hypertension can be strongly suspected in this patient. Catheterization calculations of elevated pulmonary vascular resistance could be used to confirm a diagnosis of pulmonary hypertension.

How Is Pulmonary Vascular Resistance Calculated?

Reminiscent of Ohm's Law in physics (V = IR), vascular resistances can be calculated. Resistance equals change in pressure divided by flow. In the case of pulmonary vascular resistance (PVR), the change in pressure driving blood from the pulmonary artery to the left atrium is divided by pulmonary flow (or right-sided cardiac output).

$$\text{PVR} = (\text{mean PA pressure} - \text{mean LA pressure})/\text{Qp}$$

For our patient, mean PA pressure is approximately 36 torr and mean LA pressure is approximately 3 torr. Qp is 4.6 L/min/m^2 from the previous calculation. PVR = 7.17 Wood units/m^2.

Are Outcomes Following Congenital Heart Surgery in Children with Down Syndrome any Different than Other Children?

From a large retrospective cohort study, patients with Down Syndrome had similar mortality following cardiac surgery compared to their euchromosomal counterparts. The Down syndrome cohort did, however, have increased length of hospital stay if they underwent ASD, VSD or tetralogy of Fallot repair. Patients who underwent VSD closure also had higher rates of heart block.

Suggested Reading

Fudge JC Jr, Li S, Jaggers J, et al. Congenital heart surgery outcomes in Down syndrome: analysis of a national clinical database. *Pediatrics.* 2010;126(2):315–22. PMID: 20624800.

Lam JE, Lin EP, Alexy R, et al. Anesthesia and the pediatric cardiac catheterization suite: a review. *Paediatr Anaesth.* 2015;25 (2):127–34. PMID: 25331288.

Chapter 64

Tetralogy of Fallot

Kriti Puri and Adam C. Adler

A four-week-old infant presents to the emergency room with agitation and cyanosis. His mother says he has been doing this for shorter periods of time for the past couple of weeks whenever he cries for food. These episodes resolve when she takes him in her lap and breastfeeds him. However, he started running a fever yesterday and had a few episodes of diarrhea this morning. And this current episode has been going on for several minutes and he is only getting more agitated and inconsolable.

Vital signs are: blood pressure unmeasurable due to worsening agitation as the cuff inflates, heart rate 180/min, respiratory rate 60/min, oxygen saturation reads 40–50% during times of agitation but improves when the patient is calm.

What Condition Are You Most Worried About? What Are Tet Spells?

This child is experiencing a hypercyanotic "tet" spell characteristic of tetralogy of Fallot (ToF).

Tetralogy of Fallot is the most common cyanotic congenital heart disease. Often, ToF is prenatally diagnosed or detected by the newborn congenital heart defect (CHD) screen. However, occasionally ToF may present with worsening spells of cyanosis, also known as hypercyanotic or "tet" spells, during which there is severe obstruction of blood flow to the lungs. In conditions that increase the pulmonary vascular resistance, more blood shunts from right-to-left through the VSD, resulting in worsening cyanosis. Tet spells are ominous indicating the acute need for palliative intervention to provide pulmonary blood flow and improve oxygenation.

What Is the Underlying Anatomy in Tetralogy of Fallot?

The tetralogy in ToF develops due to anterior deviation of the interventricular septum or infundibular tissue (Figures 64.1 and 64.2). The remainder of the tetralogy occurs following this movement. The anterior movement of the infundibulum compresses the right ventricular outflow tract (RVOT). This shift also results in an anterior malalignment VSD for which the aorta "overrides" or sits over the VSD. The compression of the RVOT ultimately results in compensatory right ventricular hypertrophy (RVH) (Figure 64.3).

Identify the Anatomic Spectrum That Is Encompassed by Tetralogy of Fallot

Tetralogy of Fallot is a spectrum of anatomy and physiology manifestations, depending on the degree of the obstruction to the right ventricular outflow tract, and the subsequent pulmonary blood flow limitation. ToF can include varying degrees of pulmonary stenosis (mild to severe). In its most extreme form, there is complete pulmonary atresia in which no blood flows from the RVOT; hence the patient is dependent on a patent ductus arteriosus (PDA) to supply blood to the lungs. If not detected prenatally, these patients may present with worsening cyanosis and may be found to have a closing PDA on echo. This cohort of patients will benefit from prostaglandin infusion and usually undergo either a modified Blalock–Taussig shunt (BTs) or PDA stent placement in the catheterization laboratory, to provide stable pulmonary blood flow. After a few months the patient will undergo completion of the repair with a takedown of the shunt or stent, and closure of the VSD, and placement of a conduit from the right ventricle (RV) into the main pulmonary artery, to create normal septated anatomy.

Considering a slightly lower less degree of pulmonary outflow obstruction, there may be a very small amount of blood flow through the pulmonary valve but this may not be adequate in the absence of supplementation from the PDA. These ToF patients with severe pulmonary stenosis (PS) follow the course of the ToF with pulmonary atresia and undergo shunting or stenting initially, prior to complete septation and repair later in infancy.

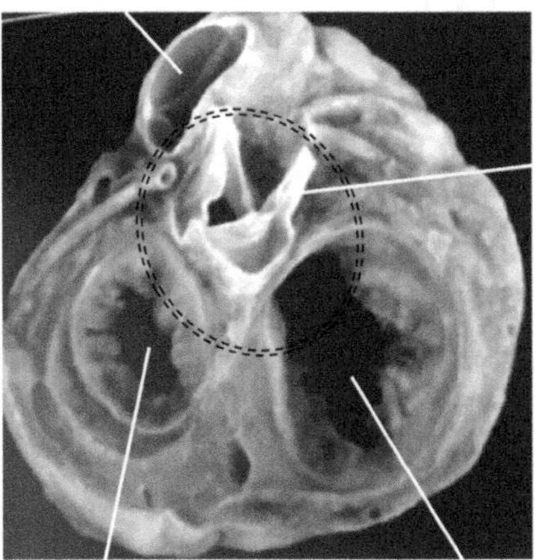

Figure 64.1 Cardiac specimen highlighting the infundibulum region (dashed circle). The region between the aortic valve and right ventricular outflow tract (RVOT) is underdeveloped leading to anterior shift of structures.

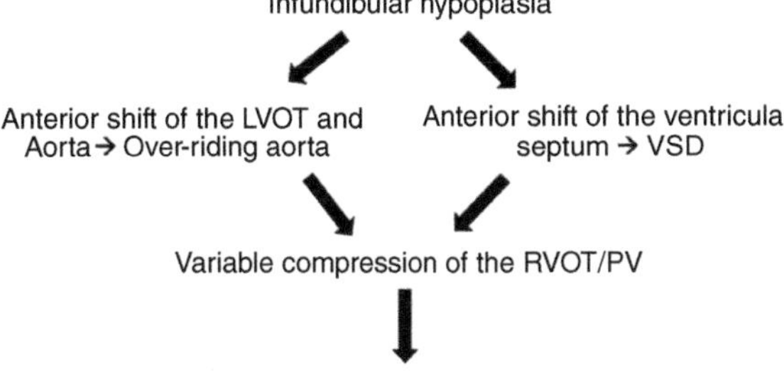

Figure 64.2 Schematic identifying the primary and compensatory changes seen in patients with tetralogy of Fallot. LVOT, left ventricular outflow tract; RVOT, right ventricular outflow tract; PV, pulmonary valve; VSD, ventricular septal defect.

Moving further along the spectrum, there are patients that may have mild to moderate obstruction initially and be able to manage without a PDA. However, as time passes the RV muscle hypertrophy just under the narrow pulmonary valve worsens and adds a dynamic component of RV outflow obstruction to the mix. This dynamic obstruction is worse when the patient is dehydrated and volume deplete, as the hypertrophied RV does not have adequate preload and generates dynamic obstruction from all the thick muscle bundles collapsed together. It is also worse when the heart rate is higher, and the RV is unable

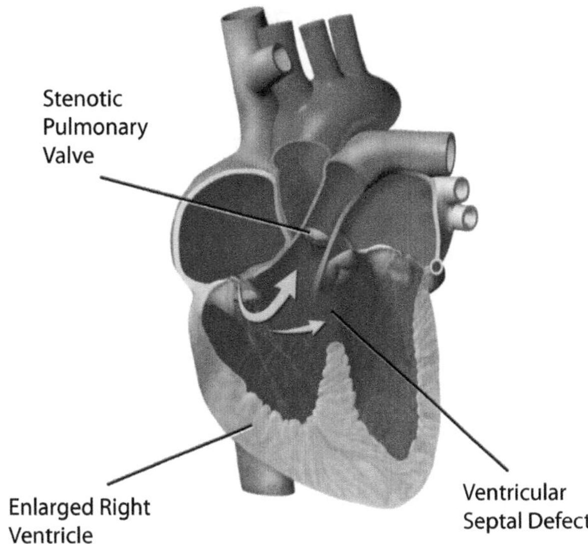

Figure 64.3 Drawing of characteristic components of tetralogy of Fallot: Reproduced from Blausen.com staff (2014). "Medical gallery of Blausen Medical 2014". *WikiJournal of Medicine* 1 (2) under CC BY-SA 4.0 license https://creativecommons.org/licenses/by-sa/4.0/.

to relax completely in diastole and fill. Episodes of agitation and higher pulmonary vascular resistance or intrathoracic pressures would further limit the ability of the RV to push blood through the narrow outflow tract. Hence patients having a "tet" spell prefer to shunt blood across the VSD through the aorta, instead of being able to send it to the lungs. Thus, while they do not lose cardiac output, they become hypoxemic and cyanotic and more inconsolable and tachycardic, getting into a vicious cycle.

A final category of ToF, which manifests very differently from the usual cyanotic CHD, are ToF with pulmonary atresia and major aortopulmonary collateral arteries (MAPCAs). These MAPCAs originate from various spots on the descending aorta or from the aortic arch or its branches, and supply various segments of the lungs (Figure 64.4). The patients with MAPCAs will not present with cyanosis, rather they may have pulmonary overcirculation and manifest with tachypnea, tachycardia, and failure to gain weight normally. Their surgical planning is more precarious, as the MAPCAs may be physically far apart and difficult to unifocalize to a central main pulmonary artery. The MAPCAs also expose the pulmonary vascular bed to systemic blood pressures and predispose to development of pulmonary hypertension.

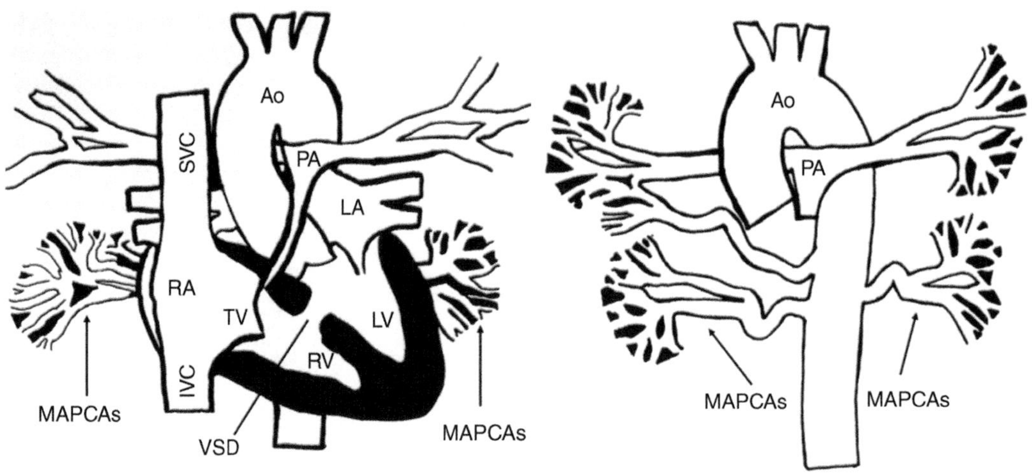

Figure 64.4 (Left) Diagram of tetralogy with pulmonary atresia and major aortopulmonary collaterals. (Right) Image demonstrating the major aortopulmonary collaterals coming off the aorta. LV and RV, left and right ventricles respectively; LA and RA, left and right atria respectively; IVC and SVC, inferior and superior vena cava respectively; VSD, ventricular septal defect; PA, pulmonary artery; Ao, aorta; TV, tricuspid valve; MAPCAs, major aortopulmonary collaterals. Illustration by Adam C. Adler MD

How Are "Tet Spells" Managed?

Acute "tet spells" are managed by firstly helping calm the patient (e.g., by handing the child to the mother to hold, allowing to feed, or sedation if needed), placing the child in a knee-chest position (to increase systemic vascular resistance, and may be achieved by mother holding the baby in her arms and cradling the knees and chest together), initiating oxygen (preferably through the least noxious route for the child, e.g., blow-by or face-mask), administering a bolus of intravenous fluids, and finally intravenous metoprolol (to slow down the heart rate) and phenylephrine (to increase systemic vascular resistance). Some will require anesthesia (on the way to the operating room). Obtaining a blood pressure may be further annoying to the child and is hence not necessary at this time. Instead a minimal intervention strategy to allow the child to recover is prudent, while remaining alert to act in case of needing more support. Rate control, volume repletion, sedation, and peripheral vasoconstriction all come together to boost blood flow through the narrow RV outflow tract.

What Are the Classic Exam Findings of a ToF Patient?

ToF patients manifest a harsh ejection systolic murmur loudest over the pulmonic area and radiating into axillae, indicating pulmonic stenosis. As the stenosis becomes worse, initially the murmur is slightly louder, but eventually it starts becoming softer as the obstruction increases. For example, during a ToF spell, the pulmonary stenosis murmur may not be audible at all. Higher saturations indicate less RV outflow obstruction. "Tet spells" may become a vicious cycle and require a combination of heart rate control and vascular resistance manipulation to break. The murmur during a hypercyanotic or "tet spell" becomes softer due to decreased pulmonary flow. Iron deficiency anemia will accelerate the onset of these spells.

Management

The time of presentation and intervention for ToF is determined by the degree of RV outflow obstruction, and the limitation of pulmonary blood flow. These clinical indicators are the O_2 saturation levels and the development of hypercyanotic spells. The Doppler-echocardiographic indicators are the pressure gradients observed across the RV outflow tract. Children with saturations less than 80% or those having hypercyanotic spells are scheduled for surgery. Surgical management includes palliative procedures like a modified Blalock–Taussig–Thomas shunt (mBTT shunt) to help provide consistent pulmonary blood flow in the setting of significant stenosis or atresia at the pulmonary valve.

Complete repair of the heart comprises closure of the VSD as well as resection of the RV obstruction, resulting in normal saturations. Complete repair is replacing the palliative approach in many centers. Even after complete ToF repair, the patients need lifelong cardiology follow up, as their pulmonary valve may become more regurgitant (depending on the surgical approach and the intervention on the valve annulus itself) leading to RV dilation.

They may also develop arrhythmias due to the RV dilation/hypertrophy and scarring (as a result of the pulmonary valve regurgitation as well as the primary surgery), with an increase in risk of sudden cardiac death in pediatric patients with QRS > 170 ms on the EKG. Cardiac MRI is used to estimate the volume of the RV to determine the time for pulmonary valve replacement (catheter-based or surgical). While complete ToF repair ensures that these children have normal saturations, a majority of patients have a prolonged QRS and features of right bundle block on the EKG due to the intervention on the interventricular septum.

> A two-week-old 3 kg female infant was diagnosed with ToF with pulmonary atresia and underwent right-sided 3.5 mm mBTT shunt placement through a lateral thoracotomy. Her saturations were around 85–90% after this surgery. You respond to a code that is called as the baby is "fussy and cyanosed" over the past 20 minutes, and now her saturations are in the 40s.

What Is the First Medication You Would Like to Administer? What Exam Finding Would Be Concerning for You?

This child may have a clotted shunt, which is limiting her pulmonary blood flow. The shunt is especially critical for her, as she has pulmonary atresia, making the shunt her solitary source of pulmonary blood flow. The first medication, which has hopefully already been administered by the time you arrive, is 100 U per kilogram of a heparin bolus to try and open up the shunt. A volume bolus of colloid or crystalloid may also be considered. The lack of a loud harsh murmur on exam is extremely concerning for a shunt obstruction.

What Are the Major Anesthetic Considerations for ToF Surgery? What Are the Differences of Shunt or a Complete Repair?

ToF surgery has some unique considerations based on the procedure planned. For any ToF patient, it is imperative to have checked an ionized calcium level preoperatively, as ToF falls in the category of conotruncal anomalies that are commonly associated with DiGeorge syndrome.

Further, for a ductal stent, it is important to turn the prostaglandin infusion off a few hours prior to the procedure if possible to help the PDA constrict a little and allow the stent to fit well. During ductal stenting, there may be spasm of the PDA when the wire crosses it, hence the team must always be prepared with a stent on the wire to prevent the PDA from collapsing entirely.

A complete repair is done through a median sternotomy, with its usual considerations. In the perioperative transesophageal echocardiography, it is very important to assess for residual VSDs.

What Are the Most Common Complications Associated with ToF Surgeries?

The complications after ToF surgery vary with the kind of surgery.

- After a mBTT shunt, the patient may have significant symptoms of pulmonary overcirculation (tachypnea, tachycardia) along with lower diastolic pressures as the shunt offers runoff for the systemic flow. If the shunt is performed from a lateral thoracotomy, they can be more painful. A ductal stent may have similar features.
- A shunt (surgical or catheter-based) can never be trusted. Clotting of a shunt causing limitation of pulmonary blood flow is a dreaded complication, and usually patients are started on at least low dose heparin or other anticoagulation, and anti-platelet therapy once feeds are tolerated.
- A complete repair with a VSD patch may be complicated by arrhythmias postoperatively. While heart block of varying degrees may be

possible due to the proximity of the patch to the normal conduction system of the heart, one of the classic arrhythmias after ToF repair is junctional ectopic tachycardia (JET). JET is often attributed to the physical stretching of the junction during the VSD repair; however, it has also been seen in patients without any intra-cardiac surgery, so a component of intrinsic arrhythmogenicity is suspected. Due to the potential for arrhythmias, patients benefit from being left with atrial as well as ventricular wires for the perioperative period.

- ToF patients have very hypertrophied RVs which have significant diastolic dysfunction. Hence it is not uncommon to see higher than usual central venous pressure (CVP) being tolerated for these patients. One must resist the urge to diurese a number, since the RV hypertrophy is still a set-up for dynamic outflow tract obstruction if the patient is volume depleted and the RV is under filled. Similarly, a volume depleted ToF will be tachycardic which also does not bode well for dynamic RV outflow tract obstruction. The tachycardia may be more prominent in patients who have been on a beta-blocker preoperatively.
- If there has been significant manipulation and augmentation of branch pulmonary arteries, especially if they were discontinuous to begin with, always be suspicious of desaturations, unilateral oligemia on the chest x-ray or a widening end tidal-pCO_2 gradient. Residual ductal tissue or scarring and inflammation may cause stenosis of a branch PA and may need catheter-based intervention if clinically significant.
- ToF with pulmonary atresia and MAPCAs is a unique condition in the ToF family. After a MAPCA unifocalization, patients may have very non-compliant lungs that have borne the brunt of the imbalanced Qp:Qs for so long. They may also demonstrate pulmonary hypertensive crises as the MAPCA vascular architecture is abnormal with thicker media and has also been exposed to systemic blood pressures for so long.
- Thoracic duct injury can lead to chylothorax, which manifest as the child starts feeding more after surgery.

What Is the Management of Junctional Ectopic Tachycardia (JET)?

JET is a classic postoperative arrhythmia manifesting in the first 72 hours after ToF repair. The initial management is to minimize the sympathetic stimulation with cooling and sedation. If the rate of JET is within normal limits of heart rate for age, one may elect to wait and watch, or intervene with overdrive pacing at a few beats above the JET rate to achieve atrioventricular synchrony.

Preemptive use of dexmedetomidine by infusion and magnesium repletion may help to reduce the incidence of postoperative JET following these repairs.

What Is the Natural History of Patients with RV-PA Conduits?

Over time, the artificial conduits undergo a number of changes that may affect their function. Of course,

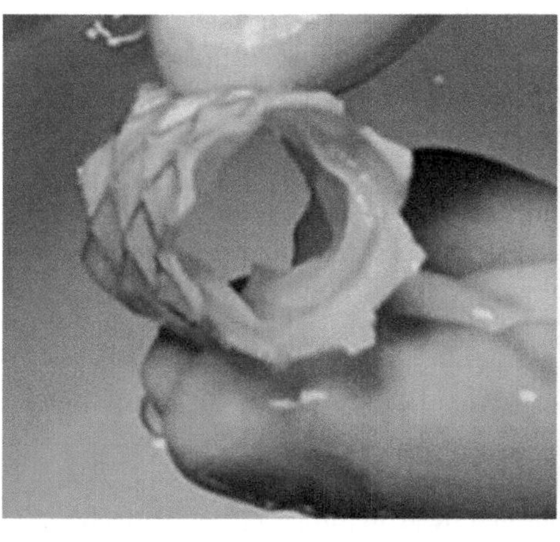

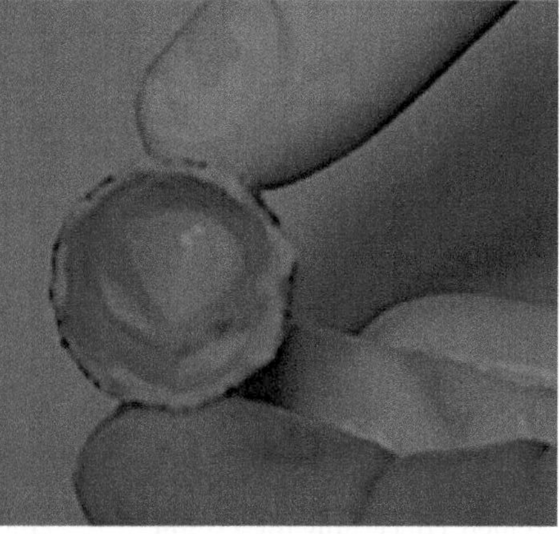

Figure 64.5 Transcatheter pulmonary valve in the open (left) and closed positions (right)

these artificial conduits do not grow over time. When placed in small children, these conduits often require replacement with larger conduits as they become flow limiting. Additionally, internal calcifications and/or narrowing at the proximal or distal end may restrict flow.

Additionally, the native valve within the conduit eventually becomes incompetent leaving pulmonary insufficiency, which can be severe or even freely regurgitant.

What Is a Melody Valve or Transcatheter Pulmonary Valve?

This device is a trans-catheter pulmonary valve that can be deployed into an RV-PA conduit. Provided the conduit is of an appropriate size and length for the patient, a Melody valve can be deployed into the conduit in cases where severe or pulmonary regurgitation exists and functions as a pulmonary valve (Figure 64.5).

Suggested Reading

Downing TE, Kim YY. Tetralogy of Fallot: general principles of management. *Cardiol Clin.* 2015;33 (4):531–41. PMID: 26471818.

El Amrousy DM, Elshmaa NS, El-Kashlan M, et al. Efficacy of prophylactic dexmedetomidine in preventing postoperative junctional ectopic tachycardia after pediatric cardiac surgery. *J Am Heart Assoc.* 2017 Mar; 6(3): e004780. PMID: 28249845.

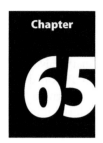

Transposition of the Great Arteries

Devyani Chowdhury and Ramesh Kodavatiganti

> A 26-year-old has a full-term delivery of a 3.8 kg male baby that has an in-utero fetal diagnosis of transposition of the great arteries (TGA). Apgar scores are 4 and 6 (at 1 and 5 min). You are called upon for help.

What Is Transposition of the Great Arteries (TGA)?

TGA is a congenital cardiac malformation accounting for 5–7% of congenital cardiac anomalies. The basic abnormality in TGA is that the aorta arises from a morphologic right ventricle, and the pulmonary artery arises from a morphologic left ventricle (Figure 65.1). The common clinical entity of "simple" TGA is associated with situs solitus atria, concordant atrioventricular, and discordant ventriculo-arterial alignment. The anatomic derangement results in systemic venous blood flow predominantly to the aorta and pulmonary venous blood to the pulmonary artery creating a circulation in parallel. The deoxygenated and oxygenated blood need to mix at atrial, ventricular, or ductal level to be compatible with life. This physiologically uncorrected entity of TGA is fatal without treatment with mortality of 30% in the first week of life and 90% mortality within the first year.

What Are Oxygen Saturations in TGA?

Oxygen saturations greater than 85% on room air are reassuring; however, if the baby is severely cyanotic it is concerning as the baby may have pulmonary hypertension or poor mixing of the oxygenated and deoxygenated blood secondary to a restricted atrial septum.

What Is the Difference between D- and L-TGA?

In D-TGA the aorta is anterior and rightward, or dextroposed, and the circulations are parallel. In L-TGA, the circulation is in series and is often referred to as "corrected transposition" or "ventricular inversion." Anatomically, there is atrio-ventricular and ventriculo-arterial discordance which causes the deoxygenated venous return coming to the right atrium to get to the pulmonary artery but via a morphological left ventricle. The oxygenated pulmonary venous blood returns to the aorta via the morphological right ventricle.

What Is the Status of the Atrial Septum?

The atrial septum is very important in patients with D-TGA. This is the site of mixing of blood and allows the patient to have a systemic circulation with improved oxygenation. Secondly, the nonrestrictive atrial septum allows the decompression of the left atrium and a decrease in left atrial pressures.

What Is the Role of the PDA in This Congenital Anomaly?

The size and patency of the PDA is important (in the setting of a restricted atrial septum) in determining the degree of mixing of systemic and pulmonary circulations, and thereby survival. The patency of the PDA becomes less important if the atrial septum is non-restrictive. Hence it is not unusual to discontinue the prostaglandin after an atrial septostomy.

What Other Anomalies Occur with TGA?

No other coexisting defects may be present in nearly half of the patients with TGA. A persistent PDA or patent foramen ovale (PFO) may be the only anomaly. However, in about 40–45% of patients with TGA, a VSD is the most common anomaly. A combination VSD with significant left ventricular outflow tract obstruction (LVOTO) is seen in about 10% of patients. The presence of these coexisting defects along with valvular anomalies may alter surgical planning.

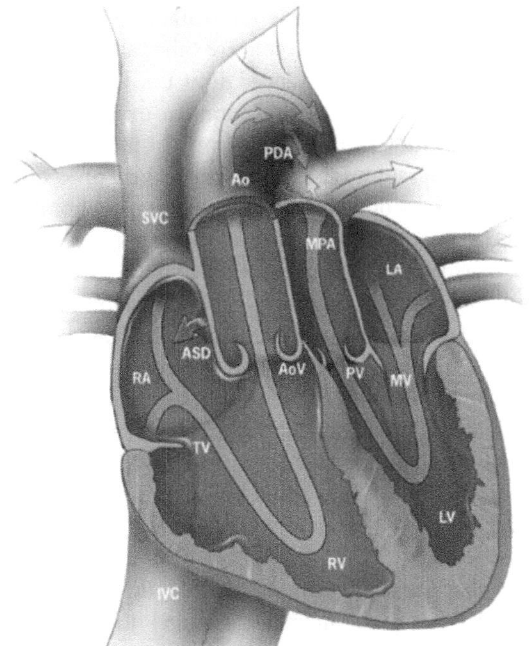

Figure 65.1 Illustration of transposition of the great vessels. RA and LA, right and left atrium; RV and LV, right and left ventricles; SVC and IVC, superior and inferior vena cava respectively; TV, MV, PV, AoV, tricuspid, mitral, pulmonary, and aortic valves respectively; MPA, main pulmonary artery; PDA, patent ductus arteriosus; ASD; atrial septal defect. Image courtesy of the Centers for Disease Control and Prevention, USA

The VSD may be small or large and located anywhere in the septum. Conoventricular or perimembranous VSDs account for 33% followed by malalignment for 30% and muscular defects accounting for 27%.

Is Pulmonary Stenosis Seen in Association with TGA?

Usually TGA with intact septum does not have pulmonary stenosis (PS).

Patients with TGA/VSD may have PS and can be extremely cyanotic.

How Is the Diagnosis of TGA Confirmed?

Echocardiography is the mainstay in confirming the diagnosis of d-TGA. The presence of a PDA, interatrial septal communication or VSD and other anomalies should be confirmed. These findings are important in surgical planning.

What Is the Difference in Circulation Physiology between a Normal Neonate and a Neonate Born with TGA?

The anatomic derangement results in deoxygenated systemic venous blood flow predominantly to the aorta and oxygenated pulmonary venous blood to the pulmonary artery creating a circulation in parallel. This means that the deoxygenated blood returns via the aorta back to the body and the oxygenated blood returns to the pulmonary circulation for re-oxygenation, causing a complete physiological right-to-left (to systemic circulation) and left-to-right shunt (to pulmonary circulation). The deoxygenated and oxygenated blood need to mix at the atrial, ventricular, or ductal level to be compatible with life. This mixing allows some deoxygenated blood to get oxygenated and some oxygenated blood to return to the systemic circulation.

How Is Survival Possible in a Parallel Circulation as Noted in TGA?

A parallel circulation is incompatible with life. There has to be mixing at the atrial, ventricular, or ductal level for the patient to survive. This physiologically uncorrected entity of TGA is fatal without treatment with mortality of 30% in the first week of life and 90% mortality within the first year.

What Are the Immediate Measures in a Neonate Born with a Confirmed Prenatal Diagnosis of TGA?

Room air oxygen saturations are one of the most important determining factors for management of the neonate. Umbilical lines may be placed as part of initial management. If the neonate is cyanotic, an atrial septostomy can be performed in the cardiac catheterization laboratory or at the bedside using echocardiography.

What Is a Typical ABG in d-TGA?

A typical arterial blood gas in room air reveals systemic pO_2 values <30 mm Hg that remain below 35–40 mm Hg during 100% oxygen administration, suggesting intracardiac mixing as the etiology of cyanosis versus a pulmonary etiology. In addition, in d-TGA the pCO_2 is also low as there is a high pulmonary blood flow which washes out the CO_2. The pH is also usually normal. In d-TGA there is no paucity of pulmonary blood flow, but it is oxygenated blood that keeps returning back to the pulmonary circulation. On the contrary, the systemic circulation receives deoxygenated blood and thus metabolic acidosis ensues due to anaerobic metabolism.

What Data on Echocardiogram Would Help Decide Medical Versus Interventional Management?

The status of the interatrial septum is the most important parameter in deciding further course of management.

What Is the Medical Management in the Newborn with TGA?

Treatment with prostaglandin to keep the ductus patent is the mainstay of medical management. Correction of metabolic acidosis and inotropic support is sometimes necessary with the goal of maintaining oxygen saturations between 75% and 85%.

What Are the Complications Associated with the Administration of Prostaglandins?

Prostaglandins can cause apnea, fever, seizures, and skin blanching.

What Is the Role of Mechanical Ventilation in This Medical Management?

Ventilation may need to be supported if the apneic spells are frequent and prolonged. The patient should be mechanically ventilated if a septostomy is performed.

What Is the Purpose of the Balloon Atrial Septostomy (BAS)? How Can It Be Performed?

The communication between the left and right atrium created by the atrial septostomy will allow for mixing of oxygenated and de-oxygenated blood.

The procedure can be performed at bedside or in the catheterization laboratory. In babies less than 48 h old, the umbilical vein can be used successfully for BAS. Percutaneous needle and catheter sheath placement via femoral vein access are other alternatives.

The catheter is advanced into the left atrium or pulmonary vein, across the foramen ovale. The catheter tip location should be confirmed – most readily by echocardiography (at-bedside–performed procedures) or by fluoroscopy (in the catheterization laboratory). The balloon is inflated with dilute angiographic contrast medium to approximately 15 mm in diameter, and then rapidly withdrawn across the septum with a short sharp tug. The procedure is repeated several times with increasing balloon volumes until balloon inflation at the level of the septum meets with minimal resistance. On echocardiography an interatrial defect of 5–6 mm represents an adequate BAS and palliation.

Complications such as tears of the atrial wall, pulmonary veins, and inferior vena cava (IVC) are uncommon. Temporary heart block which is self-limiting rarely happens and may rarely need long-term pacing.

BAS improves neonatal survival to more than 95%. However, centers that perform early arterial switch choose to perform BAS only in cases with profound hypoxemia or when surgery is delayed for other reasons.

What Are the Surgical Options for the Neonate with TGA?

If the baby is a few days old and has no other extra cardiac anomalies, the arterial switch operation, or Jatene procedure, is the surgical procedure of choice.

If the patient presents late or with other reasons to avoid cardiopulmonary bypass (CPB), the patient can be managed for a few months medically with an atrial septostomy. The patient would then be a candidate for an "atrial switch procedure" like Mustard or Senning where an atrial baffle is created to redirect the deoxygenated blood to the left ventricle, which is connected to the pulmonary artery. The atrial switch operation leaves the morphological right ventricle as the systemic ventricle.

What Are the Names of the Surgical Procedures and How Do They Differ from Each Other?

Arterial switch: Jatene's procedure (1975) – creates left ventricle as the systemic chamber and anatomically provides corrective repair.

Atrial switch: Senning (1959) or Mustard (1964), which baffles the venous return to the left ventricle and serves as the pulmonary ventricle, leaving the right ventricle as the systemic ventricle. This results in physiologic correction however with the left ventricle functioning as the pulmonary ventricle and the right ventricle as the systemic ventricle.

In the Senning procedure the atrial baffle is created from the right atrial wall and atrial septal tissue. No extrinsic tissue or materials are used.

The Mustard operation on the other hand involves resection of the atrial septum and creation of a baffle from synthetic material.

Both these procedures are performed usually between 1 month and 1 year of age. Surgical mortality from these procedures is usually between 1% and 10%.

Rastelli operation (1969): This surgical option is usually reserved for TGA with pulmonary outflow tract obstruction and VSD. The procedure entails using the VSD as part of the LVOT and placement of a baffle within the RV directing oxygenated blood from the VSD to the aorta. The pulmonary valve is oversewn and a conduit is inserted between the RV and PA. A subaortic and large VSD is suitable for this procedure as surgical enlargement carries a large risk of causing complete heart block. The biggest advantage with this procedure is that the LV becomes the systemic ventricle, however an important limitation is that multiple reoperations are needed during the patient's life.

What Prompts Correction versus Palliative Procedure?

Age. If the patient is older than six to eight weeks, then the left ventricle is de-conditioned as it is no longer pumping to the systemic circulation but instead to the pulmonary circulation. The pulmonary circulation is at a lower pressure than the systemic circulation so performing an arterial switch at a later age does not allow the LV to generate systemic pressure. The patient may need to undergo pulmonary artery banding to prepare the LV prior to a switch.

The presence of other extra-cardiac anomalies may preclude an arterial switch operation.

Other conditions like RSV infection and MRSA pneumonia may preclude CPB.

What Are Some of the Anesthetic Considerations Preoperatively in This Neonate Scheduled for TGA?

These patients are usually monitored and managed in the ICU setting. It is important to perform a complete assessment of the child for any extra cardiac anomalies which can alter further management. A review of the arterial blood gases since birth should be done to identify current ventilation, oxygenation, and acid base status. A neutral acid base status with saturations in the mid 80% is preferred for a balanced circulation hence avoiding systemic acidosis or pulmonary overcirculation.

These patients may be supported on mechanical ventilation secondary to increasing apneic spells by the institution of prostaglandin infusions to keep the PDA open for systemic circulation. An assessment of the umbilical lines if present should identify the correct depth of catheter insertion and presence of free aspiration of blood.

What Are Some of the Risk Factors for an Increased Perioperative Mortality?

A restrictive PFO or ASD, persistent pulmonary hypertension, prematurity, low birth weight and a delayed diagnosis all tend to increase mortality.

What Is the Strategy for Monitoring in These Patients during Surgical Correction of TGA?

The presence of a fresh umbilical stump makes it conducive for placement of invasive monitoring lines both venous and arterial. Normally the umbilical cord is composed of a gelatinous material – Whartons jelly – two umbilical arteries, and one umbilical vein. These blood vessels can be accessed under sterile conditions for central venous access and invasive arterial pressure monitoring. Central venous access under ultrasound guidance via the internal jugular or femoral route is another alternative.

What Are Some of the Important Intraoperative Anesthetic Considerations?

Almost all of these infants will present to the OR with an intravenous access – central (umbilical) or peripheral. A narcotic-based induction technique followed by a balanced anesthetic with narcotics and inhalational agents is often a prudent choice with better control of hemodynamics as well as blunting of the stress response.

Occasionally profound arterial desaturations may be seen during induction of anesthesia and positive pressure ventilation in the patient with TGA/IVS. It is often related to the sudden suppression of endogenous catecholamines, along with the decreased preload due to positive pressure ventilation and decreased myocardial contractility due to the high dose narcotics. Inadequate ventilation may cause hypercarbia and pulmonary hypertension.

Ensuring adequate ventilation, oxygenation, anesthetic depth and volume status are the steps to ensuring recovery from these critical moments failing which cardiopulmonary bypass may need to institute rapidly.

Is the Cardiopulmonary Bypass Different for Correction of TGA?

The conduct of CPB is unique to each institution and may include flow rates of 200 mL/kg/min, moderate hypothermia of 28–32°C, blood cardioplegia, and modified ultrafiltration at the termination of CPB. The use of antifibrinolytics (aminocaproic acid) is useful in control of coagulopathies.

What Are Some of the Critical Issues Soon after Termination of Cardiopulmonary Bypass?

As soon as CPB is terminated, global ventricular function and regional myocardial wall motion abnormalities should be assessed by transesophageal echocardiograph (TEE). The presence of regional wall motion abnormalities (RWMAs) may alert to kinking or spasm of the coronary ostia which may require repair of anastomosis and/or infusion of nitroglycerin to maximally dilate the coronaries.

The presence and persistence of arrhythmias is an indicator of abnormal myocardial perfusion and coronary artery problems must be ruled out.

Neonates with TGA/intact ventricular septum (IVS) usually will not tolerate acute and significant changes in preload and afterload due to a deconditioning of the LV. Transfusion of blood and vasodilators should be carefully titrated to intracardiac filling pressures (LA or RA) along with maintenance of systolic blood pressure in the range of 50–70 mmHg and RA pressures in the range of 5–6 mmHg.

Chest closure may sometimes become difficult due to myocardial edema, hemodynamic instability, coagulopathy, and need for transfusion of blood products.

Is Inotropic Support Mandatory for the Termination of Bypass?

Inotropic support is needed in situations where global ventricular function is depressed and coronary arterial abnormalities have been excluded. Infusions may include either or a combination of dopamine 3–10 mcg/kg/min, epinephrine 0.03–0.05 mcg/kg/min or milrinone 0.25–0.75 mcg.kg/min. Nitroglycerin infusion at 1–2 mcg/kg/min may be added to aid in coronary vasodilation and relief of increased afterload.

Increasing dosage of inotropic support with increasing systemic acidosis and hemodynamic instability warrant re-exploration and correction of the coronary anastomosis.

Is There a Need for Intraoperative Transesophageal Echocardiography?

Intraoperative TEE is useful in the assessment of ventricular function and regional wall motion abnormalities after switching of the great vessels and reimplantation of coronaries to the neoaorta. TEE is also useful in the assessment of de-airing of the ventricles after completion of the surgical repair and cessation of cardiopulmonary bypass. TEE is also useful in assessment of the anastomotic sites of the neoaorta and neopulmonary artery.

What Are the Immediate Postoperative Concerns in the Intensive Care Unit after Correction of TGA?

Arrhythmias, depressed ventricular function, and ongoing coagulopathy are critical issues during the early postoperative period. Cardiac catheterization for assessment of coronaries and surgical reexploration is warranted if myocardial function continues to be depressed or deteriorating. Circulatory support with extracorporeal circulation should be warranted if hemodynamic instability continues.

What Are the Common Complications after an Arterial Switch Operation (ASO)?

Arrhythmias, LV dysfunction, sudden cardiac death, pulmonary artery stenosis, and neoaortic valve regurgitation are common late sequelae after ASO. Symptoms of myocardial ischemia are atypical due to the denervation of the heart at the time of the ASO. It is therefore important to be aware of this complication and remain vigilant.

Suggested Reading

Boris JR. Primary care management of patients with common arterial trunk and transposition of the great arteries. *Cardiol Young*. 2012;22 (6):761–7. PMID: 23331600.

Anomalous Pulmonary Venous Return

Jamie W. Sinton

A one-hour-old male is severely tachypneic. He is the product of a full-term spontaneous vaginal delivery to a healthy 27-year-old G1 now P1 mother with good prenatal care. In the delivery room, Apgar scores were 7 at one and five minutes. Central and peripheral cyanosis were present and did not improve with supplemental oxygen.

DIAGNOSIS

What Are the Important Diagnoses to Consider?

Differential diagnosis for this patient is broad and includes:

- transient tachypnea of the newborn;
- meconium aspiration;
- pulmonary hypertension;
- congenital heart disease.

Life-threatening diagnoses such as total anomalous pulmonary venous return (TAPVR) should be ruled out prior to evaluation for less severe disorders.

Is Routine Newborn Pulse Oximetry Screening Useful in Identifying TAPVR?

Not necessarily. Neonates with TAPVR may not be cyanotic at birth. However, pulse oximetry will detect even suboptimal oxygen saturation without frank or severe cyanosis.

Screening pulse oximetry is performed to detect infants with potentially life-threatening duct-dependent lesions or lesions requiring an invasive procedure within the first 28 days of life.

What Clinical Signs and Symptoms are Present in Children with TAPVR?

The signs and symptoms depend of the presence or absence of pulmonary venous obstruction. In patients with obstruction they may include:

- Soft murmur over the vertical vein;
- Cool to cold extremities;
- Cyanosis;
- Tachypnea;
- Hepatomegaly (infracardiac location of anomalous veins);
- Hypotension.

Describe the Anatomy of Pulmonary Venous Drainage in TAPVR

Total anomalous pulmonary venous return is a rare condition in which all pulmonary venous blood empties into the systemic circulation or directly into the right atrium. A right-to-left shunt at the atrial level maintains systemic cardiac output. This may be in the form of a patent foramen ovale (PFO) or atrial septal defect (ASD).

There are four anatomic variants of TAPVR and these are classified according to their relationship with the systemic veins.

Supracardiac TAPVR. The pulmonary veins retain their connection to the embryologic cardinal veins. Pulmonary veins from the left and right lung coalesce and continue as a vertical vein that drains into the right superior vena cava (SVC), azygous vein, or the left SVC. Supracardiac location is the most common variant and is present in nearly 50% of patients with TAPVR (Figure 66.1).

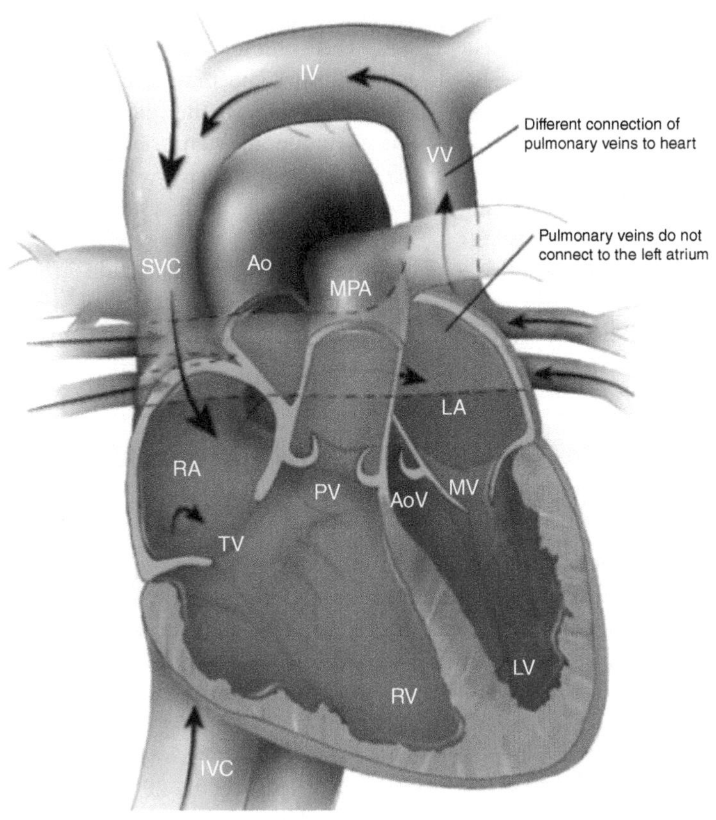

Figure 66.1 Drawing of supracardiac anomalous venous return. The pulmonary veins coalesce posterior to the heart and travel cranially via the vertical vein, eventually draining into the right atrium: IVC, inferior vena cava; SVC, superior vena cava; RA, right atrium; TV, tricuspid valve; RV, right ventricle; PV, pulmonary valve; MPA, main pulmonary artery; LA, left atrium; AoV, aortic valve; LV, left ventricle; MV, mitral valve; PVs, pulmonary veins; VV, vertical vein; IV, innominate vein. Image courtesy of the Centers for Disease Control and Prevention, USA

Cardiac TAPVR. The PVs retain their connection to the embryologic cardinal veins. The veins drain into the right heart directly via the right atrium or via the coronary sinus.

Infracardiac TAPVR. The pulmonary veins (PV) retain their connection to the embryologic umbilicovitelline veins. Pulmonary veins from the left and right lung coalesce and continue as a vertical vein that travels inferiorly through the mediastinum, through the diaphragm, and inserts into the portal vein or inferior vena cava (IVC) below the diaphragm. Due to their lengthy course, infracardiac TAPVR has the highest risk of becoming obstructed.

Mixed TAPVR. Sites of pulmonary venous drainage in mixed TAPVR are variable as the name suggests. Commonly the left and right pulmonary veins have separate drainage patterns. These drainage patterns may involve supra-cardiac, cardiac, or infracardiac locations.

What Anatomic Anomalies Are Associated with TAPVR?

Atrial septal defects (ASD) are nearly universally present, as they allow pulmonary venous blood to enter the left atrium and maintain systemic cardiac output. If a paucity of blood has entered the left-sided heart structures in utero, left-sided heart structures may be small in size. Other associated lesions include: patent ductus arteriosus, ventricular septal defect, and pulmonary stenosis.

Heterotaxy with poly- or asplenia is also common in patients with TAPVR.

What Are the Clinical Presentations of TAPVR?

Clinical presentation is patient dependent and based on the anatomic variant and presence or absence of obstruction. A neonate with obstruction of any of the anatomic variants of TAPVR will be critically ill, severely cyanotic, and have severe pulmonary edema.

Supracardiac TAPVR. Clinical presentation is usually with tachypnea alone as these veins are less commonly unobstructed. An ASD is usually present and allows right-to-left shunting (and left heart filling). The patients are often not markedly cyanotic as the larger shunt from the lesion is left to right (pulmonary veins to right atrium).

Cardiac TAPVR. As pulmonary veins of cardiac TAPVR are least likely to be obstructed, presentation may be subtle. Saturated blood from the pulmonary veins usually drains into the left atrium via an unroofed coronary sinus (CS) or ASD.

Infracardiac TAPVR. Pulmonary veins of infracardiac TAPVR are very likely to be obstructed. Clinical presentation is often of a tachypneic, cyanotic infant in significant respiratory distress with pulmonary edema.

Mixed TAPVR. As expected, presentation is usually dictated by degree of obstruction of pulmonary venous drainage.

How Is the Diagnosis of TAPVR Established?

Pre- or postnatal echo can suggest the diagnosis. Transesophageal echocardiography is not performed as placement of the echo probe may compress any pulmonary venous confluence posterior to the left atrium and result in rapid cardiovascular collapse.

How Is Pulmonary Venous Obstruction (PVO) Defined?

Suboptimal oxygen saturation in addition to nonphasic flow velocity (on echo) greater than 1.8 m/s define PVO.

What Are the Physiologic Consequences of PVO?

Veins that are obstructed have consequent pulmonary venous hypertension. This increases pulmonary capillary pressure and very quickly leads to pulmonary edema. At this point, chest roentgenogram reveals bilateral infiltrates and may be confused with intrinsic lung disease. After the development of pulmonary edema, pulmonary arteries constrict to prevent further edema. Subsequently, right ventricular (RV) pressures increase, and systemic hypoxia ensues.

Hypoxic pulmonary vasoconstriction further increases pulmonary vascular resistance (PVR), exacerbates RV hypertension, and worsens physiologic trespass.

What Is the Natural History of TAPVR?

The clinical course of TAPVR depends on the presence and degree of obstruction.

Patients with severe obstruction require emergent surgical intervention.

Patients with restrictive intra-atrial communication (small ASD) require intervention to enlarge this communication and maintain cardiac output and oxygenation.

For those who survive infancy, repair of TAPVR has a good prognosis (Reddy et al., 2011). In each of the 26 patients reported, there were no early deaths or postoperative complications. None in this series had infracardiac TAPVR. Of those with significant RV dysfunction, a 5 mm ASD was left open postoperatively. Factors attributed to survival beyond infancy include a large ASD and near normal pulmonary vascular resistance.

Patients with unobstructed veins may go unrecognized with mild symptoms. These patients generally suffer from chronic right heart failure due to overcirculation and may develop pulmonary hypertension.

What Is the Short-Term Outcome of Infants Born with TAPVR?

Postoperative survival is reduced in neonates by the presence of pulmonary venous obstruction, mixed TAPVR, single ventricle physiology, or heterotaxy. Early mortality postoperatively occurs in about 5% of patients. Patients with single ventricle anatomy have a high mortality and morbidity due to chronic pulmonary vein stenosis requiring reoperation.

What Is the Long-Term Outcome of Infants Born with TAPVR? What Cardiac Interventions Are often Required Years Following the Initial Repair?

Severe and recurrent pulmonary vein obstruction is a leading cause of late mortality. After correction of TAPVR, pulmonary venous confluence stenosis remains a long-term complication. While percutaneous interventions have been successful in the form of PV stents, chronic obstruction remains a major source of morbidity.

What Are the Specific Anesthetic Concerns Related to Patients with TAPVR?

Patients with TAPVR require management of pulmonary blood flow as they generally have some degree of pulmonary overload. This may result in chronic pulmonary venous congestion and reduced lung compliance. High inspired oxygen concentration is often required in addition to higher levels of positive end-expiratory pressure (PEEP). Avoidance of metabolic acidosis is important and attempts to correct base deficits should be considered when appropriate.

For a variety of reasons (circulatory overload, small left ventricle, associate anomalies) these patients may require inotropic support.

Transesophageal echocardiography is usually avoided as it may worsen obstruction by external compression, especially in neonates.

Pre-bypass, inhaled nitric oxide is avoided as this may increase pulmonary blood flow and worsen cyanosis. Post-bypass, inhaled nitric oxide is often used and should be immediately available to reduce pulmonary vascular resistance.

Post-bypass, the left heart, which is often small, may be ill-prepared to accept the full complement of pulmonary venous return.

In patients post repair of anomalous veins, recurrent venous obstruction should be considered.

How Is TAPVR Different from PAPVR?

PAPVR or partial anomalous pulmonary venous return is where one or more (but not all) of the pulmonary veins drains outside the left atrium. Most commonly a single vein drains into the SVC and is a source of persistent left-to-right shunt. Chronic right heart overload can, over time, lead to symptoms of congestion however PAPVR, especially single anomalous veins, is often an incidental finding and does not require treatment.

What Are the Specific Anesthetic Concerns Related to Patients with PAPVR?

Patients with one or more anomalous veins (especially supracardiac veins entering the SVC) are considered for a Warden Procedure. This procedure involves removing the portion of the SVC with the anomalous veins connected and baffling this blood to the left atrium. The SVC flow is reestablished with the use of a small conduit. As such, issues related to the baffle as well as the SVC conduit may occur, especially stenosis.

Suggested Reading

DiBardino DJ, McKenzie ED, Heinle JS, et al. The Warden procedure for partially anomalous pulmonary venous connection to the superior caval vein. *Cardiol Young.* 2004;14 (1):64–7. PMID: 15237673.

Mahle WT, Newburger JW, Matherne P, et al. Role of pulse oximetry in examining newborns for congenital heart disease: a scientific statement from the AHA and AAP. *Pediatrics.* 2009;124(2):823–6. PMID: 19581259.

Reddy KP, Nagarajan R, Rani U, et al. Total anomalous pulmonary venous connection beyond infancy. *Asian Cardiovasc Thorac Ann.* 2011;19: 249–52. PMID: 21885551.

Shi G, Zhu Z, Chen J, et al. Total anomalous pulmonary venous connection: the current management strategies in a pediatric cohort. *Circulation.* 2017;135(1):48–58. PMID: 27881562.

Chapter 67

Truncus Arteriosus

Devyani Chowdhury and Ramesh Kodavatiganti

A four-day-old term baby boy is transferred from an outside hospital with a postnatal observation of a murmur. There was no prenatal care prior to delivery. The baby had some peripheral cyanosis at birth which corrected with supplemental oxygen. His tachypnea is more pronounced with feeds.

Vitals BP 63/39, Pulse 166, Temp 36.9°C, Resp 49/min at rest and 60–70 per min with feeds, Wt 2.8 kg, SpO_2 94% on 1L nasal cannula.

Physical examination reveals a cleft palate, coarse respiratory sounds, and a continuous precordial murmur. Subcostal retractions are present when the child is fed. The abdomen is soft with a fullness appreciated over the hepatic border. Bounding pulses are present throughout.

What Is a Truncus Arteriosus (TA) Anomaly?

Truncus arteriosus (TA) is a rare congenital anomaly characterized by a common arterial trunk from which the ascending aorta and the pulmonary arteries originate distal to the coronary arteries but proximal to the first brachiocephalic branch of the aortic arch (Figure 67.1).

The common arterial trunk arises from normal ventricles and the semilunar valve is labeled as a truncal valve. In patients with a normal aortic arch, the ductus arteriosus may be either absent or diminutive.

How Is TA Classified?

The pulmonary artery arises from the TA in many different patterns and is the basis used to classify subtypes of TA. There are two classifications commonly used: Collett and Edwards (1949) and Von Praagh (1965).

The earliest classification, developed by Collett and Edwards, includes TA types I–IV, as follows:

- Type I TA is characterized by origin of a single pulmonary trunk from the left lateral aspect of the common arterial trunk, with the left and right pulmonary branches arising from the pulmonary trunk.
- Type II TA is characterized by separate but proximate origins of the left and right pulmonary arterial branches from the posterolateral aspect of the common arterial trunk.
- Type III TA occurs when the branch pulmonary arteries originate independently from the common arterial trunk or aortic arch, most often from the left and right lateral aspects of the trunk.
- Type IV TA, originally proposed as a form of the lesion with neither pulmonary arterial branch arising from the common trunk, is now recognized to be a form of pulmonary atresia with ventricular septal defect.

The Van Praagh classification includes four primary types of TA variants:

- Type A1 is identical to the type I of Collett and Edwards.
- Type A2 includes Collett and Edwards type II and most cases of type III, namely those with separate origin of the branch pulmonary arteries from the left and right lateral aspects of the common trunk.
- Type A3 includes cases with origin of one branch pulmonary artery (usually the right) from the common trunk, with pulmonary blood supply to the other lung provided either by a pulmonary artery arising from the aortic arch (a subtype of Collett and Edwards type III) or by hyphenate arterial collaterals.
- Type A4 is defined not by the pattern of origin of branch pulmonary arteries, but rather by the coexistence of an interrupted aortic arch. In the

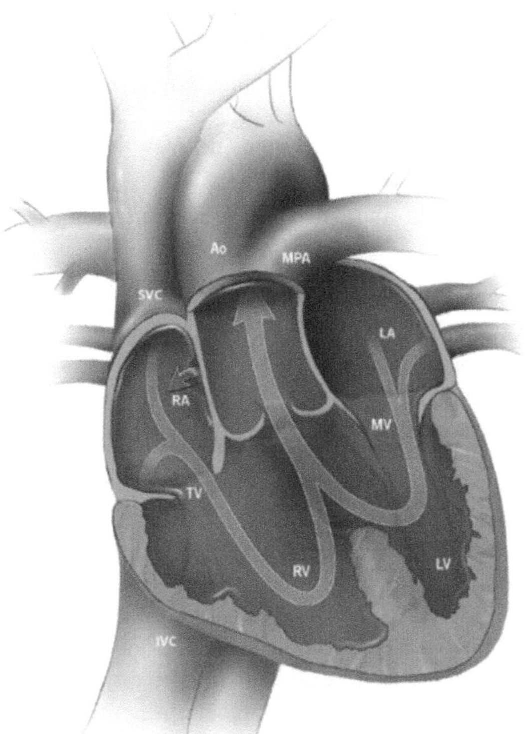

Figure 67.1 Illustration of truncus arteriosus (TA). RA and LA, right and left atrium; RV and LV, right and left ventricles; SVC and IVC, superior and inferior vena cava respectively; TV, MV, tricuspid, mitral, valves respectively; MPA, main pulmonary artery; Ao, aorta. Image courtesy of Centers for Disease Control and Prevention, USA

vast majority of cases of type A4, which fall into the type I of Collett and Edwards, the pulmonary arteries arise as a single pulmonary trunk that then branches. In any of these patterns, intrinsic stenosis, hypoplasia, or both may be present in one or both branch pulmonary arteries, which may have an effect on management and outcome.

What Are the Presenting Signs and Symptoms?

Poor feeding, diaphoresis, tachypnea, and cyanosis are common presenting symptoms with TA although many are prenatally diagnosed by echocardiography.

What Is the Embryological Basis for This Anomaly?

The failure of complete or incomplete septation of the embryonic TA leads to this uncommon anomaly. Because the common trunk originates from both the left and right ventricles, and pulmonary arteries arise directly from the common trunk, a ductus arteriosus is not required to support the fetal circulation.

Is There a Genetic Abnormality Associated with TA?

As with other congenital cardiac anomalies of the conotruncal region, a substantial number of patients with TA (approximately 30–40%) have microdeletions within chromosome band 22q11.2. This particular type of chromosomal deletion is thought to affect migration or development of cardiac neural crest cells and may contribute to the pathogenesis of TA.

Is TA Associated with Any Other Congenital Heart Defects?

Structural abnormalities of the truncal valve, including dysplastic and supernumerary leaflets including truncal valve regurgitation (moderate or severe) may be present in 20% or more of patients. Approximately one third of patients will have a right-sided aortic arch.

Coronary artery abnormalities are common and may include as single coronary artery with an intramural course as the most important variation.

Interrupted aortic arch is a commonly noted anomaly, which almost always occurs between the left common carotid and subclavian arteries (type B).

Other uncommon associations include: persistent left superior vena cava, aberrant subclavian artery, and atrial septal defects. Complete atrioventricular septal defect, double aortic arch, and various forms of functionally univentricular heart are some rare associations.

What Is the Typical Pathophysiology of the Anomaly?

Cyanosis and systemic ventricular volume overload are the two hallmarks of TA.

The cardiac output from both ventricles is directed into the common arterial trunk – arterial trunk. The amount of pulmonary blood flow derived from this combined ventricular output is dependent on the ratio of resistances to flow in the pulmonary and systemic vascular beds. The mixing of left and right ventricular output at the level of the arterial trunk (during systole) is the reason for cyanosis.

Infants with TA may present in shock because of high output heart failure with significant pulmonary overcirculation. This may resemble the presentation of neonatal sepsis, especially when the ratio of Qp:Qs is sufficiently high that the patient is not cyanotic.

What Is the Natural History of TA Anomaly?

In numerous earlier series, the median age at death without surgery ranged from two weeks to three months, with almost 100% mortality by age one year. Cardiac arrest or multiple organ failure secondary to systemic hypoperfusion, progressive metabolic acidosis, and myocardial dysfunction are causes of death in the unrepaired patient with TA.

Currently, for patients undergoing complete repair in the neonatal period or early infancy, early postoperative mortality is generally less than 10%. Among patients surviving the initial postoperative period, the survival rate at a 10- to 20-year follow-up is higher than 80%, with most deaths resulting from sequelae of late repair (pulmonary vascular obstructive disease), reinterventions, or residual/recurrent physiologic abnormalities.

Is This a Surgical Emergency? What Is the Surgical Approach?

The degree of pulmonary overcirculation leading to congestive heart failure dictates the urgency and need for medical management versus surgical repair.

Early neonatal repair is the recommendation. However, a delay of up to two to three months is based on the individual. Early repairs avoid the development of severe pulmonary vascular occlusive (from pulmonary overcirculation) disease and the increase in mortality.

The repair involves removal of the pulmonary arteries, and closure of the defect either directly or with a patch, closure of the VSD, and a conduit from the RV to the pulmonary arteries to supply pulmonary blood flow.

What Are the Preanesthetic Concerns in This Child with TA Scheduled for Surgery?

DiGeorge syndrome, now referred to as 22q11 deletion syndrome and velocardiofacial syndrome (Shprintzen syndrome) is associated in 30–35% of patients with TA. The patients have variable, microdeletions of chromosome 22q11 or CATCH-22 syndrome.

The CATCH-22 acronym denotes the common associated anomalies:

C – Cardiac anomalies – especially interrupted aortic arch, TA, and tetralogy of Fallot

A – Abnormal facies (velocardiofacial syndrome)

T – Thymic aplasia

C – Cleft palate

H – Hypocalcemia/hypoparathyroidism

22 – Deletion of the 22nd chromosome

Patients with 22q deletion syndrome (previously DiGeorge syndrome) have thymic aplasia and parathyroid dysfunction and are at risk for developing hypocalcemia and immune deficiencies. They also have characteristic facies consisting of a cleft palate, long narrow face, prominent maxilla and a retruded chin. A careful airway assessment is necessary as these patients are often difficult intubations.

Other noncardiac anomalies found sporadically in patients with TA include renal abnormalities, vertebral and rib anomalies, and anomalies of the alimentary tract.

The association of the above syndromes requires vigilant monitoring of the serum calcium levels to avoid the risk of hypocalcemia. The possibility of immune deficiencies requires blood products to be irradiated.

Is There Any Role for Observing Infection Precautions in These Patients?

Thymic absence poses a risk for immune deficiencies in the form of T cell mediated immunity. This requires that all blood products be irradiated and serum calcium levels monitored when citrated blood products are administered. Sterile techniques should be employed during the placement and conduct of procedures.

How Is Anesthesia Managed in These Critically Ill Patients?

The patient's age and anatomy of the lesion dictate the anesthetic management. Patients with severe congestive heart failure (CHF) may require preoperative inotropic support, and anesthetic induction in these patients is aimed at maintaining systemic vascular resistance (SVR) and preserving myocardial function.

Some of these patients may be intubated in the ICU because of cardiopulmonary compromise.

The goal is to balance pulmonary to systemic blood flow by manipulating factors that enhance or reduce pulmonary blood flow. This becomes more critical after the first few days of life when a natural reduction in pulmonary vascular resistance (PVR) occurs promoting excessive pulmonary blood flood.

These infants are ventilated with an FiO_2 of 21% and $PaCO_2$ maintained around 45–50 mmHg targeting an arterial pH of 7.25–7.35. Transporting these patients to the operating room requires that the FiO_2 is maintained around 21%, with hypoventilation to achieve hypercarbia. Analgesia and muscle relaxants should be chosen to avoid tachycardia and hypotension. Inotropic support should be continued during transport to the operating room in infants with CHF.

The non-intubated infant must be managed very carefully. Intravenous induction is preferred with a synthetic opioid and muscle relaxant. Mask ventilation with 100% oxygen may be used immediately prior to intubation, however, once the trachea is intubated the FiO_2 should be decreased to 0.21 targeting a saturation of 75–85%. Minute ventilation should be controlled to maintain a $PaCO_2$ of 45–50 mmHg.

Maintenance of anesthesia and ventilation should be carefully titrated to optimize a balance between PVR and SVR, and a Qp:Qs ratio of 1:1 (see Chapter 62). Hyperventilation and high inspired oxygen concentrations should be avoided as they promote a decrease in PVR and will exacerbate pulmonary blood flow and lower diastolic perfusion pressure. In patients with truncal valve regurgitation this may precipitate myocardial ischemia.

Some patients may present in late infancy and may have developed significant pulmonary hypertension from chronic pulmonary overcirculation. Ironically these patients will require higher concentrations of FiO_2 to maintain SaO_2 between 75–85%.

These patients will require inotropic support and afterload reduction upon weaning from cardiopulmonary bypass. Transesophageal echocardiography aids in assessment of ventricular volumes and pulmonary artery pressures with the intent to improve right heart function. Pulmonary hypertension is frequently noted after weaning from cardiopulmonary bypass and may continue into the postoperative period.

What Are the Postoperative Concerns Following Repair of TA?

These patients should be sedated, paralyzed, and ventilated in the intensive care unit during the first 24 hours to avoid and/or minimize pulmonary hypertensive crises. Right heart inotropic support (milrinone), hyperventilation, 100% oxygen FiO_2, correction of acidosis, and nitric oxide are used as needed to treat any pulmonary hypertensive crisis. Residual VSDs, truncal valve anomalies (stenosis/regurgitation), or right ventricular incision (VSD closure, RV-PA conduit) may also cause right heart dysfunction. A bedside transthoracic echocardiography may be helpful in resolving this treatable clinical dilemma. Postoperative arrhythmias such as right bundle branch block, complete heart block, and atrial or junctional ectopic tachycardia can cause ventricular dysfunction. Supplemental calcium infusions may be beneficial due to the common association of TA with DiGeorge syndrome and after administration of citrate anticoagulated blood products.

What Are the Sequelae of TA Repair?

Residual VSD, truncal valve regurgitation, and stenosis of RV-PA conduits are late sequelae of truncus repair.

Suggested Reading

Boris JR. Primary care management of patients with common arterial trunk and transposition of the great arteries. *Cardiol Young.* 2012;22(6):761–7. PMID: 23331600.

Martin BJ, Karamlou TB, Tabbutt S. Shunt lesions part II: anomalous pulmonary venous connections and truncus arteriosus. *Pediatr Crit Care Med.* 2016;17(8 Suppl 1):S310–4. PMID: 27490615.

Chapter 68

Pulmonary Hypertension in Children

Yang Liu

A three-year-old female, former 29-week preterm infant, presents for direct laryngoscopy and bronchoscopy due to stridor at rest. She has a history of chronic lung disease, bronchopulmonary dysplasia, small perimembranous ventricular septal defect, patent foramen ovale, moderate patent ductus arteriosus (PDA) (s/p coiling closure), pulmonary hypertension (on sildenafil), subglottic stenosis, and previously tracheostomy dependent.

Current vital signs include: BP 86/42 mmHg; heart rate 112/min; respiratory rate 25/min; SpO_2 98% on room air. Auscultation reveals a loud systolic murmur. ECG shows sinus tachycardia, ST abnormality and T-wave inversion in inferolateral leads. Transthoracic echocardiography reveals a residual PDA with continuous left-to-right shunting with a peak velocity of about 2 m per second; sometimes has evidence of minimal right-to-left shunting in systole. Patent foramen ovale with left-to-right shunting. Mild tricuspid regurgitation, peak velocity ~4.7 m per second, consistent with right ventricular systolic pressure of 88 mmHg + right atrial pressure. Blood pressure 93/48. Mild right ventricular hypertrophy with qualitatively normal right ventricular size and systolic function.

What Is the Incidence of Pulmonary Hypertension in Pediatric Patients?

Pulmonary hypertension (PH) is defined as a resting mean pulmonary artery pressure (mPAP) >25 mm Hg in children under three months of age in term infants at sea level.

In utero, pulmonary artery pressure is similar to systemic arterial pressure. After birth, pulmonary artery pressure decreases rapidly. By two to three months of postnatal age, the pressure generally achieves adult values. The annual incidence of idiopathic PH and congenital heart disease (CHD) associated PH is 0.7% and 2.2, respectively.

What Are the Causes of Pulmonary Hypertension in Pediatric Patients?

In the majority of pediatric patients, PH is idiopathic or associated with congenital heart disease. PH is classified into five major groups:

Group 1: PH associated with CHD. PH associated with CHD is most commonly seen among patients with large left-to-right shunts, such as a ventricular septal defect (VSD), patent ductus arteriosus (PDA), complete atrioventricular canal, truncus arteriosus, and transposition of the great arteries. The size of the shunt, the blood flow through the shunt and the location of the shunt are the most important risk factors for the development of pulmonary arterial hypertension.

Group 2: PH due to left-sided heart disease. Left-sided heart diseases that can lead to PH include left ventricle systolic and/or diastolic dysfunction, valvular disease, congenital/acquired left heart inflow/outflow tract obstruction, and cardiomyopathy.

Group 3: PH caused by chronic lung disease or hypoxemia. Chronic lung diseases that can cause PH include bronchopulmonary dysplasia (BPD), lung hypoplasia, congenital diaphragmatic hernia (CDH), or other lung lesions.

Group 4: PH caused by chronic thromboembolic disease.

Group 5: PH with unclear or multifactorial mechanisms. A combination of many rare diseases that infrequently causes PH is still seen in children.

What Is the Pathophysiology of Pulmonary Hypertension?

Increased pulmonary artery pressure (PAP) can be caused by decreased cross-sectional area of the pulmonary vascular bed. Although pulmonary veins may be the primary site of the problem, small pulmonary arteries are most affected in cases of PH. The diameter of small pulmonary arteries or veins may be narrowed by active vasoconstriction and/or pathological remodeling of small vessels through medial hypertrophy, proliferation of "neointimal cells" and deposition of connective tissues. Medial hypertrophy can resolve when the inciting stimulus is removed.

Increased PAP can also be caused by increased pulmonary blood flow (most commonly due to CHD) and/or increased pulmonary venous pressure (most commonly due to elevated left atrial pressure).

What Is a Pulmonary Hypertensive Crisis?

A PH crisis is characterized by a rapid increase in pulmonary vascular resistance (PVR) that results in pulmonary pressure exceeding systemic arterial pressure. Hypercarbia, hypoxemia, acidosis, and noxious stimuli from pain or airway manipulation can all cause a sudden increase in PVR, resulting in pulmonary hypertensive crisis and/or right heart failure. A sudden increased pulmonary pressure will compromise cardiac output from the right ventricle. Left ventricular stroke volume will also decrease, as there is limited volume available for left ventricular filling. Without rapid and effective treatment, a pulmonary hypertensive crisis can soon escalate to circulatory collapse and death.

Review the Clinical Presentation and Investigation of a Patient with PH

Persistent and/or progressive PH are commonly associated with CHD, chronic lung disease, and idiopathic/heritable PH in children. Transient PH is also relatively common in newborns with persistent pulmonary hypertension or congenital diaphragmatic hernia. Children with PH often have chromosomal abnormalities and syndromes. Children with syndromes such as Down syndrome, DiGeorge syndrome, Pierre–Robin syndrome and Noonan syndrome are commonly found to have PH.

Symptoms of PH are often similar to other less severe childhood diseases. Common presentations include fatigue, difficulty breathing, or shortness of breath with activity, dizziness, fainting, swelling in the lower extremities, or chest pain. Because the symptoms are so common, the diagnosis for childhood PH is often delayed by several months.

PH should be suspected in any child with respiratory distress, labile oxygenation, and/or cyanosis. The physical examination may be unremarkable. The primary findings on physical examination include tachypnea, retractions, grunting, desaturation unresponsive to supplemental O_2, and cyanosis. Cardiac examination may have altered heart sounds, such as a loud P2, split S2, a systolic murmur secondary to tricuspid regurgitation, or a diastolic murmur of pulmonary valve regurgitation and the signs of right heart failure, such as hepatomegaly. The initial assessments include chest X-ray, electrocardiography (ECG), and echocardiography.

Describe the Appearance of a Chest X-Ray and ECG in a Patient with PH

The chest X-ray may be normal or may demonstrate changes of underlying disease. Radiographic signs of PH include right ventricle enlargement and enlarged main and hilar pulmonary arterial shadows with peripheral attenuation of peripheral pulmonary vascular markings. The ECG is abnormal in most cases, with right ventricular predominance. However, the findings from ECG are somewhat nonspecific.

What Echocardiographic Findings Are Suggestive of PH?

There are a host of echocardiographic signs suggestive of pulmonary hypertension. Enlargement of the right ventricle can be seen in the parasternal long axis view (Figure 68.1). Classically, a "D" shaped septum can be seen in the parasternal short axis view. Due to elevated right ventricle pressure, the interventricular septum bows toward the left ventricle (Figure 68.2). Cardiologists estimate the RV pressure by assessing the degree of regurgitation. RV pressure is always assessed in comparison to systemic blood pressure. RV pressure that is one-quarter to one-half of systemic is seen as mild to moderate. Pressures exceeding three-quarters of systemic blood pressure and certain RV pressure that is systemic or suprasystemic increases the risk for patients requiring anesthesia.

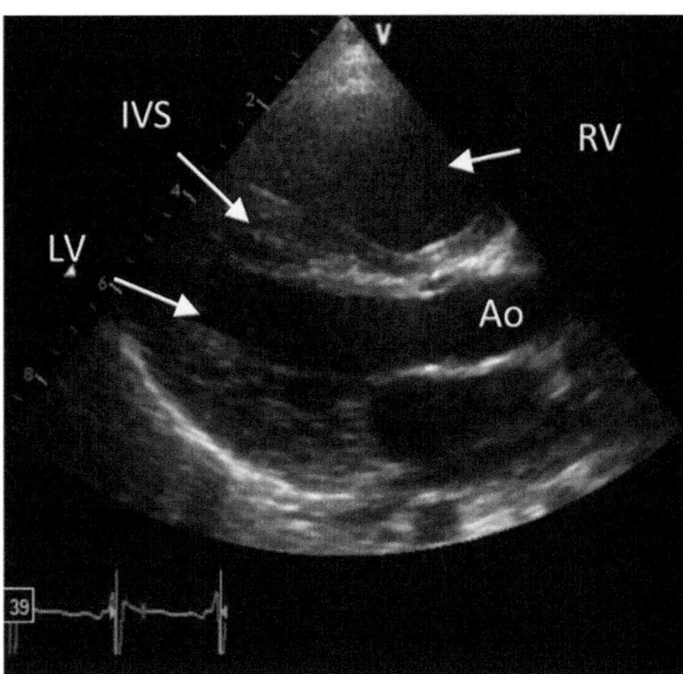

Figure 68.1 Parasternal long axis view of patient with severe pulmonary hypertension demonstrating a large right ventricle (RV), and bowing of the interventricular septum (IVS) into the left ventricle (LV) during systole. Ao, aorta. Courtesy of Adam C. Adler, MD

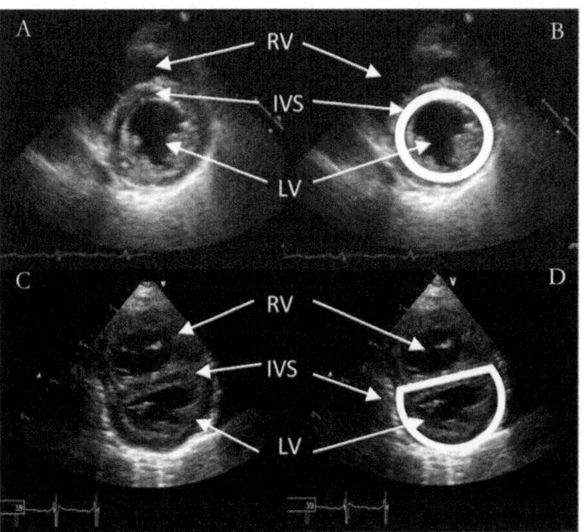

Figure 68.2 Parasternal short axis view demonstrating: (A) the normal position of the interventricular septum (IVS) and crescent shaped right ventricle (RV). (B) Schematic showing the normal relationship between the RV, IVS, and left ventricle (LV) in short axis. (C) Short axis view in the setting of severe pulmonary hypertension with large RV with downward displacement of the IVS. (D) Schematic showing the characteristic "D" shaped septum present with elevated RV pressures. Courtesy of Adam C. Adler, MD

How Is PH Diagnosed?

When PH is suspected, transthoracic echocardiography should be used to confirm the presence of pulmonary hypertension and provide additional information about the cause of PH. By measuring the systolic regurgitation of tricuspid flow velocity, Doppler echocardiography is able to estimate pulmonary artery systolic pressure. Pulmonary pressure obtained by Doppler echocardiography correlates with the values directly measured during right heart catheterization. Echocardiography is also useful to rule out congenital heart disease and to directly assess ventricular systolic and diastolic function. Cardiac catheterization is the gold standard to provide a definitive diagnosis of PH, and to determine the severity of PH. An acute vasoreactivity test is a particularly important component of cardiac catheterization to obtain the information for prognosis and to guide future treatment.

Review the Most Common Treatment Strategies for PH

The treatment of PH depends on the etiology of the original disease, the severity of PH, the cardiac and

Table 68.1 Target pathways and mechanism of action for the commonly used antipulmonary hypertensive agents

Agent	Pathway	Mechanism
Sildenafil	Phosphodiesterase inhibitor (PDE-5)	Promotes smooth muscle relaxation through increased cGMP
Milrinone	Phosphodiesterase inhibitor (PDE-3)	Promotes smooth muscle relaxation through increased cAMP
Nitric Oxide	Guanylate cyclase pathway	Promotes smooth muscle relaxation through increased cGMP production
Bosentan	Endothelin receptor blocker	Reduced vasoconstriction by blocking endothelin receptor
Treprostinil	Prostacyclin (PGI_2)–Adenylate cyclase pathway	Direct vasodilation of pulmonary and systemic arterial vasculature/ inhibition of platelet aggregation
Iloprost	Prostacyclin (PGI_2)–Adenylate cyclase pathway	Direct vasodilation of pulmonary and systemic arterial vasculature/ inhibition of platelet aggregation
Epoprostenol	Prostacyclin (PGI_2)–Adenylate cyclase pathway	Direct vasodilation of pulmonary and systemic arterial vasculature/ inhibition of platelet aggregation

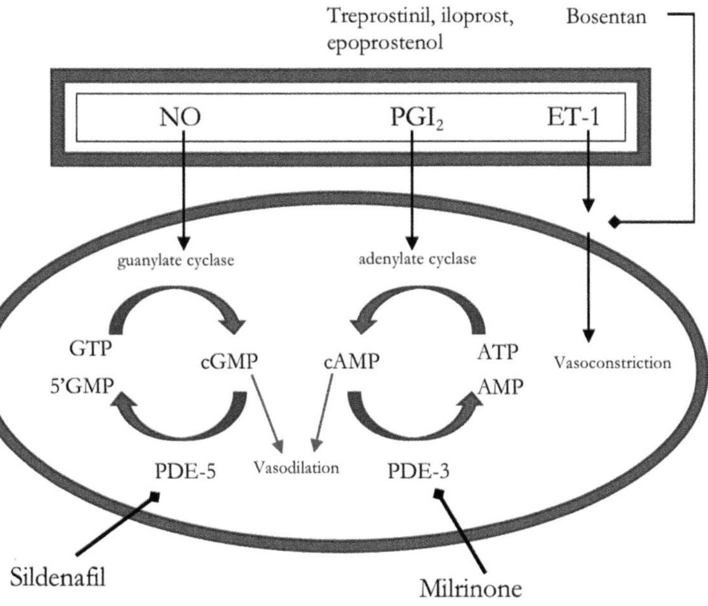

Figure 68.3 Depiction of the pathway and mechanism of action of the primary agents used to treat pulmonary hypertension. Courtesy of Adam C. Adler, MD

respiratory function, and the response to treatments. The treatment includes the management of the underlying disease, the maintenance of adequate systemic and pulmonary arterial blood pressure, the maintenance of adequate oxygenation, the mechanical ventilation to retain normocapnia, and the administration of medications to decrease pulmonary vascular resistance (Figure 68.3; Table 68.1).

Commonly used vasodilators include inhaled nitric oxide (iNO), sildenafil, milrinone, and calcium channel blockers and others. Extracorporeal membrane oxygenation (ECMO) may be considered in critically ill children with persistent PH who do not respond to the above therapies.

What Are the Major Anesthetic Considerations for Patients with PH?

The anesthetic management of children with PH is a great challenge for anesthesiologists. Intubation, surgical stimulation, inadequate oxygenation, and ventilation can cause pulmonary artery vasoconstriction and induce a pulmonary hypertensive crisis. Children with PH undergoing anesthesia have a higher morbidity and mortality from cardiovascular complications. The goals of anesthetic management in patients with PH are (1) to provide an adequate depth of anesthesia and analgesia to minimize the autonomic response to surgical stimulation and airway manipulation; (2) to maintain adequate central venous pressure and right ventricle stroke volume; (3) to optimize myocardial function; (4) to choose a ventilation and oxygenation strategy that decreases pulmonary vascular resistance (PVR); and (5) to be prepared to treat a pulmonary hypertensive crisis and cardiac collapse.

What Are the Best Anesthetic Agents to Use for Patients with PH?

No single anesthetic agent or technique has been proven superior to others for patients with PH. A balanced anesthetic technique combining volatile agents, opioids, ketamine, and/or muscle relaxants is commonly used to provide adequate anesthesia and analgesia.

All medications to treat pulmonary hypertension and heart failure MUST be continued before, during, and after the procedure, and specific medications for the treatment of pulmonary hypertensive crisis such as iNO should be immediately available.

Propofol and inhalational agents can reduce both pulmonary and systemic vascular resistance and should be carefully titrated to facilitate induction and maintenance of anesthesia. Opioids have minimal pulmonary and systemic hemodynamic effects and are the mainstay of anesthetic medication for children with PH.

Maintaining adequate intravascular volume and preload to the right ventricle is also critically important. Hypotension caused by induction agents should be treated promptly with fluid administration and inotropic support of the circulation.

Review the Treatment Strategies for an Intraoperative Pulmonary Hypertensive Crisis

Treatment of PH crisis includes: (1) The administration of 100% oxygen to maintain adequate oxygenation; (2) Correction of metabolic and respiratory acidosis. PVR is directly related to H+ concentration and PCO_2 level. Metabolic acidosis should be promptly corrected with sodium bicarbonate. Hyperventilation to generate respiratory alkalosis may also help reduce PVR. (3) Administration of fentanyl will help suppress endogenous catecholamine release and subsequently reduce pulmonary artery pressures. (4) Administer pulmonary vasodilators. iNO provides selective pulmonary vasodilatation and is the first line of medication used intraoperatively because of its rapid onset and effectiveness. (5) Support cardiac output with adequate preload and inotropic support with dopamine, epinephrine, and/or milrinone.

Suggested Reading

Abman SH, Hansmann G, Archer SL, et al. Pediatric pulmonary hypertension: guidelines from the American Heart Association and American Thoracic Society. *Circulation.* 2015;132(21):2037–99. PMID: 26534956.

Berger RM, Beghetti M, Humpl T, et al. Clinical features of paediatric pulmonary hypertension: a registry study. *Lancet.* 2012;379 (9815):537–46. PMID: 22240409.

Berger S, Konduri GG. Pulmonary hypertension in children: the twenty-first century. *Pediatr Clin North Am.* 2006;53(5):961–87. PMID: 17027619.

Carmosino MJ, Friesen RH, Doran A, et al. Perioperative complications in children with pulmonary hypertension undergoing noncardiac surgery or cardiac catheterization. *Anesth Analg.* 2007;104(3):521–7.

Ivy DD, Abman SH, Barst RJ, et al. Pediatric pulmonary hypertension. *J Am Coll Cardiol.* 2013 Dec 24;62 (25 Suppl):D117–26. PMID: 24355636.

Stayer SA, Liu Y. Pulmonary hypertension of the newborn. *Best Pract Res Clin Anaesthesiol.* 2010;24 (3):375–86. PMID: 21033014.

Chapter 69

The Fontan Patient

Premal M. Trivedi

A 16-year-old male status post-Fontan completion presents to the emergency room with a two-day history of abdominal pain and emesis. Radiography reveals a small bowel obstruction. Surgery is consulted with the plan being a laparoscopic enterostomy. Following initial resuscitation, his vitals are T: 38.4, HR: 110, BP: 90/58, RR 22, and SpO_2: 88% RA.

During preoperative evaluation, the patient is 170 cm and 70 kg, and appears comfortable. He has 1–2+ pitting edema in the bilateral lower extremities, clear respirations, and a strong pulse. His abdomen is tender in the right lower quadrant and his airway exam is unremarkable. Hepatosplenomegaly is appreciated.

On assessment of the patient's exercise tolerance prior to illness, he tolerates day-to-day activities, but doesn't exercise.

Labs are significant for a leukocytosis of 22,000/UL with an elevated neutrophil count. His C-reactive protein (CRP) is 4.

His primary cardiac disease was tricuspid atresia with associated pulmonary atresia and a ventricular septal defect. He initially underwent a modified Blalock–Taussig shunt in the first week of life, followed by a bidirectional Glenn at age three months. He underwent lateral-tunnel Fontan with fenestration at three years. His post-Fontan course has been complicated by episodes of supraventricular tachycardia for which he is on sotalol.

An echocardiogram performed in the emergency room reveals normal ventricular function with mild-to-moderate atrioventricular valve regurgitation and right-to-left shunting visualized across the fenestration.

What Are the Different Types of Fontan Procedures, and What Are Their Associated Issues?

Different surgical techniques have been used over time to restore a series circulation in patients with single ventricle physiology (Figure 69.1). Initially, atriopulmonary Fontan repairs were most common in which the right atrium would be anastomosed to the pulmonary artery. The rationale for this procedure was that the right atrium would become "ventricularized" and serve as a subpulmonic pumping chamber. With time, it became evident that such remodeling did not occur, and that complications such as atrial arrhythmias and thrombus formation were prevalent.

To minimize the risk of atrial dilation, de Leval et al. introduced the total cavopulmonary anastomosis. Initially conceived as the intracardiac lateral tunnel, this repair brings the superior vena cava to the pulmonary artery, and baffles the inferior vena cava blood to the inferior aspect of the pulmonary artery using an intraatrial conduit. While a small amount of native atrium is retained in this repair to provide growth potential, the risk of atrial arrhythmia and thrombosis is theoretically minimized.

The most recent modification to the Fontan repair has been the introduction of the extracardiac conduit. Here, an interposition graft is placed outside of the heart connecting the transected inferior vena cava and the underside of the pulmonary artery. The impetus for this repair was to avoid pulmonary or systemic venous obstruction in patients with small atria or anomalous venous return. Due to its ease of placement, it has become widely adopted as the technique for Fontan completion. Drawbacks to the extracardiac conduit include a lack of growth potential and a theoretic risk of thrombosis due to the prosthetic graft. Outcomes between the lateral tunnel and extracardiac Fontan have essentially been equivalent.

What Is the Time Frame for Fontan Completion Surgery?

The usual time frame for Fontan completion is between the ages of two to five years. As the patient

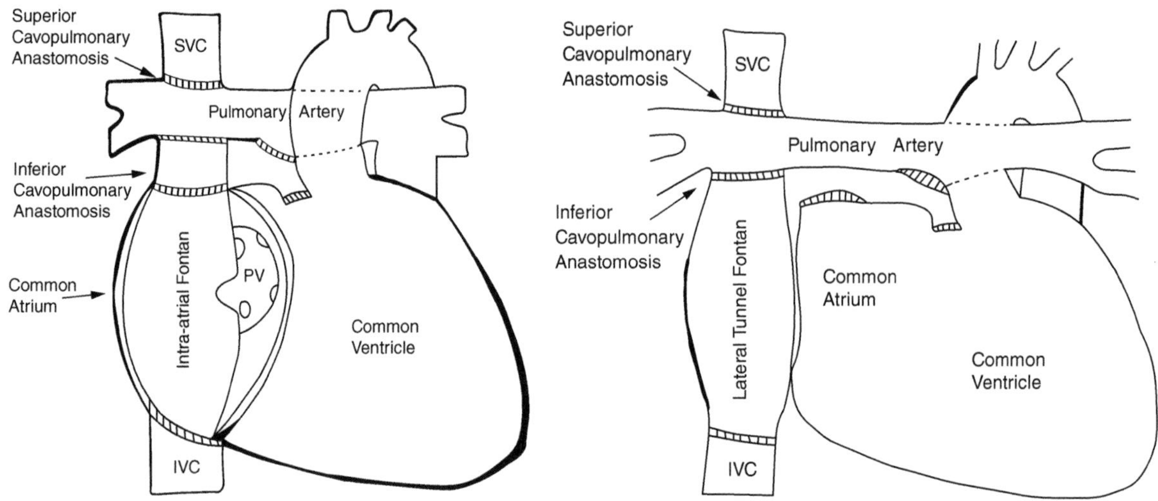

Figure 69.1 Illustration of intra-atrial Fontan (right) and lateral tunnel Fontan (left). SVC and IVC, superior and inferior vena cava, respectively. Illustration by Adam C. Adler, MD.

grows, the percentage of blood return from the lower extremities increases. The blood returning to the lungs from the upper extremities and head becomes a smaller percentage of total venous return and the patient becomes progressively more cyanotic. The ideal age for Fontan completion varies, but attempts to balance the years the patient is cyanotic and the need for revisions, as these conduits do not grow with the patient.

What Is the Purpose of Fenestrating a Fontan, and What Implications Does This Have on Saturation?

A fenestration is a hole created at the time of the Fontan completion between the conduit and the pulmonary venous atrium. This can be accomplished with both the lateral tunnel and extracardiac Fontan. The goal of the fenestration is to maintain cardiac output at the expense of a decrease in saturation in those patients who may be at risk of having significantly elevated Fontan (pulmonary arterial) pressures. This may be the case in patients with elevated pulmonary vascular resistance, ventricular dysfunction, or atrioventricular valve regurgitation.

Because filling of the systemic ventricle is dependent on passive blood flow through the pulmonary vasculature, any factor that adds resistance to this pathway can lead to a decrease in cardiac output and further elevations in both the Fontan and central venous pressures. The fenestration in this setting can be thought of as a "pop-off" valve in situations where these pressures increase. During a period of increased peak inspiration pressure, blood can return to the ventricle through the fenestration which serves as a right-to-left reversible shunt.

Saturations should be in the high 80s to low 90s in patients with fenestrations, with some variability due to the extent of right-to-left shunting across the fenestration.

What Are Other Unique Causes of Desaturation in a Fontan?

Beyond a fenestration, resting saturations <90% may indicate intrapulmonary arteriovenous shunting or the development of systemic venous-to-pulmonary venous collaterals. Both act as extracardiac right-to-left shunts.

Is There Such a Thing as a "Good" Fontan?

The ideal Fontan circulation would have normal sinus rhythm, low atrial pressures, and a low transpulmonary gradient (the difference between the pulmonary arterial pressure and the pulmonary wedge or left atrial pressure).

Implicit in this setting would be preserved systolic and diastolic ventricular function, and no residual inflow or outflow obstructions. Examples of such obstructions to flow include:

- pulmonary arterial or pulmonary venous stenosis
- elevations in pulmonary vascular resistance
- atrioventricular valve regurgitation or stenosis
- systolic or diastolic ventricular dysfunction
- ventricular outflow tract obstruction
- aortic insufficiency or stenosis
- recurrent coarctation of the aorta

While Fontan circulation provides a means of palliation for patients with single ventricle physiology, significant long-term sequelae remain. Over time, lack of a pumping mechanism providing active preload to the lungs leads to progressive issues. Each time the pulmonary or intrathoracic pressure is elevated (i.e., under stress, exercise, or Valsalva), stress in the form of elevated pressure is placed on the venous circulation. The physiologic consequence of the Fontan is cavopulmonary hypertension with a relative decrease in ventricular preload, stroke volume, and cardiac output. In addition, patients with single morphologic right ventricles develop complications related to a right ventricle ejecting against high pressures.

What Are the Signs of a Failing Fontan?

Fontan failure can present early after the Fontan procedure or late, but in either case is defined by an inadequate cardiac output and the sequelae of an elevated central venous pressure: pleural effusions, ascites, and peripheral edema.

Soon after surgery, failure may occur secondary to residual obstructions, myocardial injury, or underappreciated preoperative risk factors (elevated pulmonary vascular pressures). Unless addressed promptly, such situations can result in a vicious cycle in which cardiac output and pulmonary function rapidly worsen. Management options depend on the etiology of failure, and include repair of the residual obstruction, take-down of the Fontan, creation of a fenestration if not already present, or mechanical circulatory support.

Late failure following Fontan surgery may be in the form of progressive exercise intolerance and the insidious onset of multiorgan dysfunction. This may represent the cumulative effects of primary ventricular dysfunction and/or progressive increases in pulmonary vascular resistance over time. Elevated pulmonary pressure results in chronic hepatic venous congestion often progressing to resulting in portal hypertension and progression to hepatic failure or cirrhosis. Esophageal varices may be observed in 25% of patients although variceal bleeding is rare. Hepatorenal insufficiency may also develop. With the increasing number of Fontan patients surviving long term, focus on early recognition, diagnosis, and treatment and prevention of sequelae has become critical.

Describe the Sequelae of Protein Losing Enteropathy and Plastic Bronchitis in the Setting of the Fontan Circulation

Plastic bronchitis is a lymphatic flow disorder in which rubbery casts form within the pulmonary tree resulting in obstruction, coughing, and gas exchange disturbance.

Protein losing enteropathy (PLE) is a relatively common morbidity following the Fontan procedure. Symptoms include progressive dyspnea, large abdominal and/or pleural effusions, and peripheral edema including ascites. Patients often have intestinal malabsorption, hypoalbuminemia, hypogammaglobinemia, and lymphopenia. While the exact etiology is unknown, it is theorized that over time, low cardiac output results in intestinal vascular hypoperfusion and especially intestinal mucosal hypoperfusion.

The morbidity and mortality in patients with PLE remains high with treatment focusing on prevention and symptom amelioration especially in the form of inotropic support, diuretic therapy, and protein (albumin) replacement.

Does it Matter Whether the Systemic Ventricle Is a Morphologic Right or Left Ventricle in Predicting Fontan Failure?

While the right ventricle is capable of supporting the systemic circulation, clinical experience both with congenitally corrected transposition, and patients undergoing an atrial baffle repair for transposition suggests a high incidence of systemic right ventricular failure over time. In patients with single ventricle physiology, data has been mixed, but suggests that a systemic right ventricle is a risk factor not only for Fontan failure, but also death. The right ventricle is morphologically different from the left ventricle with its extensive trabeculations and thinner myocardium. Thus, the right ventricle is less apt to eject against high pressures for many years (Figure 69.2).

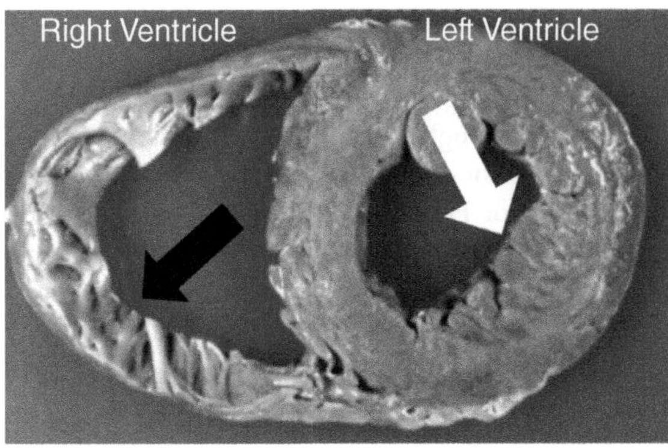

Figure 69.2 Gross cardiac specimen of the left and right ventricle demonstrating the difference in ventricular wall morphology

Is It Possible to Have Both Preserved Systolic Function and a Failing Fontan?

Yes. Two major clinical phenotypes of Fontan failure are observed: those with failure in the setting of systolic ventricular dysfunction, and those with failure in spite of preserved systolic function. This latter group accounts for up to two-thirds of adult Fontan patients who die or require transplantation. Mechanisms accounting for this paradox include elevations in pulmonary vascular resistance and the complex effects of this circulation on the liver, kidneys, vasculature, and neurohumoral system.

What Information Is Useful in the Preoperative Evaluation of a Fontan?

Thorough evaluation entails knowledge of the patient's anatomic substrate and past surgical interventions. Recent catheterization data including interventions, cardiac imaging, cardiac rhythm, and oxygen saturations should be reviewed.

Laboratory values should aim at identifying end-organ dysfunction especially cardiac, liver, and renal dysfunction. Labs of particular significance include liver function tests (including tests of coagulation), blood urea nitrogen and creatinine values to assess renal function, a complete blood count to assess platelet levels due to the risk of thrombocytopenia due to sequestration, and albumin levels if there is concern for a protein-losing enteropathy. Recent changes in functional status or excessive weight gain should raise concern for failure.

As Fontan physiology lends itself to arrhythmias, a history suggestive of rhythm abnormalities or documented arrhythmias may signal the potential need for cardioversion or pacing in the perioperative period.

Echocardiography can reveal areas of concern in the Fontan circuit, with specific attention to echocardiographic assessment of: ventricular function, the atrioventricular valve, ventricular outflow tract, and pulmonary arterial and venous flows.

Beyond the components of the normal physical exam, attention should be paid to the potential presence of pleural effusions, hepatosplenomegaly, signs of cirrhosis, ascites, or peripheral edema. Such findings suggest elevated venous pressure and potentially failing circulation. Baseline saturations should also be noted as any significant desaturation may indicate the presence of an intra- or extracardiac shunt. Lastly, as adequate hydration is critical to maintaining the hemodynamics of a Fontan, volume status should be assessed.

What Intraoperative Monitors Would You Consider Using in the Patient Described in this Chapter?

Concerns in this patient include not only his Fontan circulation, hypovolemia, and the potential for sepsis in the setting of bowel obstruction. When taken together with the need for positive-pressure ventilation, anesthesia, and laparoscopy, this patient is at significant risk for hemodynamic deterioration during this procedure. In addition to routine monitoring, one may also consider using cerebral near-infrared spectroscopy (NIRS) and arterial and central venous lines.

> Case continued: Once in the operating room, the patient undergoes a rapid sequence induction with 1 mg of midazolam, 50 mcg of fentanyl, 70 mg of propofol, and 80 mg of succinylcholine. The initial blood pressure after intubation is 92/42, but trends down to 68/40 following arterial line placement with 0.6 v/v% isoflurane.

How Would You Manage Hypotension in This Setting?

Hypotension in this patient following induction and intubation is likely multifactorial. The onset of positive-pressure ventilation in conjunction with hypovolemia are likely contributing to diminished ventricular filling, and thus a decreased cardiac output. The induction of anesthesia has also likely reduced systemic vascular resistance and increased venous capacitance, leading to a decrease in both blood pressure and preload. First-line treatment would entail volume resuscitation and the initiation of vasopressors. When time permits, volume repletion should be attempted prior to induction of anesthesia. Ventilator settings can also be reassessed to achieve the minimum peak pressures, positive end-expiratory pressure (PEEP) and rate that provide adequate oxygenation and ventilation.

What Is the Potential Impact of Laparoscopic Surgery on the Patient's Physiology?

The abdominal insufflation accompanying laparoscopy reduces lung compliance resulting in increased peak inspiratory and plateau pressures. Insufflation acts to further decreases systemic venous return, thereby decreasing cardiac output. If the Trendelenburg position is required, these effects are exacerbated. Steep reverse Trendelenburg positioning may reduce venous return on the basis of lower extremity pooling. Additionally, CO_2 used for abdominal insufflation may result in hypercapnia with a subsequent increase in pulmonary vascular resistance.

These negative effects can be mitigated if the minimal amount of insufflation pressure is used. This strategy must be communicated with the surgeon in advance of the procedure. If hemodynamic instability remains, consideration should be given to performing an open procedure.

Should This Patient Be Extubated?

Provided adequate hemodynamics, oxygenation, and ventilation, extubation is appropriate. Spontaneous ventilation improves passive venous return and therefore cardiac output.

Pain control is paramount, and can be achieved with a combination of narcotics, acetaminophen (assuming no significant hepatic derangements), ketorolac (assuming preserved renal function), and/or transverse abdominis plane blocks. Inadequate pain control results in consistently elevated PVR.

Where Should This Patient Recover?

For the first postoperative night, it may be advisable to recover this patient on a floor where the staff is familiar with the patient's physiology. If such a floor is not present, the intensive care unit may be the most appropriate.

Suggested Reading

Goldberg DJ, Shaddy RE, Ravishankar C, et al. The failing Fontan: etiology, diagnosis and management. *Expert Rev Cardiovasc Ther.* 2011;9 (6):785–93. PMID: 21714609.

Gottlieb EA, Andropoulos DB. Anesthesia for the patient with congenital heart disease presenting for noncardiac surgery. *Current Opinion in Anesthesiology.* 2013; 26(3):318–26. PMID: 23614956.

John AS. Fontan repair of single ventricle physiology: consequences of a unique physiology and possible treatment options. *Cardiol Clin.* 2015;33(4):559–69. PMID: 26471820.

Jolley M, Colan SD, Rhodes J, et al. Fontan physiology revisited. *Anesth Analg.* 2015;121(1):172–82. PMID: 26086514.

Mossad EB, Motta P, Vener DF. Anesthetic considerations for adults undergoing Fontan conversion surgery. *Anesthesiology Clin.* 2013;31:405–19. PMID: 23711650.

Chapter 70

Ventricular Assist Devices

Premal M. Trivedi

A three-month-old previously healthy infant presents to the emergency room with increased work of breathing and a two-week history of rhinorrhea and cough. Chest X-ray demonstrates severe cardiomegaly prompting an echocardiogram which reveals severe left ventricular dilation compressing the right ventricle (RV) severe mitral regurgitation, and severely depressed biventricular function. The differential includes viral myocarditis versus dilated cardiomyopathy.

Over the next week, the patient is intubated for respiratory distress and started on inotropic support to optimize cardiac output. In the past 12 hours, the infant has become increasingly tachycardic to the 180s–190s and hypotensive with blood pressures between 45–55/30–40 in spite of escalating inotropy. Labs are significant for increasing creatinine and elevations in liver enzymes. Oxygenation, ventilation, and lung compliance are stable. Due to concerns regarding impending circulatory collapse, the patient is taken to the OR for initiation of mechanical circulatory support via the Berlin Heart EXCOR ventricular assist device (VAD, Berlin Heart GmbH, Berlin, Germany).

Following device placement and stabilization of hemodynamics and bleeding, the patient is extubated, and anticoagulation is started. Two weeks thereafter, the patient becomes acutely hypotensive with decreased device filling. A large black stool is concerning for a gastrointestinal bleed. With continued instability in spite of transfusion, the patient is taken the operating room for exploratory laparotomy.

What Are the Indications for Ventricular Support in Children?

Heart failure in children can be the end result of multiple causes, with common culprits being congenital heart disease, cardiomyopathies, and myocarditis. While many of these patients can be medically or surgically managed, a minority will require mechanical circulatory support in order to maintain end-organ perfusion, either in the form of a VAD or extracorporeal membrane oxygenation (ECMO). Such support can be used as a bridge-to-recovery, bridge-to-transplantation, or bridge-to-decision.

How Is a VAD Different than ECMO?

While both a VAD and ECMO can provide short-term circulatory support, ECMO offers the additional ability to oxygenate and ventilate using the membrane oxygenator. The oxygenator, although beneficial to those in respiratory failure, also promotes an inflammatory response that can adversely affect hemodynamics as well as coagulation. A VAD functions only as ventricular support, does not use an oxygenator, and thus avoids this inflammatory insult.

VADs are better able to decompress the left ventricle (LV) in comparison to ECMO due to their placement in either the left atrium or left ventricle. A secondary goal of mechanical circulatory support is to rest the left heart by minimizing its preload. On ECMO, blood may return to the left ventricle either by inadequate venous drainage or by the presence of aortopulmonary collaterals. This leads to stretching of the left ventricular myocardium with a subsequent increase in oxygen consumption. The increase in left-sided filling may result in left atrial hypertension and worsened pulmonary dysfunction through increased pulmonary venous pressures. To manage the increase in LV pressure, some patients on ECMO require balloon atrial septostomy.

Moreover, while ECMO runs are generally limited (weeks to months) due to its associated complications, short-term VADs achieved through central cannulation can be transitioned more easily to durable VADs to allow for much longer periods of support (months to years).

In Which Situations Would ECMO Be a Better Choice than a VAD?

ECMO is most commonly deployed in the setting of cardiac arrest (extracorporeal cardiopulmonary resuscitation or ECPR) or acute postcardiotomy dysfunction. ECMO would be the preferred choice in patients with pulmonary as well as circulatory failure, or in patients with acute biventricular failure. Clinical scenarios like severe pulmonary edema in the setting of ventricular dysfunction, right ventricular failure due to pulmonary hypertension, or hemodynamic instability due to sepsis would qualify.

What Determines the Timing of Device Placement?

The ideal time to move forward with device placement remains a challenge in pediatrics. Influencing this decision are the patient's clinical course, body size, and relatedly, the device options available. The goal is to initiate support prior to the development of irreversible end-organ injury, or when medical therapy has failed. Such endpoints are difficult to define as patients can have variable clinical courses with intermittent periods of decline and improvement. Moreover, the devices available to children are not without risk. The Berlin EXCOR is the only VAD currently approved for use in neonates and infants but has a markedly higher rate of pump thrombosis compared to continuous flow VADs. And while larger children and adolescents can accommodate continuous flow VADs like the Heartmate II (Thoratec Corp., Pleasanton, CA) or HeartWare HVAD (HeartWare, Framingham, MA), the experience with these devices in children remains limited. In this setting, the medical team must weigh the risk of device placement versus the risk of worsening end-organ injury with continued medical management alone. A temporary support device or ECMO may be an option in such cases to allow for recovery of end-organ function before placement of a long-term device.

How Do We Select the Type of VAD to Place?

Different algorithms have been generated to assist with device selection. Relevant factors considered include (1) the type of support needed: cardiac-only, cardiopulmonary, left versus right ventricular support, or biventricular support; (2) the anticipated duration of support; and (3) the size of the patient. There are now many devices suitable for use in children (Figure 70.1).

What Are the Options for Temporary and Long-Term Support Devices?

Temporary VADs are deployed for settings in which myocardial function may recover within one to two weeks or if end-organ stabilization is desired prior to placement of a long-term VAD or heart transplant. Options for temporary VADs include the PediMag (Thoratec Corporation), RotaFlow (Maquet), TandemHeart (Cardiac Assist, Inc), and Impella (Abiomed), all continuous-flow devices. The PediMag and RotaFlow are extracorporeal centrifugal pumps that can support the range of pediatric sizes, assist both the right and left ventricle, and connect to centrally placed cannulas. The TandemHeart and Impella, in contrast, are percutaneously placed. Due to the size of the sheaths necessary to deploy these devices, their use is limited to large children and adolescents.

Durable or long-term VADs include both pulsatile and continuous-flow devices. They serve as bridges to transplantation, or rarely, as destination therapy. For infants and small-children, the sole device available is the Berlin Heart EXCOR, a pneumatically driven paracorporeal pulsatile pump. In adolescents and larger children, the size mismatch between "adult" devices and the patient is of lesser concern, and so continuous-flow devices such as the Heartmate II and HeartWare are chosen due to their lower risk profile. An alternative option to continuous-flow devices in larger patients is the SynCardia Total Artificial Heart (SynCardia Systems, Inc., Tucson, AZ), a pneumatically-driven device that entirely replaces the valves and ventricles of the native heart.

Which Noncardiac Procedures Are Most Commonly Performed on Patients with VADs?

The range of diagnostic and therapeutic procedures for which these patients can present is broad and include both those related to device complications and the routine management of the critically ill child. Noninvasive procedures most commonly entail

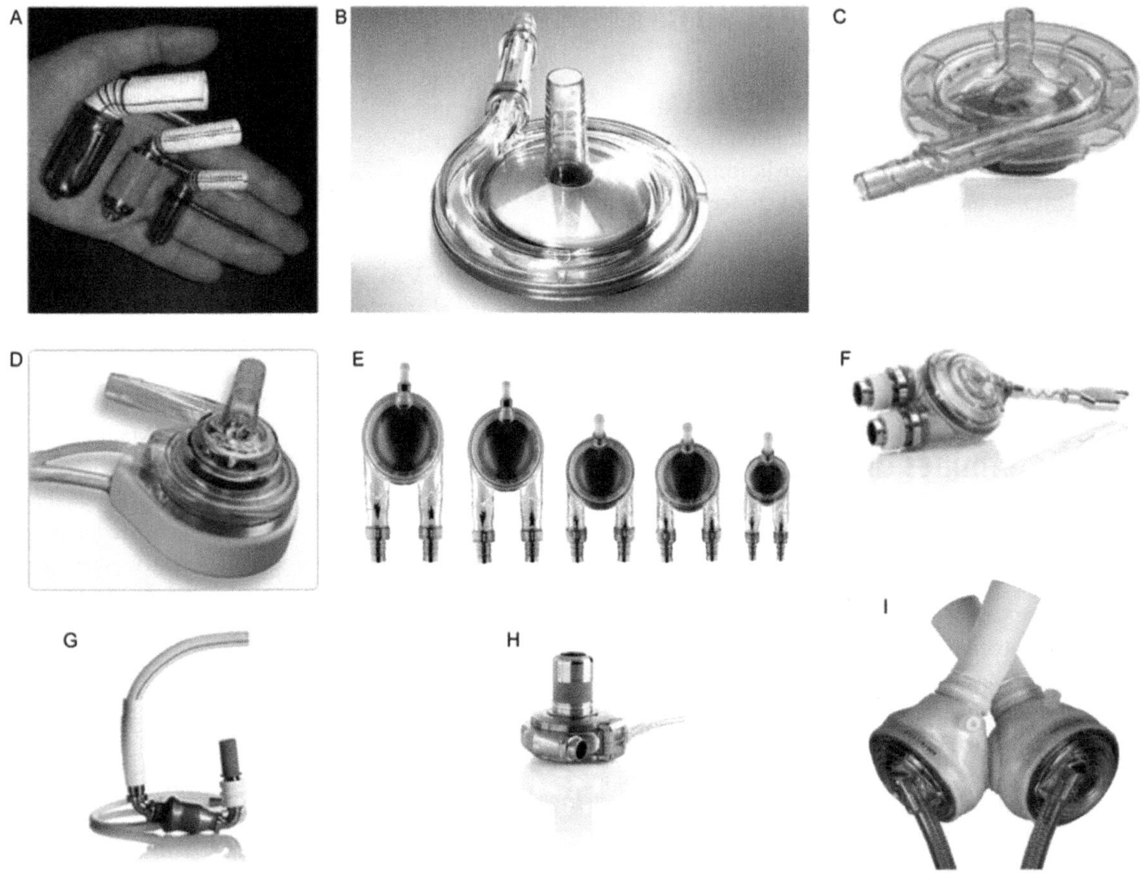

Figure 70.1 Ventricular assist devices. (A) The Jarvik 2000 devices, left to right adult, child and infant Jarvik. (B) The RotaFlow assist device. (C) The PediMag assist device. (D) The TandemHeart assist device. (E) Variety of Berlin Heart EXCOR devices from left to right 60, 50, 30, 25, 10 mL. (F) Thoratec assist device. (G) Heartmate II assist device. (H) Heartware assist device. (I) SynCardia total artificial heart. Reproduced with permission of John Wiley and Sons, from Mascio CE. *Artif Organs* 2015 Jan;39(1):14-20

imaging studies like CT (MRI is contraindicated due to the device). Invasive procedures include those needed for venous access, imaging of the heart and device via transesophageal echocardiography, or to address otolaryngologic, general surgical, or neurosurgical issues. For those patients with the Berlin Heart EXCOR, device exchange is commonly performed due to the presence of fibrin strands or clot in the pump.

What Preoperative Information Should One Collect Prior to Planning an Anesthetic?

An evaluation of the patient's underlying cardiac history, native ventricular function, end-organ dysfunction, and device type are essential. To help in this process, the input of the patient's cardiologist, cardiac surgeon, or VAD coordinator can be elicited. Complications incurred following device placement should also be sought. These can entail bleeding or thromboembolic events that can manifest as neurologic sequelae like strokes or seizures, gastrointestinal bleeds, or pump thrombosis. The balance between clotting and bleeding is tenuous in VAD patients, and a review of the patient's anticoagulation strategy and current level of anticoagulation may assist in assessing bleeding risk and in deciding which blood products to order.

Other device risks to assess include infection, which may influence the choice of perioperative antibiotics, and the presence of persistent renal or hepatic dysfunction. Even following VAD placement, patients can be anuric and require continuous renal replacement therapy or intermittent dialysis due to the extent of end-organ injury experienced in the pre-device period. Such knowledge may impact anesthetic drug choice or the type and amount of volume to be administered intraoperatively.

What Device Parameters Should One Assess in the Berlin Heart EXCOR, Heartmate II, and Heartware?

Berlin Heart EXCOR

- Pump rate
  - Operates at a predetermined rate but is adjustable
  - Pump rate × device volume = cardiac output delivered by the device
- Per cent time in systole
  - Set to mimic native physiology in which diastole is longer than systole
- Systolic pressure
  - Set higher than the native systolic blood pressure
- Diastolic pressure
  - Set higher than the native diastolic pressure
- Adequacy of pump filling and ejection
  - Assessed by direct inspection of the pump
    - Wrinkling of the chamber in diastole indicates inadequate fill
    - Wrinkling of the chamber in systole indicates impaired ejection
- Battery life prior to transport

Heartmate II

- Pump speed (RPM)
  - Optimized using echocardiography to achieve the desired physiologic response
  - Operates at the predetermined rate with the ability to decrease speed during suction events (i.e., when the LV sucks down or collapses due to hypovolemia, RV failure, or tamponade)
- Power (watts)
  - A direct measure of motor voltage and current
  - ↑ pump speed > ↑ power
- Pulsatility index (PI): 110 scale
  - Corresponds to the magnitude of pulsatility seen by the pump
    - A function of how well the native heart is contracting and pump speed
  - As the native ventricle contributes more to ejection, more pulsatility is seen by the pump
  - As the pump speed increases, the ventricle is more unloaded and pulsatility decreases
  - A higher PI thus indicates less support by the pump, whereas a lower PI indicates more support
  - Fluctuates with volume status, SVR, and biventricular function
- Flow (L/min)
  - An estimated value based on power, pump speed, and viscosity (hematocrit)
    - ↑ power > ↑ flow
    - ↑ pump speed > ↑ flow
  - Used as a trend monitor rather than an actual reflection of cardiac output
  - Low flow may be secondary to any process that impairs device filling and ejection
    - Inflow or outflow graft occlusion
    - Hypovolemia
    - Right ventricular dysfunction
    - Elevated PVR
    - Increased SVR
  - High flows in the setting of gradual increases in power should raise suspicion for pump thrombosis
    - High flows in this setting are artifactual as they are based on power
- Battery life prior to transport

Heartware

- Pump speed (RPM)
  - Operates at the predetermined rate, but speed does not decrease during suction events

Table 70.1 Examples of commonly used parameters in selected support devices

Heartmate II			
RPM	**Power (watts)**	**Pulsatility Index**	**Flow (L/min)**
9600 (6000 – 15000)	7	3.6 (1–10)	4.5
Berlin Heart EXCOR			
Rate / **% Time in systole**		**Systolic Pressure**	**Diastolic Pressure**
80 / 40%		220 mm Hg	-40 mm Hg
Heartware			
RPM	**Power (watts)**		**Flow (L/min)**
2400–3200	2.5–8.5		3–8

- Power (watts)
- Flow (L/min)
- Flow pulsatility (amplitude)
  - Similar to the pulsatility index in the Heartmate II
    - Difference between the peak and trough flows
    - Recommended >2 L/min in order to avoid retrograde flow or suction events
    - Reflects pump speed as well as LV preload, afterload, and native contractility
- Battery life prior to transport

Examples of device-specific parameters are identified in Table 70.1.

What Are the Physiologic Principles to Consider When Anesthetizing a Patient with a VAD?

Device filling is dependent on adequate preload and sufficient right ventricular function. As such, efforts should be made to attain euvolemia and minimize pulmonary vascular resistance (PVR) via adequate oxygenation, ventilation, and analgesia while avoiding acidosis. For those patients who have pre-existing depressed right ventricular function or elevations in PVR, inotropic support can be used to bolster the ventricle in the perioperative period while inhaled nitric oxide can be used to further decrease PVR. Spontaneous ventilation can also be considered if the procedure allows for its beneficial effects on PVR, venous return, and hemodynamic stability compared to positive pressure ventilation, especially for the RV.

Maintenance of systemic vascular resistance (SVR) is also necessary to minimize periods of hypotension. Anesthesia-induced vasodilation leads to a decrease in SVR and increased venous capacitance that can produce hypotension out of proportion to that expected with standard anesthetic dosing. This hypotension further reduces preload to the right heart, thereby diminishing both left ventricular and device filling. Vasopressors such as phenylephrine, norepinephrine, or vasopressin are often required to counteract these effects.

What Monitors, Special Equipment, and Personnel Should One Plan For?

Standard monitors are often sufficient for noninvasive procedures or for those in which significant fluid or hemodynamic shifts are not anticipated. Of note, the ECG in patients with the Berlin Heart reflects native contractions and not the device rate selected on the console. The native rhythm merits monitoring, nonetheless, as arrhythmias may influence right ventricular function, and thus device filling.

In patients with continuous-flow devices, a noninvasive blood pressure cuff can provide an accurate measurement due to the native contractility of the left ventricle. Exceptions include those patients with severely depressed left ventricular function and minimal pulsatility. Arterial line placement using ultrasound or Doppler guidance is then indicated. Consideration should also be given to the accessibility of the patient's arms should arterial access be needed during the case. Given these patients' propensity to develop hypotension with anesthesia, the threshold to place an arterial line should be low if the arms are to be tucked or draped.

For more involved procedures, central venous catheters and transesophageal echocardiography can be used to guide fluid management and inotropy, particularly when response to traditional measures to improve hemodynamics has failed. Cerebral perfusion can also be trended using near-infrared spectroscopy probes.

Critically, a perfusionist or member of the institution's VAD team should be available to help with device management and transport whenever a patient is in need of an anesthetic.

What Blood Pressures Should Be Targeted with These Devices?

A reasonable target may be the patient's baseline pressures following stabilization on the device and recovery of end-organ function. For continuous-flow devices, target mean arterial pressure should be comparable to age-appropriate goals and can be adjusted to the perfusion needs of the individual. Pulsatile devices, similarly, should aim to generate an age-appropriate systolic and diastolic pressure. Factors that may skew the patient's pressures include patient-pump size mismatch or persistently elevated SVR following implantation.

Which Induction and Maintenance Regimens Result in the Least Hypotension?

Clinical experience and study suggest that ketamine may offer the most hemodynamically stable anesthetic induction in patients with VADs. This is likely secondary to its ability to maintain SVR through increasing circulating levels of catecholamines. For maintenance, age-appropriate levels of anesthetics often lead to hypotension, suggesting a minimal therapeutic window. Specifically, significant hypotension has been observed with sevoflurane >1%, desflurane >2%, propofol >50 mcg/kg/min, and remifentanil >0.01 mcg/kg/min. Compared to remifentanil, fentanyl, or sufentanil may better preserve SVR. Such data underscores the frequent need for volume resuscitation and pressor support simply to provide a minimal anesthetic in this patient population.

Can a Patient with a VAD Be Externally Cardioverted or Defibrillated in the Event of a Malignant Arrhythmia?

Yes. While an left ventricular assist device (LVAD) will continue to function during an arrhythmia, the filling of the left heart may be impaired by the decreased right ventricular output. During attempts at external cardioversion or defibrillation, the patient can remain connected to the device and the pads should be placed such that they do not directly overlie the implanted pump. In patients who have been fibrillating for an unknown or long period of time, the risk of thromboembolism due to the development of thrombus must be considered.

Can Chest Compressions Be Performed on Those with VADs?

Yes. Though there is a risk of device and cannula dislodgement or malposition, chest compression should be performed if indicated by pediatric advanced life support. Supporting this practice is one retrospective review which found no dislodgement and 50% return of neurologic function in eight LVAD patients who received chest compressions while in cardiac arrest. Additional therapy in the setting is aimed at supporting the right ventricle by providing oxygenation, ventilation, and pharmacologic assistance.

Algorithm for Managing Perioperative Hemodynamic Changes

The perioperative management algorithms for patients with VAD support are summarized in Tables 70.2 and 70.3.

Berlin Heart EXCOR

Table 70.2 Perioperative management algorithms for patients supported by the Berlin Heart

	Potential etiologies	HR (native)	CVP	Device inspection	Treatment
Hypotension	Hypovolemia	↑	↓	Wrinkling/ poor fill in diastole	Give volume; increasing device rate not recommended (will decrease fill time)
	Vasodilation	↑	↔	Chamber may fill completely	Alpha-agonists, vasopressin
	RV failure	↑↑	↑↑	Wrinkling/ poor fill in diastole	Inotropy, iNO, maneuvers to decrease PVR
	Tamponade	↑↑	↑↑	Wrinkling/ poor fill in diastole	Surgical exploration
Hypertension	Pain	↑↑	↑, ↔	Wrinkling/ poor emptying in systole	Analgesia; avoid increasing systolic driving pressure > 195 mm Hg
	Awareness	↑↑	↑, ↔	Wrinkling/ poor emptying in systole	Sedation, analgesia
	Hypervolemia	↔	↑↑	Full fill in diastole, poor emptying in systole	Increase device rate, diuresis
Thrombus	Inadequate anticoagulation	↔, ↑↑ if large/occlusive, cardiac output would be determined by native cardiac function	↔, ↑↑ depending on severity of occlusion	Fibrin strands on valves or larger clot	Pump change

Continuous-Flow Devices

Table 70.3 Perioperative management algorithms for patients supported by the continuous flow devices (e.g., Heartware)

	Potential etiologies	HR (native)	CVP	Heartmate II	HVAD	Treatment
Hypotension	Hypovolemia	↑	↓	↓ Pulsatility Index (PI); ↓ in RPMs (lowest 6000) beyond which the device will stop until volume is replete	↓ amplitude RPMs do not decrease as in the Heartmate II unless changed manually	Give volume, ↓ RPMs in the HVAD to prevent a suction event
	Vasodilation	↑	↔	↑ flow with ↔ in RPM	↑ flow with ↔ in RPM	Alpha-agonists, vasopressin
	RV failure	↑↑	↑↑	↓ PI and watts	↓ amplitude and watts	Inotropic support, iNO, maneuvers to decrease PVR
	Tamponade	↑↑	↑↑	↓ PI and flow	↓ amplitude and flow	Surgical exploration
Hypertension	Pain	↑↑	↑, ↔	↓ flow with ↔ in RPM	↓ flow with ↔ in RPM	Analgesia
	Awareness	↑↑	↑, ↔	↓ flow with ↔ in RPM	↓ flow with ↔ in RPM	Sedation and analgesia
	Hypervolemia	↔	↑↑	↓ flow	↓ flow	Increase RPMs and diuresis
Thrombus	Inadequate anticoagulation	↔, ↑↑ depending on severity of occlusion	↔, ↑↑ depending on severity of occlusion	↑ watts and flow (artifact of increased watts)	↑ watts and flow (artifact of increased watts)	Heparin or pump exchange

Suggested Reading

Cooper DS, Pretre R. Clinical management of pediatric ventricular assist devices. *Pediatr Crit Care Med.* 2013;14:S27–36. PMID: 23735982.

Jaquiss RDB, Bronicki RA. An overview of mechanical circulatory support in children. *Pediatr Crit Care Med.* 2013;14(5 Suppl 1):S3–6. PMID: 23735983.

Mascio CE. The use of ventricular assist device support in children: the state of the art. *Artif Organs.* 2015;39(1):14–20. PMID: 25626575.

Mossad EB, Motta P, Rossano J, et al. Perioperative management of pediatric patients on mechanical cardiac support. *Paediatr Anaesth.* 2011;21(5):585–93. PMID: 21332879.

Pratap JN, Wilmshurst S. Anesthetic management of children with in situ Berlin Heart EXCOR. *Paediatr Anaesth.* 2010;20(12):1137–8. PMID: 21199125.

Stein ML, et al. Ventricular assist devices in a contemporary pediatric cohort: Morbidity, functional recovery, and survival. *J Heart Lung Transplant.* 2016; 35:92–98. PMID: 26210751.

Noncardiac Surgery in a Glenn Patient

Jaime Bozentka and Laura Diaz-Berenstain

A three-year-old female is scheduled for laparoscopic appendectomy. She has been vomiting for the past 24 hours and has had minimal oral intake. She has a history of hypoplastic left heart syndrome and her last cardiac surgery was a Glenn procedure performed at six months of age. Her mother states that she is normally active and has no trouble keeping up with her five-year-old brother. They are regularly seen by a cardiologist at a hospital two hours from home.

Her current vital signs are: heart rate 140 beats/min; respiratory rate 20 breaths/min; SpO_2 78% on room air. Her abdomen is tender, but not distended. Her hemoglobin is 15 and her hematocrit is 45%. All other laboratory work is within normal limits. A bedside echocardiogram in the emergency department shows normal ventricular function and trace atrioventricular valve regurgitation.

What Is the Anatomical Name and Description of a Bidirectional Glenn Procedure? Why Is It Described as "Bidirectional?"

First introduced in 1958 by William Glenn, superior cavopulmonary anastomosis (SCPA) is a procedure in which the superior vena cava (SVC) is disconnected from the atrium and anastomosed to the right pulmonary artery (Figure 71.1). The main pulmonary artery, if not atretic, is disconnected from the heart, and other surgically created sources of pulmonary blood flow, such as an existing systemic to pulmonary shunt, are removed. It is referred to as "bidirectional" because blood from the SVC flows to the right pulmonary artery as well as across to the left pulmonary artery, thereby supplying both lungs.

What Type of Cardiac Lesions Require SCPA?

SCPA is typically the second stage in the palliation of single ventricle cardiac lesions. Patients may require single ventricle palliation for a variety of pathologies including hypoplastic right heart lesions (tricuspid atresia, pulmonary atresia with intact ventricular septum, severe forms of Ebstein's anomaly with tricuspid dysplasia), hypoplastic left heart lesions (aortic atresia or stenosis, mitral atresia, or stenosis), or lesions which do not permit surgical septation of the heart into two ventricle physiology (unbalanced atrioventricular canal defects, double inlet ventricle, some forms of heterotaxy).

The Flow of Blood to the Heart in the Glenn Patient

All blood flow to the pulmonary circulation is passive and supplied from the upper body via the SVC anastomosis to the pulmonary arteries. Because patients have had a complete atrial septectomy as part of their first stage procedure, when oxygenated blood returns to the heart from the pulmonary veins, it mixes with deoxygenated blood returning from the lower body via the inferior vena cava (IVC) and then proceeds to the single ventricle.

What Are Typical Hemoglobin–Oxygen Saturations for a Patient with SCPA Physiology?

Typical hemoglobin–oxygen saturations for a patient with Glenn physiology are between 75 and 85%.

What Is the Typical Hematocrit in a Patient with SCPA Physiology?

Due to the cyanotic nature of the physiology and the need to maximize oxygen delivery, the hematocrit of

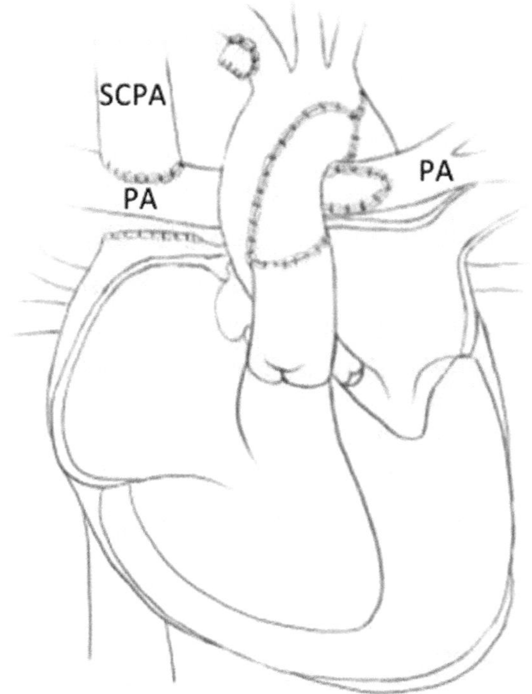

Figure 71.1 A schematic of hypoplastic left heart syndrome following superior cavopulmonary anastomosis (SCPA) or the Glenn procedure highlighting connection of the SVC and pulmonary artery (PA). Printed with permission from Texas Children's Hospital

SCPA patients is generally expected to be maintained between 40% and 45%.

At What Age Is SCPA Generally Performed? Why Is It Not Performed on Newborns?

The SCPA/Glenn procedure is usually performed at two to six months of age, as pulmonary vascular resistance (PVR) continues to fall after birth and passive pulmonary blood flow becomes possible. It cannot be performed earlier due to high PVR in newborns that would preclude successful passive pulmonary blood flow.

What Physiologic Advantage Does SCPA Offer Over Native Circulation or a Systemic-to-Pulmonary Arterial Shunt?

Prior to SCPA, blood exits the single ventricle via an outflow tract that then provides flow to both the systemic and pulmonary vascular circulations, with their relative resistances determining the amount of flow to each. This arrangement, known as *parallel circulation*, places a volume burden on the ventricle. SCPA places the two vascular beds in series by making pulmonary blood flow a diversion of systemic venous return. This effectively reduces the volume load on the ventricle, which in turn allows ventricular remodeling to occur, improving ventricular function and lowering end diastolic pressure. In addition, the transition to a *series circulation* also eliminates reliance on the balance between systemic and pulmonary vascular resistance to provide adequate flow to each system.

In comparison to a modified Blalock–Taussig (BT) shunt, which is made of synthetic Gore-Tex, the native tissue of the SVC provides a more stable source of pulmonary blood flow that is able to grow with the patient and is less likely to be compromised by thrombosis.

What Is the Final Stage in Single Ventricle Palliation?

At two to five years of age, the patient will undergo total cavopulmonary anastomosis (TCPA), also known as the Fontan procedure. This surgery results in all systemic venous return being diverted passively to the pulmonary system by connecting the inferior vena cava (IVC) to the pulmonary artery, most often via an extracardiac conduit. After undergoing the Fontan procedure most single ventricle patients will have hemoglobin-oxygen saturation in the high 90s.

Why Is SCPA Considered More Stable for Noncardiac Surgery than TCPA?

In comparison to TCPA, cardiac output after SCPA is not entirely dependent on pulmonary blood flow because the IVC remains directly connected to the heart, providing venous return. Therefore, should pulmonary blood flow be compromised by an increase in PVR, such as during bronchospasm or light anesthesia, cardiac output can be maintained via IVC flow. After TCPA, an abrupt increase in PVR could result in a precipitous decrease in pulmonary blood flow and preload to the single ventricle, unless a fenestration was created at the time of surgery, which allows IVC blood to potentially divert from the extracardiac conduit to the atrium. In TCPA patients with a fenestration, blood can shunt from the conduit to the single ventricle, as the resultant decrease in hemoglobin-oxygen saturation is better tolerated than low cardiac output. These patients may have hemoglobin-oxygen saturation in the 85–95% range.

If SCPA Is More Stable, Why Is Completion of the TCPA Necessary?

Total cavopulmonary anastomosis becomes necessary because of a progression in cyanosis that is inevitable following SCPA. The cause of this increased cyanosis is two-fold. Firstly, as the child ages and begins walking, the ratio of blood flow through the SVC to that in the IVC begins to favor the IVC, resulting in a greater proportion of deoxygenated blood return to the heart. Secondly, due to the lack of hepatic blood flow to the lungs, all SCPA patients form pulmonary arteriovenous malformations (AVM) which result in increased intrapulmonary shunting.

What Should I Tell Parents about Anesthetic Risk?

According to the Pediatric Perioperative Cardiac Arrest Registry data, children with heart disease, including those who have undergone SCPA, have a higher incidence of cardiac arrest during anesthesia than those without heart disease. In addition, more than half of these cardiac arrests occurred in the general OR rather than the cardiac OR or cardiac catheterization laboratory. For this reason, a comprehensive preoperative evaluation is critical in order to identify and anticipate any situations that would incur additional risk in this already compromised population.

Are Patients with SCPA Physiology Appropriate for Outpatient Surgery, or Surgery at a Surgery Center?

An SCPA patient who is developing normally, without functional restrictions, and undergoing regular evaluation by a pediatric cardiologist can be an appropriate candidate for same day surgery for low-risk procedures where there is minimal expectation for postoperative pain or functional limitations. However, common post-anesthetic complications will be less well-tolerated in this patient population compared to healthy children. Even mild bleeding or vomiting can lead to dehydration and a reduction in pulmonary blood flow. Similarly, increased pulmonary vascular resistance with a resultant increase in hypoxemia can result from unrecognized upper respiratory infection (URI), bronchospasm, or surgical complications. Therefore, planned outpatient procedures should be done at a hospital which allows postoperative monitoring and admission if necessary, rather than at a surgery center.

What Information Should Be Gathered in a Preoperative Cardiac Evaluation in an SCPA Patient?

The history should focus on determining whether any degree of functional limitation exists due to the cardiac disease. In younger patients, this may manifest as tachypnea, diaphoresis with feeds, or failure to thrive. In older children dyspnea on exertion or the inability to keep up with peers may be noted. Preoperative vital signs, in particular the hemoglobin-oxygen saturation while on room air, will help to establish baseline values to maintain during the perioperative period. The most recent report from the patient's cardiologist should be sought, as well as a recent electrocardiogram and echocardiogram. Gather a complete medication history as patients may be on a variety of agents such as antihypertensives, diuretics, or anticoagulants, and occasional patients may be on anti-arrhythmic medications.

When Reviewing the Electrocardiogram and Echocardiogram, What Are the Most Significant Indicators of Cardiac Status?

Single ventricle patients generally do not tolerate cardiac arrhythmias. Therefore, normal sinus rhythm should be ensured on electrocardiogram. When reviewing the echocardiogram, the two most important pieces of information are the systolic function of the single ventricle and the atrioventricular valve competence. Other things of importance include the presence of any residual ventricular outflow tract obstruction and any previously noted or currently abnormal pulmonary artery anatomy.

What NPO Considerations Exist?

The American Society of Anesthesiology NPO guidelines of eight hours for solids, six hours for formula, four hours for breastmilk, and two hours for clear liquids should still be followed. However, as these patients are reliant on preload to drive pulmonary blood flow, emphasis should be placed on ensuring that clear liquid intake is continued until the two-hour cutoff. If fasting is prolonged, strong consideration should be given to preoperative institution of intravenous fluids in order to minimize dehydration and its adverse effects.

How Should Upper Respiratory Tract Infection (URI) Symptoms Be Evaluated in These Patients?

The increased PVR and airway hyperreactivity that accompanies URIs can result in life-threatening cyanosis and hypoxemia in these patients that rely on passive flow of blood through the pulmonary system. Therefore, extra caution should be utilized in the presence of any signs of URI and strong consideration should be given to rescheduling the case, if at all possible, after resolution of symptoms and return to baseline status has occurred.

What Is the Minimum Workup That Should Be Ensured Prior to Emergency Surgery?

If a child presents emergently to a hospital other than the one where he or she normally receives cardiac care, every attempt should be made to obtain the most recent cardiac data from the home institution. If such information cannot be obtained, a cardiology consult should be obtained in addition to an ECG and echocardiogram. In many cases of emergency surgery the child may be dehydrated from decreased oral intake and vomiting prior to presentation. As pulmonary blood flow is dependent on adequate preload, particular attention should be paid to the volume status and induction should be delayed until adequate hydration is achieved.

What Are Current AHA Recommendations for Subacute Bacterial Endocarditis (SBE) Prophylaxis?

The AHA recommends SBE prophylaxis for cardiac conditions with the highest risk of adverse outcomes from endocarditis. These conditions include:

- Prosthetic cardiac valves or valve material
- Previous history of endocarditis
- Unrepaired cyanotic congenital heart disease (CHD)
- Completely repaired CHD with prosthetic materials during the first six months following repair
- Repaired CHD with residual shunts or valvular regurgitation adjacent to prosthetic material
- Cardiac transplant patients with valvulopathy

As a cyanotic lesion, SCPA meets the criteria for SBE prophylaxis prior to dental procedures that manipulate the oral mucosa as well as invasive respiratory tract procedures.

What Methods Are Appropriate for Induction of Anesthesia?

The child with SCPA physiology may be appropriate for either intravenous or inhalational induction. The decision should be based on the preoperative evaluation as well as the needs of the case being performed while keeping in mind caveats specific to SCPA patients. If the preoperative workup reveals any compromise in cardiac function, an intravenous induction should be performed. Additionally, if there is a possibility of dehydration, intravenous access should be obtained for fluid resuscitation prior to anesthetic induction. In a patient with no cardiac symptoms, inhalational induction is generally well tolerated. It should be noted that induction will be slower than in non-SCPA patients due to the interventricular mixing of pulmonary and IVC blood. In addition, any coughing or breath-holding will decrease pulmonary blood flow and lead to increased desaturation. Consideration should also be given to the fact that as these children have already had many interventions, intravenous access may be difficult and premedication may be necessary.

What Respiratory and Ventilatory Considerations Exist for These Patients?

SCPA patients function optimally during spontaneous ventilation, when negative intrathoracic pressures help to draw blood into the pulmonary circulation. When positive pressure ventilation is necessary, conservation of passive pulmonary blood flow requires maintenance of normal to low PVR. A ventilation strategy that uses moderate tidal volumes and short inspiratory times will result in low mean airway pressure and PVR. Positive end expiratory pressure (PEEP) should be utilized to maintain functional residual capacity, but high PEEP should be avoided as this will decrease pulmonary blood flow.

Maintain slight hypercarbia, targeting an end-tidal carbon dioxide level between 40 and 50 mmHg. This will increase cerebral blood flow, thereby increasing flow through the pulmonary vascular system. However, excessive hypercarbia should be avoided as the associated increase in pulmonary vascular resistance will begin to outweigh the benefits of increased cerebral blood flow. Inspired oxygen should be used as needed to maintain baseline preoperative oxygen saturation.

Can a Laryngeal Mask Airway (LMA) Be Used in SCPA Patients?

While the use of an LMA offers the advantage of allowing spontaneous ventilation, care must be taken to avoid hypoventilation which could lead to atelectasis and intrapulmonary shunting. Additionally, some anesthesiologists prefer not to use LMAs in younger patients. With vigilant observation an LMA may be employed for shorter surgeries, such as urologic procedures, where the anesthesiologist has full access to the airway and conversion to general endotracheal tube anesthesia is possible if necessary.

What Considerations Exist When Placing Invasive Lines in Patients with SCPA Physiology?

Due to the multitude of previous surgeries and catheterizations, both arterial and central venous access may prove difficult to obtain in the child with SCPA physiology. At the site of previous Blalock–Taussig (BT) shunt, the possibility of residual subclavian arterial narrowing can occasionally negatively impact arterial pressure readings in that extremity. For central venous access, institutional preferences vary, and many would advocate avoiding both internal jugular and subclavian catheters, as the potential for SVC thrombosis could prove catastrophic to pulmonary blood flow. A femoral line may be preferable if central venous access is necessary. Caution must be taken against the introduction of air bubbles through any lower extremity catheter as the IVC flows directly to the systemic circulation, introducing the risk of cerebral and coronary air embolisms.

Are SCPA Patients Candidates for Laparoscopic Surgery?

There is a risk that the reduction of functional residual capacity associated with pneumoperitoneum could compromise pulmonary blood flow. However, laparoscopic surgery has been shown to be safe in the single ventricle population. With the use of low insufflation pressures, constant vigilance, and a low threshold for conversion to open surgery, laparoscopic procedures may be attempted in the SCPA patient.

What Concerns Exist during the Maintenance of Anesthesia?

In a well-compensated SCPA patient, both inhaled and intravenous maintenance anesthetics may be well tolerated. If any cardiac compromise exists, a high-dose narcotic and muscle relaxant-based technique may provide a more stable hemodynamic profile. Care should be taken to maintain adequate intravascular volume. When appropriate, intraoperative hematocrit levels should be followed and kept above 40–45%; with ongoing blood loss these patients will require a more aggressive transfusion strategy than healthy children. It is particularly important to formulate a plan that will minimize nausea/vomiting, pain, and agitation in the postoperative period, as these all may lead to an increase in PVR and decreased pulmonary blood flow. Antiemetics should be administered prior to emergence. Consideration should be given to regional anesthetic techniques when possible, keeping in mind that the child may have previously been on anticoagulants. Postoperative agitation can be mitigated with dexmedetomidine, narcotics, and if necessary, benzodiazepines.

When Is It Safe to Discharge a Patient with SCPA Physiology?

Children with SCPA physiology poorly tolerate common postoperative issues such as vomiting, decreased oral intake, hypoventilation, and pain. It is therefore of utmost importance that these factors are well controlled prior to considering discharge from the day surgery/hospital environment. Additional aspects, such as the distance the family must travel (should the need to return to the hospital occur), and parental comfort with discharge should be considered. If any question exists as to the safety of discharge, the child should be admitted to the hospital overnight for observation and monitoring.

Suggested Reading

Gottlieb EA, Andropoulos DB. Anesthesia for the patient with congenital heart disease presenting for noncardiac surgery. *Current Opinion in Anaesthesiology*. 2013; 26(3):318–26. PMID: 23614956.

Ramamoorthy C, Haberkern CM, Bhananker SM, et al. Anesthesia-related cardiac arrest in children with heart disease: data from the pediatric perioperative cardiac arrest (POCA) registry. *Anesthesia & Analgesia*. 2010;110(5):1376–82. PMID: 20103543.

Veyckemans F, Momeni M. The patient with a history of congenital heart disease who is to undergo ambulatory surgery. *Current Opinion in Anaesthesiology*. 2013; 26(6):685–691. PMID: 24126690.

Wilson W, Taubert K, et al. Prevention of infective endocarditis: guidelines from the American Heart Association, by the Committee on Rheumatic Fever, Endocarditis, and Kawasaki Disease. *Circulation*. 2007;116:1736–54. PMID: 17446442.

Yuki K, Casta A, Uezono S. Anesthetic management of noncardiac surgery for patients with single ventricle physiology. *Journal of Anesthesia*. 2011;25(2):247–56. PMID: 21197552.

Index